School Violence and Primary Prevention

Thomas W. Miller

Editor

School Violence and Primary Prevention

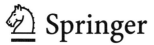 Springer

Prof. Thomas W. Miller
Department of Psychiatry
College of Medicine
University of Kentucky, KY
USA
tom.miller@uconn.edu

ISBN: 978-0-387-75660-8   e-ISBN: 978-0-387-77119-9
DOI: 10.1007/978-0-387-77119-9

Library of Congress Control Number: 2008921387

Printed on acid-free paper

9 8 7 6 5 4 3 2 1

springer.com

It is to the victims and families of victims and perpetrators of school related violence, that this volume is dedicated. May we provide herein, important steps toward the prevention and elimination of school violence and violence at all levels.

Contents

Contributors

Elizabeth A. Barton, Ph.D., is an Assistant Professor (Research) and Associate Director of the Center for Peace and Conflict Studies at Wayne State University. Barton is an internationally and nationally recognized trainer on violence by, toward, and against youth and on cross-cultural conflict. She is the author of numerous publications, including Leadership Strategies for Safe Schools and Bully Prevention: Tips and Strategies for School Leaders and Classroom Teachers. She currently implements comprehensive violence prevention program in 17 Detroit Public Schools and directs a statewide assessment of youth violence prevention programs in Michigan.

Allan L. Beane, Ph.D., is an internationally recognized expert, speaker, and author on bullying. His first book, *The Bully Free Classroom*, has been published in eight languages. He has over 30 years experience in education, which includes teaching special education, teaching regular education, serving as vice president of a university, and serving as Director of a School Safety Center. He has served as an expert witness in criminal cases involving bullying and has served as a consultant in law suites involving bullying. His program *The Bully Free Program* (www.bullyfree. com) has been adopted around the USA.

Elissa P. Benedek, M.D., is Professor of Psychiatry at the University of Michigan, School of Medicine. She is a consultant for the Center for Forensic Psychiatry (Ann Arbor, Michigan), is an examiner for the American Board of Psychiatry and Neurology, and has a private practice in child, adolescent, and forensic psychiatry. She served as president of the American Psychiatric Association from 1990 to 1991 and as Director of Research and Training at the Center for Forensic Psychiatry from 1980 to 1997. Dr. Benedek has published six books, written more than 60 papers, and led over 300 presentations at scientific meetings. Having authored or edited over 100 publications, including Principles and Practice of Child and Adolescent Forensic Psychiatry, and led over 300 presentations at scientific meetings, Dr. Benedek is a distinguished expert in child and adolescent forensic psychiatry. She served as a past president of the American Psychiatric Association and as training director for the Center for Forensic Psychiatry in Michigan for over 20 years. Currently, she is in private practice, remaining a consultant to the Center for Forensic Psychiatry, a mentor for trainees, and now an Adjunct Clinical Professor at the University of Michigan.

Christian Berger, M.S., is Assistant Professor in the School of Psychology at Universidad Alberto Hurtado, Chile. He is currently a doctoral candidate in educational psychology at the University of Illinois at Urbana-Champaign. His research focuses on the role that aggression plays within peer ecologies in adolescent populations, and particularly its associations with the social standing of the individual within his or her social context. He has served as consultant for several Chilean educational institutions regarding school climate improvement and staff training on well-being promotion.

Paul Boxer, Ph.D., is Assistant Professor of Psychology at Rutgers University in Newark, New Jersey. He received his Ph.D. in Clinical Psychology from Bowling Green State University after completing internship training at Wayne State University. Boxer directs the Social Development Research Program at Rutgers. Research in this program focuses on the development and prevention of antisocial behavior under high-risk environmental conditions and in atypical populations. Boxer's current projects examine relations between aggressive behavior and social–contextual risk, with an emphasis on the effects of exposure to violence in the community and in the media and the experience of maltreatment.

Bobbie Burcham, Ph.D., is currently employed as a school psychologist for the Fayette County Public Schools in Lexington, Kentucky, and is an Adjunct Professor at Georgetown College in Georgetown, Kentucky. She earned a master's degree at Ohio University and the doctoral degree at the University of Kentucky. In addition to serving in the public schools since 1979, she was employed for 4 years at the University of Kentucky Medical Center, Department of Outpatient Psychiatry, where, in addition to clinical work, she developed and directed a summer program for children with disruptive behavior disorders. Dr. Burcham has seven publications and has directed two grants from the Office of Special Education Programs, US Department of Education, focused on interventions for children and youth with disruptive behavior.

Connie Callahan, Ph.D., holds a doctorate in Counseling from the University of New Mexico and a master's degree in Psychology from Pittsburg State University. From 1987 through the present, she has practiced as a Licensed Professional Clinical Counselor and as a university professor. She is currently a full professor and the Chair of the Counseling and Educational Psychology at Eastern Kentucky University. Dr. Callahan has taught 57 different university and college courses and publishes and presents nationally on a variety of topics.

Noel A. Card, Ph.D., is an Assistant Professor in the Division of Family Studies and Human Development at the University of Arizona. He received his Ph.D. in Clinical Psychology from St. John's University and completed a postdoctoral fellowship in quantitative and developmental psychology at the University of Kansas. His research focuses on social development during childhood and adolescence, especially on peer relations and aggressive behavior, and has been published in Developmental Psychology, International Journal of Behavioral Development, and Social Development. His quantitative interests are in structural equation modeling, longitudinal analysis, and interdependent data analysis; he recently coedited the book Modeling Ecological and Contextual Effects in Longitudinal Studies.

Dorothy L. Espelage, Ph.D., is a Professor of Educational Psychology at the University of Illinois, Urbana-Champaign. She was named University Scholar and has fellow status in Counseling Psychology of the American Psychological Association. A Ph.D. in Counseling Psychology from Indiana University in 1997, she has conducted bullying research for the last 14 years. She is coeditor of a 2004 published book entitled "Bullying in American Schools: A Social-Ecological Perspective on Prevention and Intervention." She has served on editorial boards for the *Journal of Counseling Psychology*, *Journal of Educational Psychology*, and *Journal of Youth and Adolescence*.

William P. French, M.D., is completing his 5th year residency in the Department of Psychiatry, College of Medicine, University of Kentucky, and the Chandler Medical Center, University of Kentucky. He received his M.D. from University of Kentucky College of Medicine in 2003 graduating with high distinction. He completed his fellowship in child and adolescent psychiatry in 2004–2006 at the UK Medical Center, Lexington, Kentucky. His professional interests include developing integrative medical models (e.g., biopsychosocial), investigating neurobiological substrates of psychiatric disorders, developing digital animations for teaching purposes, and researching the role of mindfulness-based meditation practices in promoting health and healing.

Sara E. Goldstein, Ph.D., is Assistant Professor of Family and Child Studies at Montclair State University in Montclair, New Jersey. She received her Ph.D. in Developmental Psychology from Bowling Green State University. Goldstein's research centers on developmental and social-cognitive factors underpinning the expression and maintenance of relationally aggressive forms of behavior, particularly during adolescence. Her current work examines the prevalence and effects of relational aggression in different interpersonal relationships, as well as intergenerational continuities and discontinuities in this type of aggressive responding.

Ernest V. E. Hodges, Ph.D., is an Associate Professor in the Department of Psychology at St. John's University in New York City, New York. He received his Ph.D. in Psychology from Florida Atlantic University and completed postdoctoral training at the Research Unit on Children's Psychosocial Maladjustment in Quebec, Canada. His research interests broadly include social and personality development during middle childhood and adolescence, and he has published on a variety of topics (e.g., parenting dimensions, parent–child attachment, social cognitive evaluations, emotion dysregulation, and gender identity) in relation to behavioral (e.g., internalizing and externalizing) and social (e.g., peer rejection, victimization, and enemies) maladjustment.

Thomas F. Holcomb, Ed.D., is a Professor of Counseling and Chair of the Department of Educational Studies, Leadership and Counseling at Murray State University. He has been highly involved with the Kentucky Counseling Association and has held numerous leadership positions in the organization. He also served several terms on the Kentucky Board of Licensed Professional Counselors. His major interest lies primarily in the area of School Counseling and he has published numerous articles on the subject. He has been a former elementary school teacher and elementary school counselor. He has been a Counselor Educator at Murray State University since 1971.

Jenny Isaacs, Ph.D. Dr. Isaac's research examined why middle-school students might carry weapons to school. Subjects were 414 children—primarily Latino, sixth- to eighth-grade boys and girls in some of New Jersey's inner cities who completed two self-report measures, one assessing weapon carrying and a peer-nomination inventory assessing the connection between aggressive behavior and weapon carrying. The study covered a 4-year period, enabling the students to be queried when in middle school and high school. The results of her research indicated that students' aggression levels and whether they had been threatened with a weapon both independently predicted their thoughts about weapons and weapon-carrying behavior. Dr. Isaacs is an Assistant Professor of Psychology at Yeshiva College of Yeshiva University, New York.

Dana L. Johnson, M.A., is the Interim Title III Director at Central State University in Wilberforce, Ohio (2007–present) after serving as Interim Principal Investigator (2005–2007), the national prevention specialist, and Deputy Director of the FCVP Program between 2000 and 2005. Her professional and personal focus has been on supporting youth and community programs through mentorship as well as serving as a court-appointed special advocate/guardian ad litem (CASA/GAL). She is also a certified True Colors Facilitator who conducts workshops to increase communication and team-building relationships among community-based organizations.

Praveen Kambam, M.D., is a child and adolescent psychiatry fellow at the UCLA Semel Institute for Neuroscience and Human Behavior. At the time of writing, Praveen was a general psychiatry resident at the University of Michigan. He has longstanding interests in forensic psychiatry as well as medical education. Other academic interests include media impacts on children and adolescents and physician wellness. His immediate career plans include completing a fellowship in forensic psychiatry. Along with his supervisor, Dr. Elissa P. Benedek, Professor of Psychiatry at the University of Michigan School of Medicine, he shares an interest in acute cases of psychiatric trauma related to school violence.

Ramin Karimpour is a doctoral student in educational psychology at the University of Illinois at Urbana-Champaign. Mr. Karimpour specializes in social–ecological bullying prevention programs, with a particular interest in field implementation opportunities and challenges. A former primary school teacher and secondary school principal, he served 7 years as an educator for the Tohono O'odham Nation of southwest Arizona.

Robert F. Kraus, M.D., is Professor of Psychiatry and Anthropology, Associate Residency Director of Training and former Chair of the Department of Psychiatry at the University of Kentucky. His career has involved clinical and academic administration, teaching, clinical practice, and research. Recently he was the recipient of the Lifetime Achievement Award of the Society for the Study of Psychiatry and Culture of which he is a charter member. The award was given for outstanding and enduring research contributions to the field of Cultural Psychiatry. It is the highest honor bestowed by the Society

Ken Kyle, Ph.D., is an Assistant Professor of Public Affairs and Administration at California State University, East Bay, and currently serves as editor of *Social Problems Forum: The SSSP Newsletter*. He holds an M.A. in Political Science and a Ph.D. in Justice Studies from Arizona State University. His scholarly interests revolve around the application of critical social theories to concrete public policies in the pursuit of social justice. He has published in a variety of academic journals including *Administrative Theory & Praxis, Educational Studies, Humanity & Society, Social Justice* and *Sociological Practice.*

Janet Lane, M.S., graduated from the University of Kentucky in 1987 and 1988 with a B.A. in Psychology and a B.A. in Elementary Education, respectively. Before pursuing a master's degree, she taught sixth and fifth grade in Houston, Texas. In 1997, she graduated from Murray State University with an M.S. in Clinical Psychology. Clinical practice included working with adolescents who were referred to a day treatment program for behavioral problems. Janet has provided neuropsychological and psychological assessments within a forensic setting and currently provides crisis intervention and therapy to children aged 5–12 within an elementary school setting. Targeted are children referred through the school due to truancy issues and/or behavioral problems as these children often have witnessed domestic violence in the home. Wraparound services are offered to the families of these children.

Amy Lawson, M.S.W. Candidate, is a graduate student in social work at the University of Kentucky and will graduate in December 2007. She has worked in the family resource centers at two local elementary schools and with the therapists at the University of Kentucky, Department of Psychiatry Outpatient Clinic. Following graduation, she plans to obtain her LCSW through continued education and supervision so that she can continue to treat children and families. She received a bachelor of arts in psychology from Asbury College in 2002. During her undergraduate studies, she presented research findings at the Kentucky Psychological Association Conference and worked at Boys and Girls Country, a residential facility for at-risk youth in Texas. She also led and mentored youth in two church groups throughout her 4 years in college.

Kathy McLaughlin, M.A., has been in education for over 30 years with the Fayette County Public Schools, University of Kentucky, and the Bluegrass Boys' Ranch. She has been a special education teacher, a diagnostician/school-based consultant, and currently teaches math to seventh and eighth graders. Kathy has been recognized as a most effective teacher based on her passionate love for teaching kids, knowledge of math, and achievement results. In her classroom, learning is mandatory.

She specializes in classroom management and motivation, problem solving teaching, and relationship building. She lives in Lexington, Kentucky, with her husband and has three grown children.

J. Robert McLaughlin, Ed.S., has recently retired from the Fayette County Public Schools after 31 years of service. He taught special education, was a principal, a district special education coordinator and director, and spent the last 12 years supervising principals as an Elementary School Director. He taught 2 years in Galveston, Texas, in an alternative middle school. He currently works as an independent consultant and trainer for Safe and Civil Schools (Eugene, Oregon) specializing in Classroom Management, School wide Discipline, and Leadership development for principals and district staff. He is married, has three grown children, and continues to live in Lexington, Kentucky.

Thomas W. Miller, Ph.D., has been Professor, Senior Research Scientist, Master Teacher, and University Teaching Fellow during his 36-year tenure at the University of Kentucky, University of Connecticut, and Murray State University. He received his Ph.D. from the State University of New York at Buffalo, is a Diplomate of the American Board of Professional Psychology in Clinical Psychology, and Fellow of the American Psychological Association, the American Psychology Society, and the Royal Society of Medicine. The American Psychological Association recognized him with a Special Achievement Award for his contributions to education, prevention, and clinical services for victims of abuse. He is a Distinguished Alumnus from the State University of New York and the recipient of the 2007 APA Distinguished Professional Contributions to Practice Award.

Amy Nigoff, M.S., earned her Master's in Clinical Psychology from Ohio University. She currently works with youth in a state-funded wraparound services program. Ms. Nigoff is interested in studying the long-term effects of bullying on kids and how these aggressive styles continue into adulthood. A new area of interest for her is in identifying effective interventions for children who grow up in a subculture that is accepting of violence.

Philip C. Rodkin, Ph.D., is Associate Professor of child development in the Departments of Educational Psychology and Psychology at the University of Illinois at Urbana-Champaign. Rodkin investigates children's social status (popularity) and social networks (peer groups and friendships). Of particular interest is the social placement and influence of aggressive children and the positive and negative sentiments that flow between children of different genders and ethnicities. Overcoming methodological and analytic procedures in the measurement of social relations is a central challenge of this work, as is applying knowledge of childhood social dynamics in the service of creating healthy classroom climates.

Laxley W. Rodney, Ph.D., is currently serving as the Interim Dean of the Whitlowe R. Green College of Education and Visiting Professor in the Department of Educational Leadership and Counseling at Prairie View University in Prairie View, Texas, where he teaches graduate courses in research and statistics. He previously served at Central State University in Wilberforce, Ohio, as the principal investigator of the Family and Community Violence Prevention (FCVP) Program, 1994–2005; Assistant Vice President for Academic Affairs, 1999–2004; Interim Dean, College of Education, June 2002–September 2002; and Chair of Graduate Education, 2004–2005. He has authored and coauthored several articles on youth violence which have been published in refereed journals.

Mark V. Sapp, M.D., is a board-certified pediatrician who specializes in the field of child abuse and neglect and is a member of the Child Protection Team at Children's Hospital Boston/Harvard Medical School. He is a medical consultant for the Teen Prostitution Prevention Program for the local Child Advocacy Center, sits on the Boston/Suffolk County Child Fatality Review Board, and supervises nurse practitioners in the Pediatric Sexual Assault Nurse Examiner Program. He has recently begun work evaluating the medical needs of youth exploited through the sex trade industry and plans to expand this work into a comprehensive clinical program targeting teenage prostitution.

Sarah Savoy, M.A., is a doctoral student in the Department of Psychology at Rutgers University in Newark, New Jersey. She received her M.A. in Psychology from Southeastern Louisiana State University. Savoy is interested in how social and developmental factors influence weight, body image, and problem behaviors in adolescents. Her current research focuses on how victimization experiences affect self-image and adjustment problems among overweight and normal weight youth.

Rick Spurling, Ed.D. In his 24th year with the Mitchell County Schools, Dr. Richard Spurling has served as a teacher, coach, assistant principal, and principal and now currently is the Assistant Superintendent and Career Technical Education Director. He also teaches night classes at East Tennessee State University as an Adjunct Professor in the Educational Leadership Department and Principal Preparation Program. Dr. Spurling, author of *It Is Time...To Be Bully Free! An Anti-Bullying Guidebook for School Leaders* (December 2006), has been inspirational in providing schools direction in developing, establishing, and implementing anti-bullying programs. His studies have allowed him the opportunity to present his findings to over 20,000 educators detailing his program to concerned educators and school leaders in Virginia, Tennessee, and North Carolina. Spurling has keynoted at several state conferences and continues to share his findings and motivational sessions through in-service training.

Rameshwar P. Srivastava, M.S., FSS, CStat, is currently serving as Manager, Evaluation Systems, Alcohol, Drug Addiction, and Mental Health Services (ADAMHS) Board for Montgomery County, Dayton, Ohio. He Previously served as Assistant Professor in the Department of Mathematics and Computer Science at Central State University, Ohio, and was the national Evaluation Coordinator of the FCVP Program (2002–2006). He also served as Research Assistant Professor of Social Sciences/ Statistics at the University of Virgin Islands (2000–2002), Commonwealth Expert in the Eastern Caribbean (1997–2000), and United Nations Advisor in Africa (1985–1990). He was elected a Fellow of the Royal Statistical Society in 1978 and a Chartered Statistician, UK, in 1994 and has authored and coauthored several articles in the field of statistics and evaluation.

Susan M. Swearer, Ph.D., is an Associate Professor of School Psychology in the Department of Educational Psychology at the University of Nebraska—Lincoln and the co-director of the Nebraska Internship Consortium in Professional Psychology. She received her Ph.D. in School Psychology from the University of Texas at Austin in 1997 and is a licensed psychologist in Nebraska. She has conducted research on the relations among internalizing psychopathology and bullying among school-aged youth for over a decade. She is the coeditor (with Dr. Espelage) of the book *Bullying in American Schools: A Social-Ecological Perspective on Prevention and Intervention*. She is an Associate Editor for the journal *School Psychology Review*, and is on the editorial review boards for *School Psychology Quarterly* and the *Journal of Anxiety Disorders*.

Andrew Terranova, Ph.D., is a Post-Doctoral Associate in the Social Development Research Program of the Department of Psychology at Rutgers University in Newark, New Jersey. He received his Ph.D. in Applied Developmental Psychology from the University of New Orleans. Terranova's interests include psychosocial risk factors for the development of aggression, particularly "bullying" behavior. He also is interested in factors that exacerbate or protect children from the negative effects of peer victimization, especially the role of different coping styles and strategies in determining adjustment outcomes of victimization as well as psychosocial functioning more generally.

Matt Thompson, M.S., is in his 4th year as the principal at Deep Springs Elementary School in Lexington, Kentucky. Currently in his 9th year in education, he previously taught third and fourth grades for 5 years in Frankfort, Kentucky. Matt has a master's degree from the University of Kentucky and is beginning to take courses to gain his superintendent's certificate. He is most proud of the gains Deep Springs has made in student achievement and narrowing the achievement gaps for minority and low-income students. He is married to his wonderful wife, Stephanie, and is the father of one son, Andrew (with one more on the way).

Stephen Thompson, Ph.D., is an applied sociology practitioner at Pennoni Associates Inc., assisting with technology transfer and policy issues, as well as an Adjunct Instructor in the Department of Sociology, Social Work, and Criminal Justice at Messiah College in Grantham, Pennsylvania. He holds an M.A. in Community Psychology and Social Change from the Pennsylvania State University. Stephen has published in the Journal of Primary Prevention, as well as numerous research documents for governmental and private agencies. A former missionary to the Republic of Haiti, his research interests revolve around the impacts of moral development processes on human behavior.

Lane J. Veltkamp, M.S.W. ACSW, B.C.D., is a Tenured Full Professor in the Child Psychiatry Division, Department of Psychiatry, College of Medicine, University of Kentucky Medical Center. He has a Joint Faculty appointment in the College of Social Work. He did his undergraduate work at Calvin College in Grand Rapids, Michigan, and his graduate work at Michigan State University. He is Board Certified. His interests over the last 35 years have focused on family violence, child abuse, and forensic issues. He has published over 60 papers, 6 chapters, and 2 books. He has given hundreds of workshops and testified in court in six states over 300 times. He developed and directed the Child and Adolescent Forensic Clinic in the Department of Psychiatry for 30 years.

William Weitzel, M.D., is a physician and psychiatrist in private practice in Lexington, Kentucky. He has provided expert testimony in numerous forensic cases that have included cases related to school violence and those involving school shootings by adolescent students. Dr. Weitzel is also a faculty member in the Department of Psychiatry, College of Medicine, at the University of Kentucky in Lexington, Kentucky. He has taught, provided clinical supervision, and published during his career in psychiatry and psychiatric practice.

Jina S. Yoon, Ph.D., is an Associate Professor in Educational Psychology at Wayne State University. She has a doctoral degree in School Psychology and completed a postdoctoral fellowship in Child Clinical Psychology. Her research has focused on emotional and social development of behaviorally challenging children and adolescents and on school environment as an important developmental context, including victimization in school, peer relationships, and teacher–student relationships. She has published numerous publications and presented at conferences in these areas. Dr. Yoon also teaches developmental psychopathology and psycho-therapy in graduate training. She also works with children and adolescents in individual and group therapy at a private practice.

List of Tables

List of Figures

Chapter 1
School-Related Violence and Prevention: Editorial Introduction

Thomas W. Miller

In 2004, I was invited to serve as guest editor for a special edition of the *Journal of Primary Prevention* (Miller, 2005). This edition would focus on the prevention of school violence. In September 2005, a special edition of this journal produced a well-received series of articles from a national group of prevention researchers, scholars, and clinicians (Edwards et al., 2005; Thompson & Kyle, 2005). An invitation to broaden the scope and direction of this journal publication has led to this volume. It follows an excellent publication in this series dealing with cross-national and cross-cultural perspectives (Denmark et al., 2006). Our purpose in this volume is to provide to you, the reader, a compendium of papers addressing school violence and the critical ingredients in prevention interventions that contribute to reducing and/or eliminating various forms of violence in the school setting.

There are two major sections to the volume. Initially, we examine the theory, assessment, and an overview of the definition and boundary issues involved in the term "school violence" as used in research and applied prevention programs. The second section presents strategies and interventions for the prevention of school violence. As editor, the first chapter deals with the definition, scope of the problem, and the goals for prevention we have come to know. My esteemed colleague and friend Robert F. Kraus, M.D., joins me in addressing this chapter and the pathway to better understanding the definition, scope, and goals in the prevention of school violence. Robert F. Kraus is Professor of Psychiatry and Anthropology, Associate Residency Director of Training, and former Chair of the Department of Psychiatry at the University of Kentucky. His career has involved clinical and academic administration, teaching, clinical practice, and research. Recently, he was the recipient of the Lifetime Achievement Award from the Society for the Study of Psychiatry and Culture. He has served as a mentor and brings a rich understanding of the cultural issues to this definition and scope of the problem for violence in the schools.

In today's world, it is necessary to have a good understanding of human behavior. For this I turned to a colleague and friend, **William P. French, M.D.**, to address in the next chapter the theoretical issues we need to understand through the neurobiology of violence and victimization. Will is completing his fifth-year residency in the Department of Psychiatry, College of Medicine, University of Kentucky and the Chandler Medical Center, University of Kentucky. Will has brought science and practice together and has focused his professional life on

T. W. Miller (ed.), *School Violence and Primary Prevention.*
© Springer 2008

developing integrative medical models investigating neurobiological substrates of psychiatric disorders and researching the role of mindfulness-based meditation practices in promoting health and healing in psychiatric practice.

Assessing risk factors is critical to targeting prevention efforts in the schools. **Connie Callahan, Ph.D.**, focuses on the essentials of "threat assessment" in the schools. She holds a doctorate specializing in counseling with a focus on the prevention of school-related violence. She has practiced as a Licensed Professional Clinical Counselor and as a university professor with special emphasis on the developing of models of threat assessment in the schools. Dr. Callahan has been instrumental in developing threat assessment modules and presented nationally on the subject.

Communication and information processing is key to prevention efforts. A clinician, colleague, and researcher, **Amy Nigoff, M.S.**, examines communication and information processing as a critical factor in addressing the interrelationships of students, teachers, and school personnel. In her clinical practice, Amy currently works with youth in a state-funded wraparound services program. Her research and clinical interests have focused on the long-term effects of bullying on children and adolescents and how these aggressive styles continue into adulthood. A special focus of interest for her is in identifying effective prevention interventions for children who grow up in a subculture that is accepting of violence.

Understanding moral development is critical. Ken Kyle and Steve Thompson, who have published together previously on this topic, provide an examination of the roles of morality development and personal power within the context of school shootings. **Ken Kyle, Ph.D.**, is an Assistant Professor of Public Affairs and Administration at California State University, East Bay, and currently serves as editor of *Social Problems Forum: The SSSP Newsletter*. He holds an M.A. in Political Science and a Ph.D. in Justice Studies from Arizona State University. His scholarly interests revolve around the application of critical social theories to concrete public policies in the pursuit of social justice. He has published in a variety of academic journals including *Administrative Theory & Praxis, Educational Studies, Humanity & Society, Social Justice*, and *Sociological Practice*. **Stephen Thompson, Ph.D.**, is an applied sociology practitioner at Pennoni Associates, Inc., assisting with technology transfer and policy issues, as well as an Adjunct Instructor in the Department of Sociology, Social Work, and Criminal Justice at Messiah College in Grantham, Pennsylvania. He holds an M.A. in Community Psychology and Social Change from the Pennsylvania State University. A former missionary to the Republic of Haiti, his research interests revolve around the impacts of moral development processes on human behavior. Stephen has published in the *Journal of Primary Prevention* (Thompson & Kyle, 2005), as well as numerous research documents for governmental and private agencies.

Our next chapter addresses a review of the implications for prevention and intervention efforts. To address this area, three colleagues provide a team effort in examining this focus of study. **Noel A. Card, Ph.D.**, is an Assistant Professor in the Division of Family Studies and Human Development at the University of Arizona. He received his Ph.D. in clinical psychology from St. John's University, and completed a postdoctoral fellowship in quantitative and developmental psychology at the University of Kansas. His research focuses on social development during childhood and adolescence, especially on peer relations and aggressive behavior, and has been published in *Developmental Psychology, International Journal of Behavioral Development*, and *Social Development*. His quantitative interests are in structural equation modeling, longitudinal analysis, and interdependent data analysis; he recently coedited the book *Modeling Ecological and Contextual Effects in Longitudinal Studies*. Colleague **Ernest V.E. Hodges, Ph.D.**, is an associate professor in the Department of Psychology at St. John's University in New York City, New York. He received his Ph.D. in psychology from Florida Atlantic University and completed postdoctoral training at the Research Unit on Children's Psychosocial Maladjustment in Quebec, Canada. His research interests broadly include social and personality development during middle childhood and adolescence, and he has published on a variety of topics including parenting dimensions, parent–child attachment, social cognitive evaluations, emotion dysregulation, and gender identity in relation to behavioral maladjustment in school-aged children and adolescents.

The role of the pediatrician is critical in addressing school-related violence. **Mark V. Sapp, M.D.**, is a board-certified pediatrician who specializes in the field of child abuse and neglect and is a member of the Child Protection Team at Children's Hospital Boston/Harvard Medical School. He is a medical consultant for the Teen Prostitution Prevention Program for the Child Advocacy Center, Boston, Massachusetts. He also has a chair on the Boston/Suffolk County Child Fatality Review Board and supervises nurse practitioners in the Pediatric Sexual Assault Nurse Examiner Program. He has recently begun work evaluating the medical needs of youth exploited through the sex trade industry and plans to expand this work into a comprehensive clinical program targeting teenage prostitution.

The impact of trauma in school violence on the victim and the perpetrator becomes the focus of the next chapter. To address this area, we turn to our distinguished colleague **Lane J. Veltkamp, M.S.W., A.C.S.W., B.C.D.**, who is a tenured full Professor in the Child Psychiatry Division, Department of Psychiatry, College of Medicine, University of Kentucky Medical Center. His interests over the last 35 years have focused on family violence, child abuse, and forensic issues. He has published over 60 papers, 6 chapters, and 2 books. He has given hundreds of workshops and testified in court in six states over 300 times. He developed and directed the Child and Adolescent Forensic Clinic in the Department of Psychiatry for 30 years. A graduate student, **Amy Lawson, M.S.W.** Candidate, is completing her studies in social work at the University of Kentucky and will graduate in December 2007. She has worked in the family resource centers at two local elementary schools and with the therapists at the University of Kentucky, Department of Psychiatry Outpatient Clinic. She received a bachelor of arts in psychology from Asbury College in 2002. During her undergraduate studies, she presented research findings at the Kentucky Psychological Association Conference and worked at Boys and Girls Country, a residential facility for at-risk youth in Texas. Amy has worked closely with youth groups on moral, ethical, and bonding issues.

The next two chapters examine two critical areas in understanding and preventing school-related violence. Violent behavior is often influenced by others beyond the peer group, including cliques, cults, and, in some cases, school personnel. The role of cliques and cults is examined as is boundary violations in the schools. Sexual boundary violations have become another element of the school-related violence spectrum. This editor and his colleague **Tom Holcomb, Ed.D.**, provide an examination of this topic. **Thomas Miller, Ph.D.**, has published in the area of cult behavior having studied a nonschool–based cult that infiltrated a high school and college in rural America. He has also published on ethical issues including sexual boundary violations in the school setting. The American Psychological Association recognized him with a Special Achievement Award for his contributions to education, prevention, and clinical services for victims of abuse. He is a Distinguished Alumnus from the State University of New York, and the recipient of the 2007 APA Distinguished Professional Contributions to Practice Award. Cliques and cults have been a known entirety in the school setting and the editor joins colleagues **Robert F. Kraus, M.D.**, a psychiatrist and anthropologist and Thom Holcomb, Ed.D., a school and mental health counselor in rural Kentucky to address cult-related victims and perpetrators in the school environment. **Thomas F. Holcomb, Ed.D.**, is a Professor of Counseling and Chair of the Department of Educational Studies, Leadership and Counseling at Murray State University. He has been highly involved with the Kentucky Counseling Association and has held numerous leadership positions in the organization. He also served several terms on the Kentucky Board of Licensed Professional Counselors. His major interest lies primarily in the area of School Counseling and he has published numerous articles on the subject. He has been a former elementary school teacher and elementary school counselor. He has been a Counselor Educator at Murray State University since 1971. Tom Miller has published, taught, and conducted research with his colleague Tom Holcomb while serving as a tenured professor in the College of Education at Murray State University and worked closely with Professor Tom Holcomb on several areas including school violence. While at Murray State University, Miller won the Deans Award for Research focusing on the benefits of character education as a buffer against school-related violence.

In examining threat and prevention of violence in the schools, we turn to three critical professionals in the school setting for this chapter. Seeking the collaborative skills of administrators, teachers, and school psychologists, we sought the expertise of Matt Thompson, Kathy McLaughlin, and Bobbie Burchum. **Matthew Thompson, Ed.D.** (Candidate), is the principal at Deep Springs Elementary School in Lexington, Kentucky. Currently in his ninth year in education, he previously taught third and fourth grades for 5 years in Frankfort, Kentucky. Matthew has a master's degree from the University of Kentucky and is beginning to take courses to gain his superintendent's certificate. He is most proud of the gains Deep Springs has made in student achievement and narrowing the achievement gaps for minority and low-income students. He is married to his wonderful wife, Stephanie, and is the father of one son, Andrew (with one more on the way). **Kathy McLaughlin, M.Ed.**, has been in education for over 30 years with the Fayette County Public Schools,

University of Kentucky, and the Bluegrass Boys' Ranch. She has been a special education teacher, a diagnostician/school-based consultant, and currently teaches math to seventh and eighth graders. She has developed a specialized curricular approach to enhancing school and peer bonding in the classroom. Her efforts have focused on prevention interventions in the classroom that promote character development and effective communication and peer relationship for an effective learning environment. Kathy has been recognized as a most effective teacher based on her passionate love for teaching kids, knowledge of math, and achievement results. In her classroom, learning is mandatory. She specializes in classroom management and motivation, problem solving teaching, and relationship building. **Bobbie Burcham, Ph.D.**, is currently employed as a school psychologist for the Fayette County Public Schools in Lexington, Kentucky, and is an adjunct professor at Georgetown College in Georgetown, Kentucky. She earned a master's degree at Ohio University and the doctoral degree at the University of Kentucky. In addition to serving in the public schools since 1979, she was employed for 4 years at the University of Kentucky Medical Center, Department of Outpatient Psychiatry, where, in addition to clinical work, she developed and directed a summer program for children with disruptive behavior disorders. Dr. Burcham has seven publications and has directed two grants from the Office of Special Education Programs, United States Department of Education, focused on interventions for children and youth with disruptive behavior.

Bullying has become the most focused area of school-related violence. As we will see, it takes on many forms. In the school setting, the teacher is the frontline monitor and for this chapter we invited two scholars at Wayne State University to address this important area of study. **Jina S. Yoon, Ph.D.**, is an Associate Professor in Educational Psychology at Wayne State University. She has a doctoral degree in School Psychology and completed a postdoctoral fellowship in Child Clinical Psychology. Her research has focused on emotional and social development of behaviorally challenging children and adolescents and on school environment as an important developmental context, including victimization in school, peer relationships, and teacher–student relationships. She has published numerous publications and presented at conferences in these areas. Dr. Yoon also teaches developmental psychopathology and psychotherapy in graduate training. She also works with children and adolescents in individual and group therapy at a private practice. **Elizabeth A. Barton, Ph.D.**, is an Assistant Professor (Research) and Associate Director of the Center for Peace and Conflict Studies at Wayne State University. Barton is an internationally and nationally recognized trainer on violence by, toward, and against youth and on cross-cultural conflict. She is the author of numerous publications, including *Leadership Strategies for Safe Schools* and *Bully Prevention: Tips and Strategies for School Leaders and Classroom Teachers*. She currently implements comprehensive violence prevention program in 17 Detroit Public Schools and directs a statewide assessment of youth violence prevention programs in Michigan.

Developmental issues in addressing the prevention of aggressiveness and violence in the school setting is the focus of the collaborative efforts of our colleagues from Rutgers and Montclair State University. Paul Boxer serves as the leader of this effort in better understanding the critical issues in prevention of school violence. **Paul Boxer, Ph.D.**, is an Assistant Professor of Psychology at Rutgers University in Newark, New Jersey. He received his Ph.D. in Clinical Psychology from Bowling Green State University after completing internship training at Wayne State University. Boxer directs the Social Development Research Program at Rutgers. Research in this program focuses on the development and prevention of antisocial behavior under high-risk environmental conditions and in atypical populations. Boxer's current projects examine relations between aggressive behavior and social-contextual risk, with an emphasis on the effects of exposure to violence in the community and in the media and the experience of maltreatment (Boxer et al., 2005). **Andrew Terranova, Ph.D.**, is a Post-Doctoral Associate in the Social Development Research Program of the Department of Psychology at Rutgers University in Newark, New Jersey. He received his Ph.D. in Applied Developmental Psychology from the University of New Orleans. Terranova's interests include psychosocial risk factors for the development of aggression, particularly "bullying" behavior. He also is interested in factors that exacerbate or protect children from the negative effects of peer victimization, especially the role of different coping styles and strategies in determining adjustment outcomes of victimization as well as psychosocial functioning more generally. **Sara E. Goldstein, Ph.D.**, is Assistant Professor of Family and Child Studies at Montclair State University in Montclair, New Jersey. She received her Ph.D. in Developmental Psychology from Bowling Green State University. Goldstein's research centers on developmental and social-cognitive factors underpinning the expression and maintenance of relationally aggressive forms of behavior, particularly during adolescence. Her current work examines the prevalence and effects of relational aggression in different interpersonal relationships, as well as intergenerational continuities and discontinuities in this type of aggressive responding. **Sarah Savoy, M.A.**, is a doctoral student in the Department of Psychology at Rutgers University in Newark, New Jersey. She received her M.A. in Psychology from Southeastern Louisiana State University. Savoy is interested in how social and developmental factors influence weight, body image, and problem behaviors in adolescents. Her current research focuses on how victimization experiences affect self-image and adjustment problems among overweight and normal weight youth. Boxer and colleagues note that contemporary research on the development and prevention of aggressive behavior in childhood and adolescence emphasizes the importance of social-cognitive factors such as perceptual biases, problem-solving skills, and social-moral beliefs in the maintenance of aggression.

The prevention of bullying in the school setting is an essential goal of the national agenda noted in Healthy People 2010. To address these important elements in reducing school violence, two colleagues were invited to provide a pathway to change. **Philip C. Rodkin, Ph.D.**, is Associate Professor of Educational Psychology and Psychology at the University of Illinois at Urbana-Champaign. Rodkin investigates children's social status (popularity) and social networks (peer groups, friendships). Of particular interest is the social placement and influence of aggressive children and the positive and negative sentiments that flow between children of different genders and ethnicities. Overcoming methodological and analytic procedures in the measurement of social relations is a central challenge of this work, as is applying knowledge of childhood social dynamics in the service of creating healthy classroom climates. **Christian Berger, M.S.**, is Assistant Professor in the School of Psychology at Universidad Alberto Hurtado, Chile. He is currently a doctoral candidate in educational psychology at the University of Illinois at Urbana-Champaign. His research focuses on the role that aggression plays within peer ecologies in adolescent populations, and particularly its associations with the social standing of the individual within his or her social context. He has served as consultant for several Chilean educational institutions regarding school climate improvement and staff training on well-being promotion.

Paramount in addressing the most serious cases of school violence, those that involve both physical and psychological injury and pain, we looked to a well-qualified and internationally recognized expert in this area of school-related violence. **Elissa P. Benedek, M.D.**, joins a resident in psychiatry **Praveen Kambam, M.D.**, in addressing this area. Elissa Benedek is a distinguished expert in child and adolescent forensic psychiatry. She served as a past president of the American Psychiatric Association and as training director for the Center for Forensic Psychiatry in Michigan for over 20 years. At the time of publication, Dr. Kambam is a child and adolescent psychiatry fellow at the University of California, Los Angeles (UCLA) Semel Institute for Neuroscience and Human Behavior. He has longstanding interests in forensic psychiatry as well as medical education. Other academic interests include media impacts on children and adolescents and physician wellness. His interest in school violence extends to forensic psychiatry as it related to children and adolescents.

Linking school bullying research to evidence-based decision in preventing school violence became the challenge for two well-established colleagues with expertise in this area. **Dorothy L. Espelage, Ph.D.**, is an Associate Professor of Counseling Psychology in the Department of Educational Psychology at the University of Illinois, Urbana-Champaign. She was named University Scholar and has fellow status in Counseling Psychology of the American Psychological Association. She holds a Ph.D. in Counseling Psychology from Indiana University. She has conducted bullying research for more than a decade. She is coeditor of a 2004 published book entitled *Bullying in American Schools: A Social-Ecological Perspective on Prevention and Intervention*. She has served on editorial boards for the *Journal of Counseling Psychology, Journal of Educational Psychology*, and the *Journal of Youth and Adolescence*. **Susan M. Swearer, Ph.D.**, is an Associate Professor of School Psychology in the Department of Educational Psychology at the University of Nebraska-Lincoln. She received her Ph.D. in School Psychology from the University of Texas at Austin in 1997 and has conducted research on psychosocial factors and bullying among school-aged youth for over a decade. She is the coeditor (with Dr. Espelage) of the book *Bullying in American Schools: A Social-Ecological Perspective on Prevention and Intervention*. She is an Associate Editor for the journal *School Psychology Review* and is on the editorial review boards for *School Psychology Quarterly* and *Journal of Anxiety Disorders*.

In examining "risk factors" and issues in mental health assessment, I am joined by colleagues, **Bill Weitzel, M.D.**, and **Janet Lane, M.S.**, who have had considerable experience in the mental health arena in addressing the spectrum of school-related violence. Dr. Weitzel is a psychiatrist who has been involved in examining perpetrators of school shootings, as has Miller. Both have been involved in clinical evaluation of perpetrators of school shootings. Janet Lane has taught at the elementary level in Houston, Texas. In 1997, she graduated from Murray State University with an M.S. in Clinical Psychology where she worked with this editor on violence-related issues in the schools. Clinical practice has included working with adolescents who were referred to a day treatment program for behavioral problems. Janet has provided neuropsychological and psychological assessments within a forensic setting and currently provides crisis intervention and therapy to children aged 5–12 within an elementary school setting. Targeted are children referred through the school due to truancy issues and/or behavioral problems. These children often have witnessed domestic violence in the home. In her current position, she provides wraparound services for the families of these children who have witnessed and/or experienced violence in their lives.

In the next chapter, this editor and colleagues address the effectiveness of character education as a prevention strategy targeted at high-risk children (Miller et al., 2005). This chapter examines fourth-grade students in 9 of the 11 schools in a rural community. The results confirmed that the summer program participants had significant gains in school achievement, greater social competency as reported by self and teachers, greater increases in reading achievement, and a positive effect on parental–child interaction. The specialized curriculum, family program, and the experiential summer camp component contributed to the school bonding experience. Several important and substantive issues and research questions are raised by these findings. Recommendations are made for future research addressing the effects of character education programs on the predictor variables from the fourth- and fifth-grade interventions evident as youth make the transition to their next grade level in the middle school culture.

Idealistically, the goal of any school system is to have a ***Bully Free*** environment. Toward that end, we turned to experts who have been applying the evidence-based models to preventing school violence and creating a bully free environment. **Allan L. Beane, Ph.D.**, is an internationally recognized expert, speaker, and author on bullying. His first book, *The Bully Free Classroom*, has been published in eight languages. He has over three decades of experience in education, which includes teaching special education, teaching regular education, serving as vice president of a university, and serving as Director of a School Safety Center. He has served as an expert witness in criminal cases involving bullying and has served as a consultant in law suites involving bullying. His *The Bully Free Program* (**www. bullyfree.com**) has been adopted around the United States. **Rick Spurling, Ed.D.**, is in his 24th year with the Mitchell County Schools. Dr. Spurling has served as a teacher, coach, assistant principal, and principal and now currently is the Assistant Superintendent and Career Technical Education Director. He also teaches night classes at East Tennessee State University as an adjunct professor in the Educational

Leadership Department and Principal Preparation Program. Dr. Spurling is author of *It Is Time...To Be Bully Free! An Anti-Bullying Guidebook for School Leaders* (December 2006) and has been inspirational in providing schools direction in developing, establishing, and implementing antibullying programs. His studies have allowed him the opportunity to present his findings to over 20,000 educators detailing his program to concerned educators and school leaders in Virginia, Tennessee, and North Carolina. Dr. Spurling has keynoted at several state conferences and continues to share his findings and motivational sessions through in-service training. Drs. Miller and Beane have worked and published together while at Murray State University.

Cultural and individual differences play an important role in understanding school-related violence. Laxley Rodney and his colleagues consider an essential issues in their chapter that addresses a series of culturally relevant models aimed at the prevention of school violence. **Laxley W. Rodney, Ph.D.**, is currently serving as visiting professor in the Department of Educational Leadership and Counseling at Prairie View University in Prairie View, Texas, where he teaches graduate courses in research and statistics. He previously served at Central State University in Wilberforce, Ohio, as the principal investigator of the Family and Community Violence Prevention (FCVP) Program, 1994–2005; Assistant Vice President for Academic Affairs, 1999–2004; Interim Dean, College of Education, June 2002–September 2002; and Chair of Graduate Education, 2004–2005. He has authored and coauthored several articles on youth violence which have been published in refereed journals (Rodney et al., 2005). This team of researchers also includes **Rameshwar P. Srivastava, M.S.**, **F.S.S.**, **C.Stat**, who is an Assistant Professor in the Department of Mathematics and Computer Science at Central State University, Ohio, and was the national Evaluation Coordinator of the FCVP Program (2002–2006). He previously served as Research Assistant Professor of Social Science/Statistics at the University of Virgin Islands (2000–2002), Commonwealth Expert in the Eastern Caribbean (1997–2000), and United Nations Advisor in Africa (1985–1990). He was elected a Fellow of the Royal Statistical Society in 1978 and a Chartered Statistician, UK, in 1994 and has authored and coauthored several articles in the field of statistics and evaluation. Working with this team is a doctoral student, **Ramin Karimpour, Ph.D**. Candidate in educational psychology at the University of Illinois at Urbana-Champaign. Mr. Karimpour specializes in social-ecological bullying prevention programs, with a particular interest in field implementation opportunities and challenges. A former primary school teacher and secondary school principal, he served 7 years as an educator for the Tohono O'odham Nation of southwest Arizona. Finally, **Dana L. Johnson** is the Interim Title III Director at Central State University in Wilberforce, Ohio (2007–present) after serving as Interim Principal Investigator (2005–2007), the national prevention specialist, and Deputy Director of the FCVP Program between 2000 and 2005. Her professional and personal focus has been on supporting youth and community programs through mentorship as well as serving as a court appointed special advocate/guardian ad litem (CASA/GAL). She is also a certified True Colors Facilitator who conducts workshops to increase communication and team-building relationships among community-based organizations

In the final chapter, a longtime colleague and friend joins this editor in addressing a summary and series of take-home messages and lessons learned from this endeavor. **Robert McLaughlin, M.A., Ed.S.**, has recently retired from the Fayette County Public Schools after 31 years of service. He taught special education, was a principal, a district special education coordinator, and director, and spent the last 12 years supervising principals as an Elementary School Director. He taught 2 years in Galveston, Texas, in an alternative middle school. He currently works as an independent consultant and trainer for Safe and Civil Schools (Eugene, Oregon) specializing in Classroom Management, School wide Discipline, and Leadership development for principals and district staff. He is married, has three grown-up children, and continues to live in Lexington, Kentucky.

Prevention researchers, scientists, and educators hold a very special and unique position of responsibility in the realm of school-related violence. Contained in the book are a series of articles that address a spectrum of topics related to preventing school-related violence. As editor, I have searched nationally for educators', behavioral scientists, physicians, pediatricians, psychiatrists, child specialists, school principals, teachers, counselors, psychologists, most of whom are also parents with children and some with grandchildren. I challenged them to contribute to this volume. I am indeed honored by the response and the commitment and dedication of my colleagues in several disciplines, toward the contributions to the body of knowledge and to the completion of this volume. It is my sincere hope that you will find in this volume a better understanding of the issues, problems, and prevention strategies for the twenty-first century. I trust you will find, as I have, that no one person can address a topic such as this. We must recognize that this volume, along with the volumes that have preceded it, including the excellent contributions of **Florence Denmark, Ph.D.**, and her colleagues in their *Violence in the Schools: Cross-national and Cross-cultural Perspectives* (2006) and those volumes which follow us, will reflect our growth in understanding and commitment to make this a more peaceful world. The lesson clearly is that no one of us can achieve what all of us provide in our commitment to safeguarding our children and our schools in worldwide!

References

Beane, A.L. (2004). *The Bully Free Classroom. Over One Hundred Tips and Strategies for Teachers K-8*. Murray Kentucky: Bully Free Publications Inc.

Boxer, P., Goldstein, S., Musher-Eizenman, D., Gubow, E.F., & Heretick, D. (2005). Developmental issues in school based aggression prevention. *The Journal of Primary Prevention*, 26(5), 383–400.

Denmark, F., Krauss, H.H., Wesner, R.W., Midlarsky, E., & Gielen, U.P. (2006). *Violence in Schools: Cross-National and Cross-Cultural Perspectives*. New York: Springer Publishers Inc.

Edwards, D., Hunt, M., Meyers, J., Grogg, K., & Jarrett, O. (2005). Acceptability and student outcomes of a violence prevention curriculum. *The Journal of Primary Prevention*, 26(5), 401–418.

Espelage, D.L. & Swearer, S.M. (Eds.) (2004). *Bullying in American Schools: A Social-Ecological Perspective on Prevention and Intervention.* Mahwah, NJ: Lawrence Erlbaum Associates Incorporated.

Miller, T.W. (2005). School related violence and primary prevention. Guest editorial. *Journal of Primary Prevention,* 26(5), 381–382.

Miller, T.W., Veltkamp, L.J., & Kraus, R.F. (2005). Character education as a prevention strategy in school related violence. *The Journal of Primary Prevention,* 26(5), 455–467.

Rodney, L., Johnson, D., & Srivastava, R.P. (2005). Impact of culturally relevant violence prevention models on school aged youth. Developmental issues in school based aggression prevention. *The Journal of Primary Prevention,* 26(5), 439–454.

Spurling, R. (2006). *It is Time to Be Bully Free:* The Bully-Free School Zone Character Education Program. Dissertation Abstracts.

Thompson, S. & Kyle, K. (2005). Understanding mass shootings: Links between personhood and power in the competitive school environment. Developmental issues in school based aggression prevention. *The Journal of Primary Prevention,* 26(5), 419–438.

Part I
Theory, Assessment, and Forms of School Violence

Chapter 2
School-Related Violence: Definition, Scope, and Prevention Goals

Thomas W. Miller and Robert F. Kraus

The purpose of this book is to provide a compendium of papers addressing school violence and the critical ingredients in prevention interventions that contribute to reducing and/or eliminating various forms of violence in the school setting. The Center for the Prevention of School Violence developed a research-based definition of "school violence" in 1997. The definition, which emerged from a detailed microanalysis, suggests that school violence is any behavior that violates a school's educational mission or climate of respect or jeopardizes the intent of the school to be free of aggression against persons or property, drugs, weapons, disruptions, and disorder (Center for Prevention of School Violence, 2004). School violence involves a spectrum of crimes taking place within educational institutions. Ensuring safer schools requires establishing valid and reliable indicators of the current state of school crime and safety across the nation and periodically monitoring and updating such indicators. Two decades ago, the term "school violence" itself was widely used to describe violent and aggressive acts on school campuses. Today, the definition is much broader in scope.

Definition

School violence includes but is not limited to such behaviors as child and teacher victimization, child and/or teacher perpetration, physical and psychological exploitation, cyber victimization, cyber threats and bullying, fights, bullying, classroom disorder, physical and psychological injury to teacher and student, cult-related behavior and activities, sexual and other boundary violations, and use of weapons in the school environment. As resources, there are a number of state and federal agencies that include but are not limited to the U.S. Department of Education (2005), the National School Safety Center (2007), the US Department of Health and Human Services (2001), the National Center for Education Statistics (NCES), the Federal Bureau of Investigation (FBI), the Centers for Disease Control and Prevention (CDC, 2004), the Office of Juvenile Justice and Violence Prevention (2004), the U.S. Preventative Services task Force (1996), and the National Consortium of School Violence Prevention Researchers and Practitioners (2006) that provide important data in monitoring school-related violence and greater specificity to the definition of violence in schools.

T. W. Miller (ed.), *School Violence and Primary Prevention.*
© Springer 2008

Scope

Violence in American society generally and on children and adolescents specifically, who are the victims of more crimes than any other age group in the USA (Steinberg, 2000; Rennison, 2000), has become an increasingly difficult factor to control. When we speak of the scope of the problem, we realize that this problem is not uniquely our own but crosses national and international boundaries (Denmark et al., 2006). Globalization and technology and its availability to students and adults have influenced the growth of such behavior in the school environment. Suicide and homicide in the school setting is responsible for about 25% of deaths among persons aged 10–24 years in the USA (Arias et al., 2003). Epidemiological data on violence are derived from three primary sources: (1) hospital, emergency medical service, and medical examiner records; (2) police reports and arrest records (and other agency records, such as child protective services for reports of child abuse); and (3) self-report surveys and interviews. In addition, specialized studies that address the particular dynamics and contexts of violence have proven to be important to the understanding and prevention of violence. One of the more accurate markers for violence in the USA is homicide data. In our country, the overall homicide victimization rate has fluctuated during the twentieth century from fewer than 2 homicides per 100,000 in 1900 to a high of nearly 11 homicides per 100,000 in 1980. In 1998, 17,893 individuals were murdered in the USA, which translates into an average daily death toll of 49 people. The worldwide 1998 homicide rate was 12.5 per 100,000, significantly higher than the U.S. homicide rate of 6.2 per 100,000. Nevertheless, data from the 1980s reveal that among the 41 most developed countries, the USA has the third highest homicide rate (Elliott, 2001). While one does not always consider homicide as a part of school violence, it contributes to the total picture involving the scope of the problem (Blum et al., 2000; Brener et al., 2004; Thornton et al., 2000).

Risk Factors in Violence

Noteworthy in estimating the scope of violence perpetration among youth are efforts to identify *risk factors*—the characteristics that when present increase the probability that a young person will subsequently engage in violent acts. There are five important aspects of risk factors. First, risk factors tend to be additive—the more risk factors that are present, the more elevated the risk of violence. One risk factor generally has low predictive power. Even among those children and adolescents with multiple risk factors, few will become violent. Second, risk factors occur, and need to be addressed, at multiple levels, including individual, family, peer group, school, and neighborhood or community levels. Third, different risk factors pertain to different points in the lifespan, with family-level factors playing a greater role for younger children, and peer group and neighborhood factors playing a greater role for older children. Fourth, some risk factors are specific to certain types of violent behavior (e.g., risk factors for sexual violence may be quite different than those for robbery). Finally, the severity of risk-factor exposure is likely to increase or decrease risk proportionately (e.g., extreme and chronic child abuse is likely to have a more profound effect than lesser forms of child maltreatment) (Howell, 2000; Murphy, 2000).

Evidence-based information on risk factors that increase the probability that children and young teens will subsequently engage in violent behavior is emerging. These reviews have sorted out risk factors into two categories: risk factors during the childhood years and risk factors during the early adolescent years. Risk factors during infancy, and even perinatally, have also been identified, (e.g., child abuse and neglect). This entire body of research, however, is relatively new and far from exhaustive. Therefore, some factors that may in reality increase subsequent risk for violence perpetration may not have been identified in the extant literature because they have been inadequately researched or because of their complexity—the potency of a risk factor may be significantly affected by specific contextualized circumstances like neighborhood norms and personal history. Similarly, one factor may become a risk factor only, or may become a more potent risk factor, when it occurs in tandem with another factor. During childhood, the two most powerful predictors of subsequent violence perpetration are substance use and delinquency. Additional, less potent risk factors include aggressive behavior; family violence; inconsistent, overly lax, and harsh disciplinary practices; association with antisocial peers; and poor attitudes toward schooling. Media violence has been shown to increase aggression in the short term, but such exposure has not been linked directly to violent adolescent behavior. Conversely, attempts to reduce violence through media advocacy have not been shown to reduce rates of violence significantly.

During the early adolescent years, three major and interrelated risk factors have been identified: weak associational ties with nondelinquent peers; strong associational ties with antisocial and delinquent peers; and gang membership. Gang membership, in particular, appears to fulfill important psychological needs with regard to peer acceptance and belonging, as well as the need for enhanced social status, particularly for unpopular youth and for those youth who feel socially powerless. Because gangs serve these fundamental needs, efforts to dissuade young people from joining youth gangs is a more efficient strategy than trying to entice them out of the gang after they have joined, particularly since gangs typically promise to provide valued incentives such as money, power and status, excitement, and, for males, promises of sexual "favors." On the other hand, to ignore current gang members, or rely exclusively on punitive law enforcement efforts, is an inefficient and ineffective violence reduction strategy.

Community-based outreach efforts in association with community policing operations are required. Such efforts need to address the psychological, interpersonal, and economic needs of gang members; they should be based upon multiple sources of information about local gang activity and they should include collaborative efforts involving the police, schools, social service agencies, former gang members, and grassroots organizations. Other risk factors during the early adolescent years include antisocial behavior, attending a school in which gangs are prevalent, having been a victim of a violent crime, and residing in a high-crime neighborhood and/or in neighborhoods that have high levels of social disorganization. Because violence is not evenly distributed throughout the population, these overall homicide rates provide only a partial picture of homicide's toll. Most notably, homicide victimization in the USA is most prevalent among youth. In 2002, homicide was the second leading cause of death among 15- to 24-year-olds.

Prevention Goals

Healthy People 2000 and its successor Healthy People 2010 have, through a national health care policy agenda, set the goal of reducing the prevalence of physical fighting among adolescents to ≤32% and to reduce the prevalence of carrying a weapon by adolescents on school property to ≤4.9% (objective nos. 15–38 and 15–39) (U.S. Department of Health and Human Services, 2001). Schools and communities should continue efforts to establish physical and social environments that prevent violence and promote actual and perceived safety in schools. While the decline in school violence-related behaviors is encouraging, prevention efforts must be sustained if the nation is to achieve its 2010 national health objectives. In 2003, one in three high school students reported involvement in a physical fight and approximately 1 in 16 high school students reported carrying a weapon on school property. To further reduce violence-related behaviors among young persons and to have an impact on behaviors that are more resistant to change, continued efforts are needed to monitor these behaviors and to develop, evaluate, and disseminate effective prevention strategies.

As administrators, clinicians, researchers, educators, legislators, and justice department personnel continue efforts to reduce the incidence and prevalence of violence, it has generally gone unnoticed that the use and meaning of the term school violence have evolved over the past ten years. School violence is conceptualized as a multifaceted construct that involves both criminal acts and aggression in schools, which inhibits development and learning as well as harms the school's climate. School climate is important as the role of schools as a culture and as an organization has not always received attention because of different disciplinary approaches to studying the problem. Researchers have brought divergent orientations to their work, and these interests have not always been well coordinated with the primary educational mission of schools. An understanding of the multidisciplinary basis of school violence research is necessary in order to critically evaluate the potential use of programs that purport to reduce "school" violence.

Prevention scientists and practitioners hold a unique responsibility in the realm of school-based violence. Contained in this volume are a series of articles which address the spectrum of issues related to preventing the perpetration of school-related violence. They offer an understanding of theory, incidence, and prevalence and provide a forum for discussion of the need of understanding the multiple variables that must be considered in addressing prevention-based approaches to school violence as we enter the twenty-first century.

School Violence as a Public Health Initiative

The public health approach to prevention strategies for violence in the school setting and the larger community was given formal recognition in 1984 when Surgeon General C. Everett Koop stated: "Violence is every bit as much a public health issue for me and my successors in this century as smallpox, tuberculosis, and syphilis were for my predecessors in the last century." As the injury and death toll from violent behavior have become increasingly evident, multidisciplinary scholarship in the study of violence has emerged and expanded at an unprecedented pace. The most widely accepted definition of violence—sometimes termed "intentional inter-personal injury"—is: "behavior by persons against persons that intentionally threatens, attempts, or actually inflicts physical harm" (Reiss & Roth, 1993). The closely related terms "aggression" and "antisocial behavior" are generally applied to lesser forms of violence and include, but are not limited to, behaviors that are intended to inflict psychological harm as well as physical harm.

In approaching the prevention of violence, the Public Health Model advocates a four-step process: (1) data collection of violence-related problems, assets, and resources; (2) assessment of the possible causes of violence through risk-factor identification; (3) the establishment and evaluation of violence-prevention strategies; and (4) the dissemination and implementation of effective strategies. Public health, then, is inherently a research-driven and prevention-oriented science. This approach complements and overlaps with the narrower focus of criminology, which is primarily concerned with forms of violence that constitute crimes and with policies and practices that deter and punish perpetrators.

Levels of Prevention

Prevention must be considered on three levels, Primary, Secondary, and Tertiary. The U.S. Preventative Services Task Forces' Guide to Clinical Preventive Services (2nd edition, 1996) defines primary prevention measures as "those provided to individuals provided to prevent the onset of a targeted condition" (pp. xli). Primary prevention measures include activities that help avoid a given health care problem. Examples include passive and active immunization against disease as well as health protecting education and counseling promoting the use of automobile passenger restraints and bicycle helmets. Since successful primary prevention helps avoid the suffering, cost, and burden associated with disease, it is typically considered the most cost-effective form of health care.

The U.S. Preventative Services Task Forces' Guide to Clinical Preventive Services (2nd edition, 1996) describes secondary prevention measures as those that "identify and treat asymptomatic persons who have already developed risk factors or preclinical disease but in whom the condition is not clinically apparent" (pp. xli). These activities are focused on early case finding of asymptomatic conditions that occur commonly and has significant risk for negative outcome without treatment or some form of intervention. Screening tests are examples of secondary prevention activities, as these are done on those without clinical presentation of condition that has a significant latency period such as hypertension, breast, and prostate cancer. With early case finding, the natural history of disease or condition, or how the course of an illness or condition unfolds over time without treatment, can often be altered to maximize well-being and minimize the severity of the condition.

Tertiary prevention involves the care of established disease or condition, with attempts made to restore it to its highest function, minimize the negative effects of disease or condition, and prevent condition-related complications. Since the disease is now established, primary prevention activities may have been unsuccessful. Early detection through secondary prevention may have minimized the impact of the disease disorder or condition.

Major Goals and Approaches to Prevention

Prevention-oriented programs have several key goals. These include that (1) students understand their own peer culture, (2) students provide a typically untapped human resource; (3) the program is a network of involved youth; and (4) the involvement by students in implementing such programs provides an alternative for antisocial, violent, and delinquent behavior. School-based peer mediation, in which a trained student mediates a dispute between two other students with the goal of establishing a mutually agreed-upon peaceful solution, is considered to be an essential ingredient (Thompson & Kyle, 2005; Miller et al., 2005; McCord et al., 2001; Herrenkohl et al., 2000).

There are several major approaches to the prevention of school-related and other forms of violence that have been articulated: (1) the inculcation or enhancement of protective factors (factors that reduce the probability of violence perpetration among individuals exposed to known risk factors) and/or a corresponding reduction in the number or severity of risk factors, (2) the adoption of self-contained violence-prevention programs, (3) the specification of generic strategies (e.g., social skills training) derived by grouping effective and promising programs according to the approach they adopt and the specific program characteristics they utilize, and (4) the elucidation of framing principles that guide the establishment and implementation of programs.

The study of protective factors has been spurred by the long-standing observation that some children who are exposed to several known risk factors do not become violent or otherwise seriously impaired. The task, then, is to identify common characteristics or circumstances that buffer these resilient children from the ill effects of exposure to known risk factors. The scientific study of protective factors, however, is in its infancy and the evidence from this small body of literature is suggestive rather than conclusive. A well-documented protective factor is maintaining conventional values, including the rejection of aggressive or violent behavior as an appropriate means to resolve conflict. This characteristic is associated with the peer-level protective factor of associating with peers who hold prosocial values. At the family level, a warm and supportive relationship with one's parents or guardians and engagement in familial bonding activities have been associated with reduced levels of aggression (Boxer et al., 2005; Garbarino, 1999; Rodney et al., 2005).

Transitioning into the more high-risk adolescent years, family factors alone do not continue to exert a powerful protective effect. The inoculation effects of protective factors appear to require developmentally appropriate exposures at each stage of development with a firm foundation in the preschool and preadolescent phases of the life cycle. An extremely important factor involves school bonding. This is discussed in more detail in our chapter focusing on character development in this volume.

Assessments of the effectiveness of prevention programs such as these have been studied through a variety of methods. The use of scientific models of study has been recognized in the last two decades. Such scientific evaluations are costly and only a small proportion of programs now in use at schools and in communities have been evaluated using such scientific models. Those programs that have been evaluated are generally highly structured, implemented by professionals, and developed at academic institutions. While this body of research has revealed that some programs do indeed reduce rates of aggression and violence in the schools, several programs have not been studied but have realized some observable positive changes in students' behavior. It may also be wrong to conclude that programs that have been shown to be effective will necessarily work equally well in all settings, with both genders and in other contexts. There is a dearth of data on this and this must be explored in greater details so that models that are found to be effective show generalizability.

What Works Best in School-Related Violence Prevention?

During the last quarter of the twentieth century, several approaches on prevention of school violence have been documented (Edwards et al., 2005). Results of the most effective models for violence-prevention programs utilize social skills training. Social skills training programs generally utilize structured and interactive curricula (e.g., role playing) and are usually classroom based. In addition to social skills training, these programs focus on parent training, family interaction, and family dynamics. A third component involves teacher–student bonding and healthy interaction with peers in the school environment. Critical components to social skills training include emotional literacy, self-control, social competence, positive peer relations, and interpersonal problem solving. A second model involves psychoeducational strategies to reduce the likelihood of engaging in violent types of behavior. Some well-established community-based mentoring programs have been shown to be effective violence-prevention strategies. A third model offers programs involving counseling and supportive services for youth who have been exposed to violence, either as victims or as witnesses—both of which are risk factors for subsequent perpetration. Finally, a hybrid program that either combines two or more of the strategies or not fits neatly into any of the three approaches has been documented. Such a "hybrid" model is that developed by Olweus entitled Bullying-Prevention

Program (Olweus, 1993). This program has several key features, including skills-based classroom training, parent involvement, policy development, "hot spot" analysis, and counseling. Evaluations of this program suggest that it is effective in reducing levels of bullying and harassment. Indeed, multicomponent programs are generally viewed as preferable, particularly for high-risk youth.

A Pathway to Safer Schools

Prevention educators and scientists can be very helpful in consulting with school administrators, teachers, psychologists, nurses, social workers, and counselors in playing an effective role in limiting and mitigating the influence of problematic behavior, including violence in the school setting. The National School Safety Center (2007) suggests the following actions to limit violence in the schools: acknowledge the student's problem immediately and seek help from local health or mental health care professionals, police, and community resources; educate all school personnel about risk factors for both individuals and groups; establish an informed communication network with students; institute a strict visitor/trespassers policy in the schools; monitor and control points of access to the school; work closely with local police and establish procedures to share information with them. Examined in this special edition are clinical issues and case analyses of a spectrum of cases involving school violence situations in the Unites States involving lethal peer victimization by the perpetrator(s). Escape theory suggests that peer victimization is driven by the desire of the perpetrator to escape a state of painful self-awareness characterized by inadequacy, negative affect, and low self-esteem. And so in the volume, the reader will find chapters that will address critical issues and essential components of the task of preventing school-related violence and a potential pathway to safer schools.

References

Arias, E., Anderson, R. N., Kung, H. C., Murphy, S. L., & Kochanek, K. S. (2003). Deaths: Final data. *National Vital Statistics Report*s, 52, 1–100.

Blum, R. W., Beuhring, T., & Rinehart, P. M. (2000). *Protecting Teens: Beyond Race, Income and Family Structure*. Minneapolis, MN: Center for Adolescent Health, University of Minnesota.

Boxer, P., Goldstein, S., Musher-Eizenman, D., Gubow, E. F., & Heretick, D. (2005). Developmental issues in school based aggression prevention. *The Journal of Primary Prevention*, 26(5), 383–400.

Brener, N. D., Simon, T. R., Anderson, M., Barrios, L. C., & Small, M. L. (2004). Effect of the incident at Columbine on students' violence- and suicide-related behaviors. *American Journal of Preventive Medicine*, 22, 146–150.

Centers for Disease Control (2001). CDC School Health Guidelines to Prevent Unintentional Injuries and Violence MMWR 2001, 50 No. RR-22.

CDC (2004). Web-based Injury Statistics Query and Reporting System (WISQARS™). Atlanta, Georgia: U.S. Department of Health and Human Services, CDC, National Center for Injury Prevention and Control, 2004. Available at http://www.cdc.gov/ncipc/wisqars.

Center for the Study and Prevention of Violence. (2004). *Blueprints for Violence Prevention*. Boulder, Colorado: Institute of Behavioral Science, University of Colorado. Available at http://www.colorado.edu/scpv/blueprints.

Denmark, F., Krauss, H. H., Wesner, R. W., Midlarsky, E., & Gielen, U. P. (2006). *Violence in Schools: Cross-National and Cross-Cultural Perspectives*. New York: Springer Publishers Inc.

Edwards, D., Hunt, M., Meyers, J., Grogg, K., & Jarrett, O. (2005). Acceptability and student outcomes of a violence prevention curriculum. *The Journal of Primary Prevention*, 26(5), 401–418.

Elliott, D. S. (Ed.) (2001). *Youth Violence: A Report of the Surgeon General*. Atlanta, GA: Office of the Surgeon General.

Federal Bureau of Investigation (2003). *Age-Specific Arrest Rates and Race-Specific Arrest Rates for Selected Offenses: 1965–1992*. Washington, DC: Author.

Garbarino, J. (1999). *Lost Boys: Why Our Sons Turn Violent and How We Can Save Them*. New York: Free Press.

Herrenkohl, T. I., Magiun, E., Hill, K. G., Hawkins, J. D., Abbott, R. D., & Catalano, R. F. (2000). Developmental risk factors for youth violence. *Journal of Adolescent Health*, 26, 176–186.

Howell, J. C. (2000). *Youth Gang Programs and Strategies*. Washington, DC: Department of Justice.

McCord, J., Widom, C. S., & Crowell, N. A. (Eds.) (2001). *Juvenile Crime, Juvenile Justice*. Washington, DC: National Academy Press.

Miller, T. W., Veltkamp, L. J., & Kraus, R. F. (2005). Character education as a prevention strategy in school related violence. *The Journal of Primary Prevention*, 26(5), 455–467.

Murphy, S. L. (2000). *Deaths: Final Data for 1998*. Atlanta, GA: Centers for Disease Control and Prevention.

National Consortium of School Violence Prevention Researchers and Practitioners (2006). School Shootings Position Statement October 27, 2006. Author.

National School Safety Center (2007). The National School Safety Center serves as an advocate for safe, secure and peaceful schools worldwide and as a catalyst for the prevention of school crime and violence. Available at http://www.schoolsafety.us/

Office of Juvenile Justice and Violence Prevention (2004). *Promising Strategies to Reduce Gun Violence*. Washington, DC: Author.

Olweus, D. (1993). *Bullying at School*. Malden, MA: Blackwell Publishers.

Reiss, A. J. & Roth, J. A. (Eds.) (1993). *Understanding and Preventing Violence*. Washington, DC: National Academy Press.

Rennison, C. M. (2000). *Criminal Victimization 1999: Changes 1998–99 with Trends 1993–99*. Washington, DC: U.S. Department of Justice.

Rodney, L., Johnson, D., & Srivastava, E. P. (2005). Impact of culturally relevant violence prevention models on school aged youth. Developmental issues in school based aggression prevention. *The Journal of Primary Prevention*, 26(5), 439–454.

Steinberg, L. (2000). Youth violence: Do parents and families make a difference? *National Institute of Justice Journal*, 243, 30–38.

Thompson, S. & Kyle, K. (2005). Understanding mass shootings: Links between personhood and power in the competitive school environment. Developmental issues in school based aggression prevention. *The Journal of Primary Prevention*, 26(5), 419–438.

Thornton, T. N., Craft, C. A., Dahlberg, L. L., Lynch, B. S., & Baer, K. (2000). *Best Practices of Youth Violence: A Sourcebook for Community Action*. Atlanta, GA: Centers for Disease Control and Prevention, National Center for Injury Prevention and Control.

U.S. Preventative Services Task Force (1996). *Guide to Clinical Preventative Services*, 2nd edition. Baltimore: Williams & Wilkins.

U.S. Department of Education (2005). *2005 Annual Report on School Safety*. Washington, DC: Author.

U.S. Department of Health and Human Services. (2001). *Youth Violence: A Report of the Surgeon General*. Rockville, Maryland: U.S. Department of Health and Human Services, CDC, Substance Abuse and Mental Health Services Administration, and National Institutes of Health.

U.S. Department of Health and Human Services. (2000). *Healthy People 2010: Understanding and Improving Health and Objectives for Improving Health*, 2nd edition (2 vols.). Washington, DC: U.S. Department of Health and Human Services.

Violence Institute of New Jersey (2001). *Source Book of Drug and Violence Prevention Programs for Children and Adolescents*. New Brunswick: State of New Jersey, USA.

Chapter 3
The Neurobiology of Violence and Victimization

William P. French

Introduction

The primary purpose of this chapter is to provide a theoretical framework for understanding the neurobiology of violence and victimization, especially as it relates to school violence. In recent years, progress in neurobiological study designs, imaging techniques, and animal models has led to an expansion in our knowledge and understanding of the neurobiological structures, chemicals, circuits, and systems that regulate the expression of violence and victimization. However, more than simply describing the nature and function of these biological substrates, it is important to examine how environmental factors, especially early childhood experiences, influence (and are influenced by) the formation and function of these neurobiological systems. The expression of violence and victimization is best viewed within a developmental context beginning with gene expression in the embryo and continuing throughout the lifespan (Conner, 2002; Mash & Dozois, 1996). While most of the information presented in this chapter will pertain to research that is applicable to children and adolescents in their general environment, it will, for the most part, not directly be drawn from school violence literature. Therefore, while it is hoped the following discussion will provide pertinent information to the study of school violence, limits to the extrapolation of below data to the study of school violence should be kept in mind.

Key in understanding the current discussion is to keep in mind that while individuals begin the developmental process with certain innate propensities, based mainly on inherited genetic factors, the expression and direction of these propensities depends in large part on the interactions between these factors and the individual's environment. To understand the impact of these interactions, the individual's environment needs to be defined broadly enough to include the totality of environmental interactions that shape the destiny of the individual. Examples of such interactions include but are not limited to gene–protein (e.g., growth factor) interactions, gene–environment interactions, embryo–intrauterine interactions (e.g., the presence or absence of neurotoxic substances such as alcohol during gestation), infant–caregiver interactions (e.g., the quality of their attachment), adolescent–peer group interactions, and individual–community interactions. It is also important to emphasize the bidirectional nature of this process. For example, although it is true that males with high levels of testosterone have been found to display increased aggression (biology acting on environment), it has also been found that males placed in situations of social dominance experience an increase in their testosterone levels (environment acting on biology) (Conner, 2002; Rutter et al., 1997).

Note: In the remainder of this chapter, aggression and violence will be used interchangeably. Technically, aggression can only be exerted by an animate agent while violence can be produced by both animate and inanimate forces. Furthermore, the words aggression and aggressive both have potential positive meanings, which the words violence and violent do not. Therefore, it is important to note that adaptive aggression in animals and humans, if displayed in the right environmental context, is a positive trait. For example, a teenager, who fights off an intruder at home, may be aggressive, but this does not mean that he or she suffers from psychopathology. On the contrary, maladaptive aggression implies that the aggressive action being displayed is inappropriate to the context, ultimately harmful to the organism in its consequences, and represents a dysfunction of the organism, that is, it is psychopathological. Therefore, while the word "aggression" will be frequently used in the rest of the chapter, the implication is that the "aggression" being discussed is maladaptive unless otherwise noted (Conner, 2002). Additionally, when discussing victims and victimization often it will be more convenient to discuss the topic using words such as maltreatment, trauma, and traumatized.

Gene–Environment Interactions in Violence and Victimization

From a biologically oriented perspective, the study of the root causes of violence and victimization in school and in society involves attempting to understand how human biology interacts with the environment in ways that lead to maladaptive behavior. This approach inevitably brings us to discuss current concepts in the long-standing historical, philosophical, and scientific debates over the role of "nature" versus "nurture" in determining human behavior. Since the rise of the biological sciences, there have been several significant swings of the pendulum from extremes of biological determinism on the one hand to extreme behavioralism on the other (Niehoff, 1999). In recent years, however, this either/or dichotomy has been transcended (at least in certain fields such as developmental biology and neurobiology) to be replaced by a growing appreciation of the interdependent bidirectional role of *gene–environment interactions* in directing the development of organisms.

Gene–environment interactions play a role in all aspects of an organism's development from conception to death. The following example, examining the relation between developing neural cells and certain proteins called growth factors that regulate their development, illustrates the basic model of *gene–environment interactions*. Growth factors, also known as trophic factors (meaning, "to nourish"), are essential in guiding and nurturing neurons during nervous system development. By binding to receptors on the cell surfaces of young, differentiating neurons, trophic factors initiate biochemical changes that lead to selective gene expression. This process ultimately produces specialized neurons that are able to carry out the specific functions that are required in their local environments. For example, under the influence of nerve growth factor (NGF), precursor neural crest cells migrate out of the neural tube to become sympathetic neurons, which function in the autonomic nervous system (ANS). These same precursor cells, when they migrate to the adrenal gland, however, come under the influence of a different kind of trophic factor called glucocorticoid and do not develop into sympathetic neurons but into a different class of cells called Chromaffin cells, which have similar but distinct function compared to the sympathetic neurons (Niehoff, 1999). Trophic factors, thus, serve as environmental elements that interact with genetic elements to influence genetic expression. Dysregulation of trophic factors has been found in trauma victims with posttraumatic stress disorder (PTSD) and in animal and human subjects with aggression, which highlights the potential multilevel (micro to macro) influence of *gene–environment interactions* in selecting, regulating, and controlling neurobiological development. In fact, the study of *gene–environment interactions* has been able to progress beyond describing how local factors such as proteins are able to modify genetic expression. Through the work of leaders in the field of developmental psychopathology (such as Michael Rutter, Terrie Moffitt, and Avshalom Caspi), studies have conducted to show how environmental influences, as far removed from direct contact with the genome as parental treatment of children, can modulate gene expression in ways that influence the expression of behaviors such as aggression and the development of depression (see Rutter et al., 2006, for an overview of the field).

An Example of the Role Gene–Environment Interactions Play in Modulating Aggression and Violence

A number of studies have been undertaken in recent years exploring how genes interact with the environment to modify the expression of aggression and violence. One of the most interesting lines of inquiry in this regard has been into the role a class of neurochemicals called monoamines play in mediating aspects of violence. An influential study on violence in maltreated children reported by Caspi et al. (2002) highlights some of the important research findings in this area. Their study draws on a large cohort of 1,037 children born in 1972 who are part of the Dunedin Multidisciplinary Health and Development Study. The researchers looked at gene–environment interactions in children who either had or had not been exposed to maltreatment between the ages of 3 and 11 years. They were interested in determining the effect maltreatment would have in these children in predicting antisocial behavior at age 26, depending on whether the children had one of two types of polymorphisms (different versions of the same gene) for the gene monoamine oxidase A (MAOA) located on the X chromosome.

The gene product MAOA enzyme is a protein that metabolizes monoamines such as dopamine (DA), norepinephrine (NE), and serotonin. Thirty-seven percent of a subsample of 442 males in the study had a version of the MAOA gene which produces a low-activity enzyme. Sixty-three percent of the males had a version of this gene which produces a high-activity enzyme. Additionally, they categorized the children according to whether they had been exposed to severe maltreatment (8%), probable maltreatment (28%), or no maltreatment (64%). When they looked at the gene–environment interactions, they found that the 55 males who had both probable or severe maltreatment and *low* MAOA activity were twice as likely to have received a diagnosis of conduct disorder (CD) in their teens, and three times as likely to have been convicted of violent crime by age 26, as the 99 males with maltreatment and *high* MAOA activity. This subgroup of 55 boys, which was only 12% of the sample, was responsible for 44% of the violent convictions.

One conclusion which can be drawn from this study is that neither maltreatment nor genetic risk alone was associated with an appreciable level of antisocial behavior. It was only the interaction of a high-risk gene with a susceptible environment (a specific *gene–environment interaction*) that (presumably) produced a change in gene expression, which then contributed to a higher incidence of antisocial behavior.

A more recent study by Manuck (2006) investigating 531 white healthy males from the general population produced findings consistent with Caspi's original study. In this study, men with the low-activity MAOA allele were more likely to report a history of emotional reactivity, impulsive aggression, and antagonistic and confrontational behavior than those with the high-activity allele but only if they also had poorly educated fathers and were perceived as being cynical and hostile by others.

Other investigations in this area have examined the effect these polymorphisms of the MAOA gene may have on brain structure and function, especially during neurodevelopment. Meyer-Lindenberg et al. (2006), using functional magnetic resonance imaging (fMRI) to measure brain volume and activity differences, report that compared to individuals with the high-activity allele, individuals with the low-activity allele (and thus presumably with higher serotonin levels during neurodevelopment) have reduced brain volumes in several neural structures known to play crucial roles in emotional and behavioral regulation, including the anterior cingulate, bilateral amygdala, and the hypothalamus. Their results also showed increased activity in the left amygdala and decreased activity in the cingulate cortex and orbital frontal cortex (OFC), as well as decreased OFC-amygdala connectivity in males in response to emotionally provocative stimuli. These findings underscore what are thought to be the respective roles of these structures in modulating aggressive, impulsive behavior—namely, that an overly reactive amygdala, with dysfunctional inhibitory modulation by important neural structures involved in its regulation (OFC and cingulate cortex), may be playing a significant role in contributing to the pathology seen in emotionally disturbed children with impulsive, reactive aggression. While some additional studies examining how maltreatment affects the expression of the MAOA gene (including attempts to replicate Caspi's original finding) have had mixed results, a recent meta-analysis by Kim-Cohen et al. (2006) reports that the findings remain valid.

Of course, neither the above authors nor other researchers investigating the role of the MAOA gene in impulsive aggression are claiming that violence in youths and adults is caused solely by the low activity version of the MAOA gene. In contrast, most recent research in behavioral genetics stresses the probable influence of multiple genes in the etiology of any given pathological condition. Moreover, as is being suggested in this section, environmental interactions at multiple levels (biological, psychological, and social) probably impact how multiple genes contribute to the manifestation of aggression and violence (and most likely for victimization as well, though no data supporting this will be presented here).

Clinical Considerations

As the above study suggests, understanding human maladaptive behavior (in this case impulsive aggression) requires a consideration of biology, the environment, and the interaction between them. The question for care providers is not "Is it nature or nurture?" but "How do predetermined biological characteristics (genes, temperament, etc.) interact with an individual's environment (attachment experiences, exposures to violence, available resources) to influence behavior?" (Siegel, 2001).

While the use of knowledge of allelic variation of genes is currently been taken advantage of to guide treatment in some psychiatric disorders (see de Leon et al., 2006), it is, as yet, currently not being recommended or used to identify children and adolescents at risk for aggression and violence and/or to guide their treatment. Unfortunately, widespread application of behavioral genetics to societal problems like violence and mental illness unfortunately has a tainted past in the form of the eugenics movement of the early 1900s (Niehoff, 1999). In the future, though, as data on the importance genes–environment interactions in determining behavior continue to accumulate, efforts to identify youth at risk for aggression (based on genetic polymorphisms) may be critical in efforts to initiate early interventions in order to modify the risk of environmental exposure to potential pathological influences such as parental maltreatment.

While several steps removed from the level of genetic analysis, the work of Jerome Kagan (1989) is an example of how understanding nature–nurture interactions can lead to changes in developmental trajectory through first identifying unique biological traits in children and then applying targeted environmental interventions in an attempt to modify these traits. In his work with childhood temperament, Kagan has been able to show that shy children, whose parents encouraged them to be more curious in novel situations, developed more outgoing behaviors than did children whose parents did not offer this encouragement. Shy children have been shown to have larger corticosteroid responses to stress than do uninhibited children. By carefully attempting to modify inhibited children's behavioral responses through graduated, supported exposure to novel environments, these parents may be helping their children to alter corticosteroid response to stress, leading to altered gene expression in the brain, which ultimately may further influence behavior change. Victimized children, such as those who suffer from PTSD, often also show exaggerated hormonal response to subsequent stressors, which can lead to physiological symptoms that serve to maintain their hyperresponsive behavior (Siegel, 2001). Cross-fostering studies in rats where high pup licking and grooming mothers raise offspring of low pup licking and grooming parents have shown that gene expression changes in response to the cross-fostering promote changes in the function of the hypothalamic-pituitary-adrenal (HPA) axis that lead these pups to have more modest hormonal responses to stress and be less fearful as adults than those low licking and grooming pups that were not cross-fostered (Kramer, 2005).

Youth Trauma, Abuse, and Neglect

Introduction

In America, childhood and adolescent psychiatric disorders are usually diagnosed and categorized utilizing the American Psychiatric Association's *Diagnostic and Statistical Manual of Mental Disorders*, fourth edition, text revision (DSM-IV-TR, 1994). The DSM uses categorical descriptions of observable or reported signs and symptoms to define disorders. With this system, to be diagnosed with a particular psychiatric disorder, for example, PTSD, a person must meet the discreet criteria for the disorder and be experiencing impairment in daily functioning as a consequence. With the DSM, a person either has a disorder or does not. While, this chapter will discuss several DSM disorders, it focuses on understanding the neurobiological substrates associated with violence and victimization, which is not considered in the DSM. Furthermore, the approach utilized here, unlike the categorical approach in the DSM, is dimensional and assumes that behavior, if viewed as a reflection of neurobiology interacting with the environment, exists on a continuum from adaptive to maladaptive. (For descriptions of the various DSM disorders discussed, please refer to the DSM-IV-TR.)

Understanding the effects of childhood trauma, abuse, and neglect has evolved over the last three decades since Fraiberg's 1975 seminal work *Ghosts in the Nursery* (Fraiberg et al., 1987) described the multigenerational deleterious effects that occur in impaired mother–infant relationships. One of the main features of current research-driven formulations of childhood trauma is that multiple variables influence the generation and severity of psychopathology. Depending on frequency, severity, the degree to which caregivers are involved, the age of the child, and factors related to individual vulnerability and resilience, the consequences of maltreatment can range from little or no effect to profound disruptions of multiple aspects of normal development lasting across the lifespan (van der Kolk, 2003).

In current psychiatric and psychological practice, diagnoses of PTSD and acute stress disorder (ASD) are commonly employed in attempting to categorize the consequences of childhood maltreatment. However, the range and degree of potential disruption to normal development that occurs as a result of childhood trauma (especially when severe) fails to be captured in these diagnoses (Cook et al., 2005). It is not surprising, therefore, that child victims of trauma and neglect often meet criteria for multiple disorders other than PTSD and ASD, including but not limited to anxiety disorders, mood disorders, cognitive disorders such as attention-deficit hyperactivity disorder (ADHD), disruptive behavior disorders, sensory integration disorders, and reactive attachment disorders (Cook et al., 2005). In severe and chronic maltreatment cases, symptoms of PTSD may not even be prominent and may be obscured by other behavioral, affective, and cognitive concerns (van der Kolk, 2003). Child trauma experts in recent years have begun using the terms *complex trauma* and *developmental trauma* to better capture the significance of maltreatment and neglect in the young. Early trauma causes pervasive and lasting impact on the developing mind and brain, leading to disruption of developing neurobiological systems, which, in turn, manifests in the development of complex behavioral and psychological symptoms. In order to facilitate a more informed clinical approach to children whose experiences of violence, fear, and neglect play a significant role in their early development, van der Kolk argues for a new diagnostic criteria *Developmental Trauma Disorder* to guide assessment and treatment of children with complex trauma histories (van der Kolk, 2005). Alexandra Cook and colleague list seven domains affected by complex trauma, some of which are incorporated in the discussion below.

Domains of Trauma

Attachment

Mary Ainsworth and Mary Main expanding on John Bowlby's (1973) formulation of caregiver–infant attachment theory have described four patterns of relating that infants and young children use to organize their cognitive, affective, and behavioral approaches to their environments: secure, insecure-avoidant, insecure-ambivalent, and insecure-disorganized (Davies, 1999). Newborns are born with immature nervous systems that are unable to self-regulate in the face of internal and environmental stressors. Children with secure attachment receive assistance in self-regulation from attentive caregivers, who by responding caringly to their infants' needs and signals of distress help them modulate their stress responses. By responding to children with a balance of soothing and stimulation, caregivers serve as "hidden regulators" of infant physiological states of arousal and relaxation. This capacity to provide comfort and security acts bidirectionally, creating a state of "affect attunement" that reinforces the attachment process. At the same time, it creates the stable conditions necessary for the healthy maturation of the nervous system and ultimately enables the child to independently and flexibly modulate his or her stress responses (van der Kolk, 2003; Ainsworth, 1985). Caregiver–infant interactions, by contributing to the maturation of the nervous system, are one example of how interpersonal relationships influence neurobiology in the formation and function of the developing mind and brain (Siegel, 2001).

Childhood trauma, violence, and neglect often disrupt the normal attachment process; this is especially likely if the caregiver is the source of the trauma, suffers from the trauma as well, or responds to the trauma in a very disorganized, chaotic fashion (van der Kolk, 2003; McFarlane, 1988). While all the insecure attachment patterns are less than optimal, a study by Carlson found that 80% of traumatized children show the unhealthiest pattern—insecure-disorganized attachment (Carlson et al., 1989). A high percentage of parents with children who show disorganized attachment themselves have histories of abuse, neglect, and unresolved trauma. These parents are often anxious and fearful and commonly display intense emotions in the present related to unresolved traumas in the past. In interactions with their parents, children with disorganized attachment often show signs of alarm and may appear frightened by their parents' intense expression of negative emotions, inconsistent parenting, and potentially violent behavior.

Disorganized children are at high risk for the development of psychopathology for several reasons: (1) they are exposed (perhaps chronically) to frightening experiences, which produce large physiological stress responses that overcome their underdeveloped coping capacities; (2) though they are unable to cope with their stress, their caregivers not only do not serve as "hidden regulators" of physiological arousal, they often are the source of the distress; and (3) although they may feel intense anger and other negative emotions toward their attachment figures, they may be filled with conflicting feelings because they also still must rely on these caregivers as sources of security and belonging. Studies of traumatized children with disorganized styles of attachment show that they often respond to stress and perceived threat with fear-driven fight, flight, freeze reactions that (1) lead to withdrawing, self-destructive, or aggressive behaviors and (2) prevent them from developing (and learning to use) skills such as affect regulation and cognitive inhibition of impulses that enable healthy children to flexibly respond and manage stress.

The Role of Biology, Trauma, and Working Models in the Development of Psychopathology

Trauma affects multiple neurotransmitter systems, disrupts the normal development of important neural structures such as the hippocampus, impairs the connectivity and information flow between neural structures, and is implicated in producing persistent functional alterations in important stress-regulating systems such as the ANS and the HPA axis (van der Kolk, 2003).

As a child grows, modifications (e.g., as from trauma) to the biological systems that regulate functions such as arousal, behavior, affect, and cognition will, in turn, affect the way the child relates to, organizes, interprets, and responds to his or her environment. Perry and Pollard summarize this process by stating, "Experience and brain combine to determine how children interpret reality in a use-dependent manner" (Perry & Pollard, 1998; van der Kolk, 2003). Bowlby believed this process begins during the attachment period and used the term *internal working model* to describe the process in which children develop inner maps or representations of themselves, their relationships, and their environments that help them organize and regulate their responses to situations and people. Working models contribute to the development of a sense of self and play a role in a child's ability to regulate states of arousal and respond flexibly to stress. By the third year, internal working models are relatively enduring and thus tend to become stable filters through which subsequent events and relationships are experienced (Davies, 1999).

Fear conditioning in animals provides a model for understanding how childhood trauma affects internal working models, nervous system development, and development of psychopathology. Animals exposed to aversive unconditioned stimuli (e.g., an electrical shock) paired with a neutral conditioned stimulus (e.g., a light) will develop an enduring conditioned fear response to the conditioned stimulus even in the absence of a shock. This conditioning is difficult to extinguish, and depending on laboratory conditions can produce chronic alterations in biological systems involved in fear conditioning and the stress response such as the ANS and HPA axis (Conner, 2002).

Children undergoing nervous system development are especially vulnerable to developing enduring conditioned fear responses in the face of trauma. If they occur during the early attachment period, traumatic fear responses "may constitute the original organizing experience for the [children's] developing CNS" (Perry & Pollard, 1998). If trauma is ongoing, the nervous system may undergo lasting changes that "hard-wire" these fear-conditioned biological changes in a use-dependent manner, producing children who are chronically hyperaroused, fearful, and insecure and who show evidence of lasting alterations in CNS function. Heim et al. (2000) report adult women sexually or physically abused as children show abnormal HPA axis and ANS responses to mild stress, while Bremmer et al. (1997) using MRI have documented hippocampal atrophy in adult patients with PTSD who had been abused as children.

Along with changes in neurobiological function, trauma produces alterations in the working models children use to make sense of their world and organize their experiences. The working models of many severely traumatized children show a pattern of lack of self-confidence, mistrust of others, and experiencing the world as threatening. As mentioned above, working models are relatively stable after the third year, and since they are unconsciously formed, are unconsciously projected onto future relationships and situations, leading to additional dysfunctional experiences even in the absence of continuing sources of trauma. Such adaptations to traumatic experience, which then serves as a template for processing future experiences, may also occur in older children, adolescents, and adults exposed to trauma as part of a trauma accommodation syndrome (Miller & Veltkamp, 1996). Previously physically abused children who behave in ways that invite aggressive responses from otherwise well-intentioned foster parents and sexually abused woman who consistently become involved in relationships with abusive partners are examples of how past trauma acts in the present to recreate past patterns of behavior (Davies, 1999).

Cognition, Affect Regulation, and Behavioral Control: The Role of the Amygdala in the Threat Response

As discussed above, neurobiological systems that regulate arousal and stress responses, though functional, are immature at birth and therefore require caregiver intervention to modulate their activities. As development continues, however, securely attached children gain greater control in their abilities to self-soothe and control their response to stress. Part of this control is due to the gradual development of functional competencies in biological systems that regulate cognition and affect. Unlike many structures more directly involved with survival that are fully functional from birth, structures such as the hippocampus (involved in memory and emotion processing) and the prefrontal cortex (involved in executive functioning, impulse control, and affect regulation) develop their functional capacities more slowly. As these affective and cognitive (executive) capacities come "on-line" during normal development, they provide additional layers of regulatory capacity, enabling children and adolescents to fine-tune their behavioral responses to situations and people. The discussion below highlighting the role of the prefrontal cortex and hippocampus in regulating the fear pathway provides an example of how cognitive and affective input contributes to overall stress regulation.

The amygdala is a key neural structure in the limbic system that registers threat. When activated it produces fear. It functions by assigning emotional valency (or intensity) to incoming stimuli. (For example, for humans, a snake usually has more emotional valency than a stick.) When activated by a threat, the amygdala sends signals to the hypothalamus, which activates stress responses via the HPA axis and ANS, thus preparing a person for defensive action. The hippocampus begins to develop only from approximately 3 years. As it matures, it provides a child with the capacity to form context-dependent autobiographical memories, which includes the ability to organize and place sources of threat in a spatial context. It has inhibitory inputs to the hypothalamus, which serve to inhibit the activation of the stress response. This, in turn, leads to inhibition of the amygdala through feedback mechanisms involving cortisol. In fear-provoking situations, the hippocampus, through its role in memory, is able to provide greater flexibility of response and behavioral control by helping a child better interpret the emotional significance of incoming stimuli through connecting the current threatening experience to similar past emotional experiences and responses (LeDoux, 2002; Conner, 2002; van der Kolk, 2003).

The prefrontal cortex also plays an inhibitory role in relation to the amygdala and thus is able to provide additional regulatory control to the fear pathway. In situations of immediate threat, sensory information reaches the thalamus, which then directs it on two separate pathways: one to the amygdala and one to the prefrontal area (via sensory association areas), which then continues on to the amygdala (see Figs. 3.1 and 3.2). The short pathway allows for rapid responses to threats by direct amygdala activation of the fear pathway, while the long pathway permits frontal areas of the brain to gather more detailed information about the threat, which then can be used to modulate the initial response. When you come upon an object resembling a snake, the short pathway allows you to quickly move out of the way, while the long pathway, though it takes more time, allows you to gather more detailed visual information to determine if the object is really a snake or just a stick. While slower than the pathway directly to the amygdala, the long pathway, via pathways through the prefrontal cortex to the amygdala, permits cortical areas of the brain capable of reasoning, planning, problem solving, and representational memory to modulate emotional, physiological, and behavioral responses to threats and stress (LeDoux, 1999).

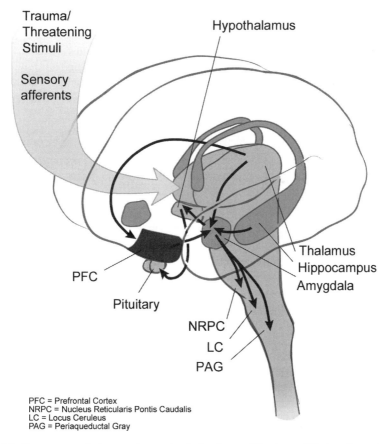

Fig. 3.1 Fear response/hot aggression anatomical pathways (Courtesy of Medmovie.com)

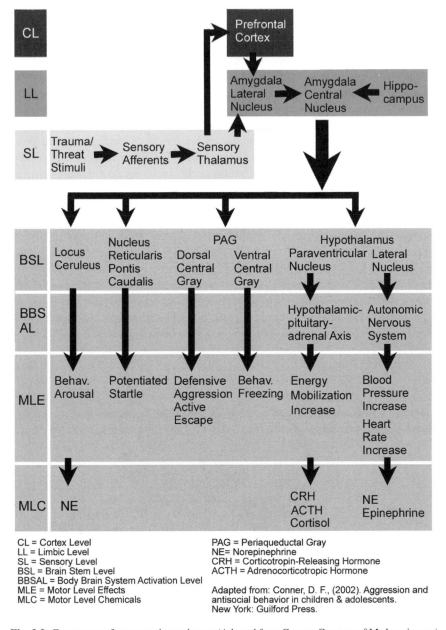

Fig. 3.2 Fear response/hot aggression pathways (Adapted from Conner, Courtesy of Medmovie.com)

In normal development, neurobiological structures and processes involving cognition, emotion, behavior, and physiology all work together in producing an integrated, functional, and flexible nervous system that enables developing children to successfully respond to their environments. As discussed above in the introduction to this section, trauma potentially produces deficits in multiple aspects of nervous system function including those that involve affect regulation, cognition, and behavioral control.

Affect

In studies involving affect regulation, maltreated children show deficits in their ability to identify and label emotional states in themselves and others, which may impair their own ability to understand, regulate, and respond appropriately to their feelings and the feelings of others (Beeghly & Cicchetti, 1996). Such deficits in important social skills often lead to social withdrawal or bullying of other children (van der Kolk, 2003). Damage to the hippocampus, as seen sufferers of PTSD, may lead to impairments in autobiographical memory impacting the ability of traumatized children to use past experiences to regulate current affective states. Studies of the long-term consequences of maltreatment on affect regulation indicate past trauma is the third most common predictor of adult depression aside from heredity and current stress (Harvard Mental Health Letter, 2005). Perhaps the most common association between childhood trauma and later problems with affect regulation, however, occurs in borderline personality disorder where a history of previous maltreatment, especially sexual abuse, is the norm rather than the exception. Such individuals commonly exhibit dysregulation of nervous system function across multiple domains including instability of emotional affect manifesting in intense mood swings, irritability, anxiety, periodic dysphoria often associated with suicidal ideation or attempts, and severe problems with anger and interpersonal relationships.

Cognition

Victimized children and adolescents also display deficits in multiple areas of cognition. Studies of maltreated children have shown decreased overall IQ; deficits in receptive and expressive language abilities; problems in learning and memory; deficits in executive functioning leading to problems in attention, impulse control, and abstract reasoning; decreased creativity, flexibility, and sustained interest in problem solving; greater need for special education services; and dropout rates three times that of the general population (Culp et al., 1991; Beers & De Bellis, 2002; Shonk & Cicchetti, 2001).

Problems with autonomic hyperarousal and affect regulation may contribute to short-term cognitive difficulties by creating physiological, emotional, social, and environmental conditions that interfere with immediate cognitive tasks; over time, these dysfunctional patterns of arousal and affect, however, can lead to permanent alterations in cognitive systems through their deleterious effects on important neural structures and circuits. Short-term impairment of cognitive capacity may occur when excessive subcortical "noise" from brain stem, autonomic, and limbic systems overwhelms cortical functioning. Hyperarousal, partly mediated by elevated epinephrine, has been associated with decreased executive functioning capacity in areas involved in working memory, attention, and impulse inhibition (Crittenden, 1997). Mezzacappa et al., (1998) showed that traumatized boys have decreased vagal modulation in parasympathetic branches of the ANS that are involved in executive control. Additional sources of cognition dysfunction in traumatized children involve (1) deficits in language due to underdevelopment of the left cortex (responsible for language function in most humans) and (2) impairments in learning and memory involving the hippocampus brought on by excess secretion of cortisol and impaired secretion of brain-derived neurotrophic factor (BDNF), a trophic factor that supports hippocampal development (Bremner, 2006).

Behavior

Childhood and adolescent trauma is associated with both overcontrolled (i.e., rigid, compulsive) and undercontrolled (i.e., impulsive, aggressive) behavior patterns. Some commonly seen behavior patterns include reenactment of the trauma (e.g., sexualized behaviors in sexually abused youth); heightened sensitivity to threat (i.e., aggressive behaviors); attempts to gain control (i.e., eating disorders); avoidance (i.e., social withdrawal); and maladaptive efforts to self-soothe (i.e., cutting) (Cook et al., 2005). Except for discussions involving the neurobiology of fear and fear-based aggression, the neurobiology involved in these complex behaviors is beyond the scope of this chapter.

Risk and Resiliency

Not everyone exposed to trauma develops PTSD or some other psychopathology. In fact, some clinicians and researchers believe that an overemphasis on the potential pathological responses to negative events places trauma victims at risk for developing maladaptive outcomes by pathologizing these experiences. In their view, such catastrophizing engenders a negative expectation concerning future outcome that can actually serve to undermine a healthy adaptive response. These researchers focus on the concept of resiliency and emphasize that stress is common, successful adaptation to stress is the norm, and overcoming stress actually can promote resiliency against future stress (Levin, 2006). Research in resiliency attempts to identify the biological, psychological, and environmental characteristics of individuals who experience stressful events and adversity but are able to recover quickly without developing maladaptive responses or dysfunction.

Animal research in rats has provided evidence as to how resiliency might occur at the neurobiological level. Amat and colleagues exposed rats to two sets of experimental conditions. In the first condition, they first exposed rats to a controllable stressor and then to an uncontrollable one; in the second condition, they first exposed rats to an uncontrollable stressor and then to an additional stressor. They were able to show that rats exposed to the controllable stressor were resistant to the development of depression-like behavior when exposed to future stressors while the rats first exposed to the uncontrollable stressor were susceptible to the development depression-like behaviors when faced with future stressors. Further experimental work showed that the ventral medial prefrontal cortex (vmPFC) and the dorsal raphe nucleus in the brain stem were both involved in this process in a way that suggests that when the rats "sense" control over stressful situations the vmPFC is able to inhibit the release of serotonin from the dorsal raphe nucleus. The clinical implication here is that perceived control is able to buffer against the deleterious effects of stress through the action of prefrontal structures inhibiting stress-responsive structures in lower brain areas such as the brain stem. This competency in the face of stress may promote resiliency by "inoculating" the organism against maladaptive responses to future stressors (Amat et al., 2006). Additional work in stress inoculation done by Parker et al. (2006) demonstrated that early stress can be beneficial in primates as well by showing that in male squirrel monkeys early, intermittent stress in infancy, such as increasing foraging demands on mothers, leads to a reduced HPA axis response in face of stress as adults.

In humans, Laura Campbell-Sills and coworkers (2006) report that individuals with childhood neglect, who also scored high on tests of resiliency, showed fewer psychiatric symptoms as adults than other individuals with high resiliency but who did not experience childhood neglect. While the neurobiological mechanism for this finding was not studied, these results echo those of the above studies in nonhuman animals and suggest that the combination of resiliency and exposure to stress creates conditions for mental health in the face of challenge.

Clinical Considerations

Paul MacLean, former director of the NIH's Laboratory of Brain Evolution and Behavior, is best known as the originator of the concept of *the triune brain* (Ploog, 2003). Introduced in 1970, the theory of the triune brain uses concepts and research findings in evolutionary theory, comparative neuroanatomy, and neurochemistry to describe how modern human brains are the result of three successive, hierarchically organized stages of animal evolution that in humans (and other closely related mammals) has led to the formation of three-brains-in-one. MacLean termed these three distinct "brains" *reptilian* (sensorimotor and autonomic systems), *paleomammalian* (limbic system), and *neomammalian* (executive system). He believed that though connected and organized to operate in an integrated fashion, because each "brain" evolved separately, each has separate distinct functions mediated through its unique anatomy and phylogeny (LeDoux, 1999).

MacLean's model provides a useful heuristic for discussing how human cognitive (executive), emotional (limbic), and behavioral (sensorimotor, endocrine, and autonomic) systems operate hierarchically to produce both adaptive and maladaptive responses to victimization. Moreover, conceiving of the brain as a triune system can be useful in assessing and devising treatment strategies, not only for victims of trauma but also for other categories of psychopathology (including maladaptive aggression) by helping clinicians analyze and breakdown complex clinical presentations into more manageable cognitive, emotional, and behavioral components. For example, in the treatment of PTSD, such a strategy can aid in selecting appropriate medications by helping categorize target symptoms (arising from a background of neurobiological malfunction) into cognitive, affective, and behavioral (including autonomic) components in order to better align medication's mechanisms of action with intended treatment outcomes (see Fig. 3.3).

Another application of the triune model is to use its hierarchical structure to separate therapeutic approaches to victimization and trauma into "top-down" or "bottom-up" interventions (Ogden et al., 2006). As discussed above, the human

ACUTE PTSD PATHOGENESIS MODEL WITH
PSYCHOPHARMACOLOGICAL INTERVENTIONS IN *BOLD*

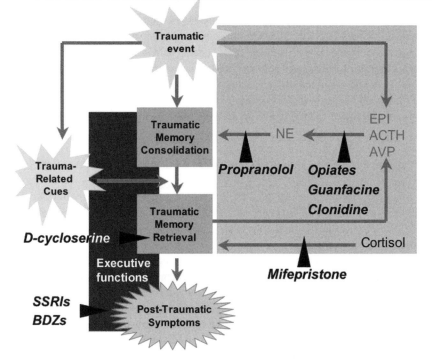

Adapted from: Pitman RK, Delahanty DL. CNS Spectr. Vol 10, No 2. 2005

Fig. 3.3 Posttraumatic stress disorder (PTSD) treatment (Adapted from Pitman, Courtesy of Medmovie.com)

brain develops through the emergence of inborn potentialities that are realized in a time-dependent developmental sequence that involves interaction with caregivers and other environmental inputs. While a child is born able to breathe and regulate many physiological processes without caregiver support, higher order capacities such as behavioral control, affect regulation, and cognitive function only develop over time through interactions with the environment.

In young people, the impact of trauma is thought to especially affect subcortical neurobiological systems, such as the limbic system and brain stem, which are critical for stress regulation and innate and learned responses to threat (van der Kolk, 2003). While top-down interventions (e.g., talk therapy) may attempt to enlist a patient's cognitive capacities in order to understand, process, or make sense of past trauma, such attempts may be misguided if the child's cognitive capacities are not yet sufficiently developed or he or she remains "stuck" in a dsyregulated physiological and emotional state that blocks effective cognitive processing of potentially curative information (Ogden et al., 2006). As such, one approach clinicians may choose to take is a bottom-up intervention using pharmaceuticals (such as a beta-adrenergic blocker or alpha 2-adrenergic agonist) to treat physiological hyperarousal through manipulating the ANS. While this approach may ameliorate some of the physiological symptoms that are contributing to suffering, it does not address the cause of the continued hyperarousal and activation of the stress response system in the absence of persisting threat.

Van der Kolk suggests that a key cause of a persistent state of conditioned fear and chronic stress in a child following trauma is the loss of a sense of safety and security, created in part by the subcortical systems responsible for responding to stress and danger having been overwhelmed and/or caregivers having been unable to intervene in their role as "hidden regulators." What needs to occur ultimately then is a restoration of a sense of security in the environment but often the child remains biologically "stuck" following the trauma in a state of chronic fear, stress, and hyperarousal and is unable to experience safe environments as unthreatening. By creating safe, predictable environments free from past trauma triggers, however, parents, caregivers, and therapists can intervene from the bottom-up by creating conditions for controllable stress responses and thus help the child to begin to modulate his or her limbic and brain stem responses to novel situations in more flexible, less frozen ways (van der Kolk, 2003). Another aspect of involvement at the bottom-up level may involve addressing, not hyperarousal, but the numbing, hypoarousal, and dissociative states of mind that often occur as a result of trauma. Here the task is to help the child begin to feel his or her body again, possibly through play or other body-focused therapies (Ogden et al., 2006).

As progress occurs and bodily sensations and feelings associated with trauma are better tolerated without creating hyper- or hypoaroused physiological states or disorganized behaviors or states of mind, top-down approaches may become more effective. At this point, therapies and interventions, such as talk therapy, that call on the children's cognitive capacities to process their traumatic experiences (and their limbic and brain stem responses reactions to them) can be better utilized to help children begin to understand and process memories and reactions to past trauma. Through being able to put feelings and sensations into words, or other symbolic representations such as drawings, children acquire the ability to objectify past experiences, understand factors outside their control that contributed to them, and gain a sense of mastery and control, which permits adaptive responses to future environmental encounters. Importantly, a child's aptitude and preference for cognitive processing of trauma needs to be monitored carefully as children who seem out of touch with their emotions and rely heavily on cognitive approaches in dealing with stress have as many problems as children who primarily rely on their emotions (van der Kolk, 2003; Crittenden, 1992).

Youth Violence and Aggression

Subtyping Aggression: "Hot" and "Cold" Aggression

Adolescent males make up 8% of the total US population but are responsible for 50% of violent crime (Fox, 1995). Research into the neurobiology and phenomenology of violence and aggression has revealed discrete patterns of aggression that arise from different neurobiological pathways and sources of pathology. Efforts to understand these different patterns have led to the segregation of aggression into different subtypes. Two important subtype groupings that have emerged are the distinctions between proactive and reactive aggression (Dodge, 1991; Dodge & Coie, 1987) and between predatory and affective aggression (Eichelman, 1987; Moyer, 1976). These two subtype groupings, though sharing different conceptual origins, overlap sufficiently to be combined for our discussion (following Steiner) into "hot" and "cold" subtypes of aggression. What follows is a brief introduction to research into the phenomenology and clinical utility of this area of aggression research (Soller et al., 2006).

"Hot" aggression comprises impulsive, aggressive, and defensive behaviors that arise in the face of actual or perceived attack or provocation. This type of aggression is best conceptualized as a defensive fear-driven response to threat and frustration often with the expectation of a negative situational outcome (see Fig. 3.2). There is high CNS autonomic arousal and irritability due to activation of the fight, flight, and freeze response, while behaviorally there is an uncoordinated, poorly modulated response to the threat with high risk of self-harm and low probability of successful outcome or reward. Children and adolescents with "hot" aggression often display biases that, in the setting of socially provocative or ambiguous situations, lead them to make inappropriate, exaggerated, and aggressive responses to peers and adults who they believe have hostile intentions toward them (Conner, 2002; Dodge, 1991; Crick & Dodge, 1996). Compared to "cold" aggression, "hot" aggression has an earlier age of onset and is more commonly associated with early developmental disturbances, such as physical abuse or social instability, and neuropsychiatric problems, such as inattention and impulsivity (Conner, 2002). Despite this seemingly greater burden of pathology, studies by Vitaro et al. (1998) and Pulkkinen (1996) showed children with "hot" aggression to be less likely than those with "cold" aggression to continue to exhibit disruptive and antisocial behaviors in adolescence and adulthood. Finally, "hot" aggression is correlated with lower IQ, greater likelihood of treatment with psychotropics, and greater likelihood of favorable response to psychotropics.

"Cold" aggression combines aspects of the proactive and predatory aggression formulations to describe a pattern of behavior and physiological arousal quite distinct from "hot" aggression. Children and adolescents with "cold" aggression typically have little CNS autonomic arousal or visible signs of fear, irritability, and anger when engaged in aggressive acts (Conner, 2002). This type of aggression is pursued in order to obtain a desired goal or favorable outcome whether for food, property, or social status. Unlike in "hot" aggression, the execution of "cold" aggressive acts occurs in an organized, patterned, goal-directed, and controlled manner, which increases the likelihood of successful outcome. "Cold" aggression models in humans postulate that this behavior is often learned and practiced in the context of social environments that provide social role modeling and external reinforcements for such behavior (Bandura, 1973).

The Connection between Victimization and Violence

If we build palaces for children we tear down prison walls.

Julius Tandler, 1938

As the tragedy at Virginia Tech attests, school violence is a national problem of critical importance and concern for ordinary citizens and professionals alike. One of the main challenges that arises in an integrative perspective that takes a developmental, longitudinal approach to behavior and emphasizes the impact of genetic–neurobiological–environmental interactions on the expression of this behavior is that it becomes difficult to attribute differences in behavior (whether adaptive or maladaptive) to simple, isolated, nondynamic linear cause and effect relationships. This is especially problematic in discussing the topic of violence and victimization because, while society would prefer to separate victims and perpetrators into distinct groups based on clear differences in biology, environment, and behavior (and assign the causes of these differences in behavior to mutually exclusive etiologic factors), the situation is much more complex than that on many levels, one of which is that there is much behavioral overlap (and interaction) between the two groups in that victims of trauma often act aggressively (both to themselves and others) while perpetrators often themselves are victims of past maltreatment and traumatization.

In the attempts to make sense of the loss and destruction at Virginia Tech, many experts from the law enforcement, mental health, education, and justice fields have been asked to provide commentary on the cause of Seung-Hui Cho's murderous actions and why the tragedy could not be prevented. One conclusion that can be drawn as one listens to the myriad voices of the "experts" is that despite the public's need for answers, the cause of this tragedy is complex, multifaceted, and resists simple explanation. While authorities continue to investigate Cho's past mental health history, school experiences, relationships, and upbringing, initial reports indicate Mr. Cho have had some life experiences similar to that of previous school shooters, including a history of being socially isolated, withdrawn, and bullied that may have contributed to building feelings of persecution, hopelessness, suicidal thoughts, rage, and desperate plans for retribution. Additionally, there is the possibility that Cho had long-standing mental illness predating his experiences of victimization and violence perpetration. Like many school shooters, Cho's actions were not done impulsively or because he "snapped" but appear to have been carefully planned and executed. In this aspect, he appears to have displayed characteristics of the "cold" aggression pattern of planned goal-directed behavior, perhaps accompanied by low physiological arousal. On the other hand, to the degree Cho was responding (possibly as a result of delusional thinking) to perceived or past actual threats from others (and even delusionally from society at large), his planned actions may have been preceded by prior feelings of victimization, accompanied by heightened physiological arousal, negative self-appraisal, and a sense of threat from and mistrust of his environment. Thus, Cho may have exhibited aspects of both patterns of aggression, and prior to his attack have been victimized by others.

Psycopathy: A Lack of Conscience and Moral Sense

Current research in the neurobiology of aggression, in delineating between "cold" and "hot" aggression, seeks to identify unique neural circuitry that leads to the separate motivational, behavioral, and physiological manifestations of each pattern. In addition, this distinction between the two patterns of aggression may aid in identifying common maladaptive pathways operating in both perpetrators and victims of violence insofar as both victims and perpetrators often show evidence of pathological adaptations to perceived or actual threat in the environment.

The concept of psychopathy, while not currently recognized in the DSM-IV-TR, is an important construct in the study of aggression and violence that further clarifies the distinction between "cold" and "hot" aggression and aid in elucidating the relationship between violence and victimization. Defined in multiple ways across different fields, the definition to be used here follows from Cleckley and Hare. Hare describes psychopaths as "intraspecies predators who use charm, manipulation, intimidation, and violence to control others and to satisfy their own selfish needs. Lacking in conscience and in feeling for others, they take what they want and do as they please violating social norms and expectations without guilt or remorse" (Hare, 1995). Research in psychopathy identifies, unlike in oppositional defiant disorder (ODD), conduct disorder (CD), and antisocial personality disorder (ASPD) populations, a fairly *homogenous* group of individuals with *stable* symptoms across childhood into adulthood. Psychopaths present with excessive use of instru-mental, proactive, predatory (i.e., "cold") behavior and have been hypothesized as having deficits in neural structures and circuitry responsible for the development of empathy and socialization (Blair, 1995; Blair et al. 1997). As a result of these deficits, individuals with psychopathy are at increased risk for learning antisocial behaviors that lead to criminal activity and to DSM diagnoses such as ODD, CD, and ASPD (Blair et al., 2006). However, as suggested above, ODD, CD, and ASPD represent a heterogeneous population and most individuals diagnosed with these disorders do not have psychopathy. Distinguishing youth who present with psychopathy versus other types of aggression has important implications for prevention and interven-tion strategies and for understanding the relationship between exposure to trauma and the development of aggression. Research in the neurobiology of psychopathy hypothesizes that at the core of the development of the disorder are genetic/molec-ular/neural circuit alterations that lead to emotional dysfunction, which impairs socialization and the development of empathy. This impairment, while increasing the risk for learning antisocial behaviors, does not necessarily mean that a child will ultimately learn antisocial behaviors, as long as other more socially acceptable means to obtain goals are available (Blair et al., 2006). However, even these individuals potentially pose harm to others through self-centered, emotionally shallow interactions with people and their environment (see Babiak & Hare, 2006, *Snakes in Suits: When Psychopaths Go to Work*).

The Role of the Amygdala in Psychopathy and "Cold" Aggression

Theories on the origins of psychopathy have speculated that early childhood mal-treatment could lead to development of psychopathy by disruption of the basic threat response system leading to heightened autonomic arousal, thereby increasing the risks of maladaptive, fear-driven responses to stress and threat. As discussed above, the amygdala plays a key role in activating endocrine and ANS responses to threat and is found to be overresponsive in many individuals previously exposed to trauma. Blair and others, however, argue that in individuals who present with pri-marily "cold" aggression, the amygdala is *not overactive* but actually shows *reduced activation* (see Fig. 3.4).

The amygdala plays a central role in both conditioned and learned responses to aversive and appetitive cues in the environment. Individuals with amygdala damage and those with psychopathic instrumental aggression show similar levels of dysfunc-tion on a number of laboratory tests designed to elicit amygdala integrity. Individuals with psychopathy show reduced autonomic responses to other individuals' sadness (Aniskiewicz, 1979; Blair et al., 1997; House & Milligan, 1976), reduced recogni-tion of the fearful expressions of others (Blair et al., 2001), impairment in aversive conditioning (Lykken, 1957), reduced augmentation of the startle reflex by threat primes (Levenston et al., 2000), deficits in passive avoidance learning (Newman & Kosson, 1986) and instrumental learning, and decreased amygdala volume as measured by volumetric MRI (Tiihonen et al., 2000).

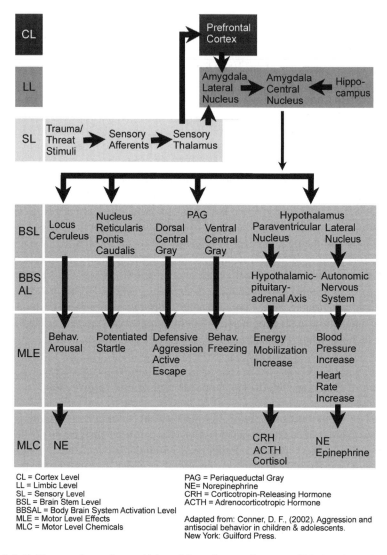

Fig. 3.4 Cold aggression pathways (Adapted from Conner, Courtesy of Medmovie.com)

Blair has suggested that amygdala dysfunction in the areas described above contributes to the formation of psychopathy by impairing normal moral development and induction of empathy. During normal development, caregivers reinforce desired behaviors and punish undesired ones. During a transgression, a victim's distress, pain, or sadness (unconditioned stimuli) results in activation (unconditioned response) of an aggressor's threat response system, which leads to autonomic arousal (and usually) postural freezing. This association of unpleasant, unconditioned cues in the victim with unpleasant, unconditioned responses in the aggressor leads a normally developing child to experience the pain of others as aversive (aversive conditioning). Caregivers then, by focusing the transgressor's attention on the victim and connecting the cause of his or her suffering (and that being experienced by the transgressor) to the act committed by the transgressor, are able (through instrumental conditioning) to promote moral socialization and the induction of empathy. As indicated above, amygdala dysfunction disrupts this process and leads to impairments in socialization (Blair, 2004, 2005). Thus, the amygdala, when normally developed, through its central role in the "fear" circuit, promotes a healthy "fearfulness," while dysfunction leads to underactivation of the threat circuitry and an inability to recognize or properly respond to fear in others, leading to the potential for development of psychopathic personality and behaviors.

Frustration: The Role of the Prefrontal Cortex in Reactive, "Hot" Aggression

While instrumental "cold" aggression appears to be the core pathology, individuals with psychopathy also present with "hot" or reactive, aggression. Whereas the display of "cold" aggression is unique to psychopathy, many other individuals with psychopathology also display reactive aggression, including children with intermittent explosive disorder, pediatric bipolar disorder (Leibenluft et al., 2003), ODD, and CD *and victims of maltreatment and violence*. The prefrontal cortex, specifically the OFC (and portions of the ventrolateral cortex), has been identified as an area that is dysfunctional both in individuals with histories of trauma and those who display reactive aggression. As discussed above, the OFC is a key regulating component of the threat response system, which includes the amygdala, HPA axis, and other areas such as the dorsal periaqueductal gray (PAG) (Gregg & Siegel, 2001; Panksepp, 1998). Overactivation of the threat, or fear, circuitry, most closely associated with overresponsiveness of the amygdala, is a core disturbance that can develop following trauma. Cortical input from the OFC to the amygdala is critical in accurately assessing and responding to environmental threats. Severe trauma, which leads to overactivation of catecholamines, has been associated with impairment of the OFC's ability to inhibit amygdala activity (Arnsten, 1998). Failure of the OFC to properly inhibit amygdala activity in the face of threatening or ambiguous environmental situations can lead to uncontrolled, maladaptive behavioral responses, including reactive aggression.

Research has targeted frontal lobe dysfunction as a potential mediator of aggressive behavior in psychopathic individuals. Damage to prefrontal areas, specifically the OFC, is associated with an increased likelihood of violence and aggression and is often seen in individuals following traumatic brain injury. This association has led to speculation that OFC dysfunction or damage may play a major role in the pathology of psychopathy (Damasio, 1994). However, patients with OFC damage show increases only in "hot" reactive aggression, not the "cold" instrumental aggression which is considered the defining characteristic of the disorder (Blair, 2005). Tests of OFC function in patients with OFC damage and/or psychopathic individuals show impairments in tasks important in controlling behavior and affect. Psychopaths with reactive aggression show impairments in OFC function related to tasks involved in response reversal. In response reversal tasks, psychopathic individuals have more difficulty than controls in changing patterns of goal-seeking behavior when contingencies arise that require alterations of behavior in order to obtain reward or avoid punishment. This impairment in the ability to modify stimulus–response associations in the face of contingency change leads to frustration-based reactive aggression, as the individuals are less able to respond flexibly to environmental demands. Patients with OFC lesions have been shown to have impairment in a related test of OFC function known as social response reversal. This test is employed as an index of OFC capacity to modify behavioral responses when confronted with actions that are in violation of societal norms or rules. Compared to controls, individuals with OFC damage show impairments in multiple parameters involving social response reversal, including the capacity to recognize facial expressions, especially anger.

These tests essentially serve as an index for an individual's ability to tolerate frustration. Frustration here is defined as resulting when an individual attempts a behavior with the expectation of obtaining a goal but then having that goal go unmet (Blair et al., 2006). Frustration is associated with reactive aggression (Berkowitz, 1993). Individuals with dysfunction in orbital frontal and ventrolateral cortex areas show impairments in their ability to achieve goals and rewards especially during situations involving contingency change (response reversal). Because of impairments in prefrontal function, subcortical systems mediating reactive aggression may be under-regulated, putting these individuals at heightened risk for displaying reactive aggression as a result of experiencing frustration in their interactions with others and their environment.

Clinical Studies Investigating the Connection Between Violence and Victimization

There are a number of clinical studies investigating the relationship between trauma and aggression. In looking at delinquent youth, the association between trauma-related environments (e.g., characterized by abuse, sexual molestation, and witnessing violence) and the development of psychopathology is well-documented (Foy et al., 1996). In such environments, it is not surprising that exposure to trauma sets up a "cycle of violence" of victim later becoming perpetrator (Ryan et al., 1996). Previous sexual molestation of male youth (often by females) leading to later sexual victimization by these males of women is one specific example. Steiner et al., (1997) investigated 85 adolescents incarcerated by the California Youth Authority for a range of offenses from first-degree murder to auto theft. The study found 32% of the youth had PTSD and 20% had PTSD symptoms but did not meet full criteria, which is significantly higher than estimates of ~9% lifetime prevalence in young adults. Fifty percent of these youth had witnessed interpersonal violence. The individuals diagnosed with PTSD had increased levels of distress, depression, and anxiety, poor impulse control, and increased levels of aggression. Another study by Ford et al. (2000) found trauma in general, but more specifically physical and sexual maltreatment, to be associated with ODD (and ADHD). In their sample, 48–73% of children diagnosed with ODD had been exposed to physical maltreatment while 18–31% had been exposed to sexual maltreatment. Investigations into the underlying biological mechanisms involved in the development of ODD reveal dysregulation of emotional and information processing (Lahey et al., 1999; Pennington & Ozonof, 1996), leading youth with ODD to (1) have negative biases toward themselves, peers, and relationships; (2) more likely experience social interactions as hostile; (3) possess rigid and limited problem solving skills; and (4) often express frustration, rage, and aggression (Dodge et al., 1997; Matthys et al., 1999). These impairments parallel findings from victimization research and are consistent with data above linking traumatization to the development of "hot" aggression.

A 2005 study involving video games highlights changes that occur in the amygdala and prefrontal regions in youths exposed to video game violence. Forty-four healthy adolescents previously exposed to a violent video game called "Medal of Honor" showed increased activation in the right amygdala and decreased activation in prefrontal areas compared to a comparison group of adolescents shown a nonviolent game called "Need for Speed" during fMRI imaging obtained during two Stroop tasks. The individuals who played the non-violent game showed more activation in the prefrontal areas, especially the anterior cingulate and the dorsolateral prefrontal cortex. These results (decreased prefrontal and increased amygdala activation in violent video game players), while not proving that watching violent media causes violence, parallel findings above that implicate exposure to previous violence in biasing the threat response system to maladaptive behavioral responses such as displays of "hot" aggression (Mathews et al., 2005).

The Connection Between Violence and Victimization: Summary

Although incomplete and speculative, the above discussion of neurobiological corre-lates of trauma and subtypes of aggression permits the following generalizations:

1. *Fear-driven Victimization*: Trauma and maltreatment produce heightened fear responses mediated partly by a dysregulated fear circuit involving an overrespon-sive amygdala. One source of the overactive amygdala may be a dysfunctional prefrontal cortex that fails to adequately inhibit the amygdala.

   "Hot" reactive aggression is one of the possible maladaptive behavioral responses that can result from dysfunction of the threat response system and may involve elements of frustration.

2. *Fearless-driven "Cold" Aggression*: "Cold" aggression involves instrumental, predatory, goal-directed aggressive behavior with little autonomic arousal; is mediated partly through a dysregulated fear circuit involving an under-responsive amygdala that prevents recognition of fear in others (via lack of

amygdala activation of the basic threat response); and is associated with a lack of socialization and empathy.

3. *Frustration-driven "Hot" Aggression*: "Hot" aggression, in the context of psychopathy, involves reactive, impulsive, frustration-driven aggression associated with dysfunction in prefrontal regions responsible for modifying responses to contingency change.

An Integrated Model of Neurobiological Function in Violence and Victimization

Jeffrey Gray's Biobehavioral Model of Brain Functioning

Jeffrey Gray has developed a comprehensive theory of how separate but interrelated neurobiological systems function in the brain to control a variety of human qualities and characteristics such as temperament, emotions, and behaviors. His theory can be used to create a relatively simple but plausible framework to facilitate an understanding of the neurobiological systems involved in controlling violence and victimization, including aspects of hot and cold aggression (Gray, 1982, 1987; Conner, 2002).

Gray's model consists of three major branches: a behavioral activation system (BAS), a behavioral inhibition system (BIS), and a fight, flight, freeze system (FFFS). By aligning these components of brain function to neurobiological findings in trauma and aggression research, the following associations are hypothesized: "Cold" aggression results when an organism displays a relative excess of behavioral activation versus inhibition. "Hot" aggression, on the other hand, is likely to arise in the context of an overactive, dysregulated FFFS, possibly from prior trauma, which is biased toward exaggerated responses to threat. Finally, in children exposed to trauma, who go on to develop the symptomatology of victimization, there is not only the risk of dysregulation of the FFFS but also the possibility of dysregulation of the BAS and BIS, leading to the development of multiple psychiatric symptoms. While trauma is not explicitly discussed in Gray's model, Gray's colleague McNaughton does discuss briefly the place of PTSD. He states that PTSD is not included in the model because, more than a single disease entity, it should be viewed as a trauma-related phenomenon that predisposes affected individuals to the development of multiple disorders, echoing conclusions presented above on the numerous possible sequelae of complex trauma (McNaughton & Corr, 2004).

The BAS is the primary system in animals that promotes behavioral approach when conditions exist such that conditioned stimuli for reward are present and conditioned stimuli for punishment are absent (McNaughton & Corr, 2004). This system is critical in producing predatory and instrumental aggression (i.e., "cold" aggression). Evidence suggests that DA and dopaminergic pathways are critical in the functioning of this system (Lara & Akiskal, 2006). This pathway begins in brain stem nuclei in fibers that ascend from the substantia nigra and the ventral tegmental area and project via the medial forebrain bundle to many areas in the midbrain and forebrain. The nucleus accumbens and the ventral striatum of the midbrain receive dopaminergic fibers that release DA, the main neurotransmitter responsible for appetitive, reward-influenced behavior.

The BIS provides a brake to the acceleration of the BAS. It works to inhibit behavioral approach in situations where conditions are present that could lead to possible danger, punishment, or frustration of nonreward. Like the BAS, it functions in response to learned conditioned stimuli; but in this case, it becomes activated, not by the promise of reward but by conditions that limit reward and predict punishment. A key concept of the BIS is that while it balances the BAS, it is still a system of approach, albeit defensive approach. That is, in conditions where both reward and punishment are present, the BIS serves as a tool of risk assessment and conflict resolution to analyze environmental circumstances and past learning in order to guide behavior. The primary emotion or felt neurophysiological experience associated with the BIS is anxiety. McNaughton identifies the septo-hippocampal system and the amygdala as being critical in the function of the BIS but also includes other important structures such as the PAG, the hypothalamus, and the prefrontal cortex. NE and serotonin (5-HT) are the neurotransmitters most active in this system.

The FFFS, unlike the BAS and BIS, is an innate (not learned) system that mediates animal responses to unconditioned stimuli such as pain, punishment, and frustration. In Gray's model, the FFFS is responsible for the generation of the emotion of fear and mobilizes an animal to attempt escape, or if that option is not available, to engage in defensive aggression. It therefore provides direction in situations where animals, confronted with threats to survival and livelihood, act defensively to avoid the source of danger. For example, cat-naïve rats when confronted with a cat respond either by freezing, fleeing, or fighting according to options available to them. While there is much overlap between the FFFS and the BIS, a key difference between them is that the FFFS involves moving away (defensive avoidance) from a negative stimulus, whereas the BIS involves a defensive approach toward the stimulus (or cues related to the stimulus). Thus, if a rat exposed to a cat is placed in the same environment but without the cat, the rat may initially remain still (but with a different posture than is seen in fear-related freezing) and then begin to cautiously explore its environment (behavioral inhibition) in a manner that has been characterized as risk assessment (Gray & McNaughton, 2000, Blanchard & Blanchard, 1990). As mentioned above, the FFFS may be overactive in some people who display reactive or affective ("hot") aggression. Such people may be subject to autonomic over-arousal and biases toward feeling threatened and fearful in situations that others find nonthreatening. The neuroanatomical substrates of the FFFS are very similar to that of the BIS. Key structures include the prefrontal cortex, the amygdala, and the PAG. Mobilization of the fear response involves elaboration of many neurochemicals including NE, 5-HT, DA, endorphins, and cortisol.

Gray's model predicts that different forms of psychopathology can result from relative deficiencies or excesses of function of any of the above three interrelated systems. In terms of different forms of aggressive behavior, the model predicts individuals with excessive BAS activity and deficient BIS activity will be especially prone to aggression, as they will be highly driven to seek rewards but also unresponsive to cues discouraging reward, such as warnings of punishment. These individuals should have low ANS arousal even in potentially aversive environments and therefore should not be easily inhibited by anxiety. Furthermore, because of their reward-dominant behavior, such individuals will be less able to learn to from punishment and therefore are likely to persist in maladaptive reward-seeking behavior despite negative consequences (Conner, 2002). Evidence for this type of aggression is present in studies of children and adolescents with CD where youth with and without CD play computerized card games in which money is either rewarded or taken away from the participants based on whether they make correct or incorrect responses. The game is set up to decrease the probability of choosing a correct response as the game proceeds. Compared to youth without CD, children and adolescents with CD are more likely to persist playing the game (and therefore lose more money) despite being able to pass on trials (Daugherty & Quay, 1991; Shapiro et al., 1988).

Gray's theory also predicts that in youth with CD and strong BIS (and therefore more prone to anxiety), the active BIS should inhibit antisocial behavior compared to youth with CD with an active BAS. In fact, several studies have provided this kind of evidence by showing that anxious boys with CD are less likely to become involved with the police than are boys with CD without anxiety (Walker et al., 1991). Additional studies looking at chemical markers of the BAS and BIS have generally supported Gray's theory with some exceptions. For example, several studies have shown decreased NE and 5-HT function to be associated with increased antisocial behavior and aggressiveness while there is yet no data available that show increased DA to be associated with increased antisocial behavior (Rogeness, 1992). Another marker used to assess BIS function is electrodermal activity (EDA), which is measured with a polygraph and increases with sweat production. In studies that measure sweating, increased EDA is used as a marker for increased peripheral sympathetic ANS arousal, which, in turn, is used as a marker for BIS activation. Gray's theory predicts that youth with CD should exhibit lower EDA production compared to controls when presented with stimuli suggestive of impending punishment or nonreward. According to Conner, seven of seven studies in youth with CD that have tested this hypothesis have results consistent with this prediction.

Clinical Considerations

While there is significant evidence to support the external and internal validity of the two distinct subtypes of aggression discussed above, there is also substantial overlap found in experimental studies. For example, in a study of 73 aggressive child and adolescent psychiatric patients, a scale describing fully predatory (+5) and fully affective (−5) patterns had bimodal peaks of −3 (predominately affective) and 1 (mixed) (Vitiello et al., 1990). One conclusion drawn from this study is that purely predatory children are less likely to receive psychiatric treatment (Vitiello & Stoff, 1997). Furthermore, both in animals and humans, the same subject at different times can display aggression more predominately in one of the two subtypes according to the circumstances that the subject is involved in (Vitiello & Stoff, 1997). Thus, clinical utility in the "cold" and "hot" formulation will likely involve a dimensional approach that respects the difficulty of identifying patients and formulating treatments purely on a clear-cut categorical basis (Vitiello & Stoff, 1997).

Clinical tools designed to aid in identifying "cold" aggression in terms of psychopathy have been developed (e.g., the Psychopathy Checklist—Revised and the Hare Psychopathy Checklist—Youth Version) but are primarily used in research settings (Conner, 2002). The implementation of these and other psychometric tools into clinical practice may aid in developing tailored treatment strategies that respect the discreet developmental etiologies of different subtypes of aggression. The identification of psychopathic tendencies in youth may have special implications for the types of environmental interventions that clinicians and other caregivers undertake with aggressive youth. As discussed above, Blair argues that the developmental pathology associated with psychopathy is the result of genetic influences that impair the function of the amygdala and OFC resulting in (1) deficits in moral development, empathy induction, and socialization and (2) increased likelihood of frustration-induced reactive aggression. Furthermore, while poor parenting has been identified as a risk factor for the development of conduct problems in previously healthy children, this association is weaker for children who show psychopathic tendencies (Blair et al., 2006; Oxford et al., 2003; Wootton et al., 1997). In fact, no studies to date have linked *any* causal environmental factor to the reduced amygdala functioning thought to be at the core of psychopathy. Therefore, it may be prudent to assume that the psychopathic child or adolescent is, regardless of the degree of supportive emotional response provided by parents, caregivers, or clinicians, going to be at an increased risk for using antisocial means for obtaining goals. Whether this occurs, however, may depend on the social/environmental conditions which that person is exposed to. For example, if there are few role models in the community or media for which to learn antisocial behaviors from, or little motivation to pursue antisocial goals (i.e., sufficient access to *legitimate* resources), then antisocial tendencies may be less likely to be acted on. Conversely, with children and adolescents primarily at risk of "hot" aggression (e.g., from prior exposure to trauma), environmental factors are implicated in both the initiation and the continuation of their maladaptive responses to their environment.

Thus, while studies demonstrating the clinical utility of developing individualized treatment strategies based on different aggression subtypes are still few in number, research does support several general guidelines. One is that, since children and adolescents with predominately "cold" aggression are at risk for using instrumental aggression to achieve goals, it is important to minimize exposure to environments where such behavior is typically modeled and rewarded (e.g., gangs) while maximizing exposure to environments where guidelines of expected behavior (to achieve rewards and avoid punishments) are clearly outlined. Treatment paradigms for this type of aggression support the use of behavioral therapy and parent education strategies that create environments where expectations for behavior are clearly outlined and consequences enforced consistently in a nonaggressive manner. Commitment to and successful implication of these strategies are especially critical in light of evidence that suggests poor response to psychopharmacological interventions in this subtype of youth aggression.

The other general guideline relates to children and adolescents who predominantly display pure "hot" or mixed aggression. Because these youth tend to be easily aroused physiologically and are biased to mistrust their environment, they are likely to react impulsively and defensively in response to threat or provocation. Such children respond favorably to interventions that create safe and predictable environments, teach social problem solving skills and the management of negative emotions, and utilize medications capable of modulating mood, anxiety, physiological arousal, and level of attention (Conner, 2002, Vitiello & Stoff, 1997).

Finally, studies examining psychiatric comorbidities associated with aggression, for example, those looking at the separate emotional and behavioral components of psychopathy, have found anxiety (and depression) to be inversely correlated with the emotional component (lack of empathy) and positively correlated with the antisocial behavioral component, especially the expression of reactive aggression. In other words, greater levels of anxiety are associated with greater levels of "hot" reactive aggression and decreased levels of "cold" aggression. One interpretation of the significance of this data is that psychopathy, to the degree that it is associated with "cold" aggression and low autonomic arousal and response to threat, while putting an individual at higher risk of expression for amoral, instrumental, goal-directed aggression, may actually protect against the development of psychiatric sequelae, which can result from environmental insults such as trauma and maltreatment. As such, *their* pathology will be experienced more through their ability to achieve goal-directed goals at the expense of *others* than through the development of emotional problems in *them* from exposure to childhood maltreatment or trauma (Blair et al., 2006, Frick et al., 1999).

References

Amat, J., Paul, E., Zarza, C., Watkins, L. R., & Maier, S. F. (2006). Previous experience with behavioral control over stress blocks the behavioral and dorsal raphe nucleus activating effects of later uncontrollable stress: Role of the ventral medial prefrontal cortex. *The Journal of Neuroscience*, 26(51),13264–13272.

Aniskiewicz, A. S. (1979). Autonomic components of vicarious conditioning and psychopathy. *Journal of Clinical Psychology*, 35, 60–67.

Arnsten, A. (1998). Catecholamine modulation of prefrontal cortical cognitive function. *Trends in Cognitve Science*, 2, 336–447.

Ainsworth, M. (1985). Patterns of infant-mother attachment: Antecedents and effects on development. *Bulletin of the New York Academy of Medicine*, 61, 771–791.

Beeghly, M. & Cicchetti, D. (1996). Child maltreatment, attachment, and the self system: Emergence of an internal state lexicon in toddlers at high social risk. In M. Hertzig & E. Farber (Eds.), *Annual Progress in Child Psychiatry and Child Development* (pp.127–166). Philadelphia, PA: Brunner/Mazel.

Beers, S. R. & De Bellis, M. D. (2002). Neuropsychological function in children with maltreatment-related posttraumatic stress disorder. *American Journal of Psychiatry*, 159(3), 483–486.

Babiak, P. & Hare, R. D. (2006). *Snakes in Suits: When Psychopaths go to Work*. New York: Collins.

Bandura, A. (1973). *Aggression: A social Learning Analysis*. Englewood Cliffs, NJ: Prentice-Hall.

Berkowitz, L. (1993). *Aggression: Its Causes, Consequences, and Control*. Philadelphia, PA: Temple University Press.

Blair, R. J. R. (1995). A cognitive developmental approach to morality: Investigating the psychopath. *Cognition*, 57, 1–29.

Blair, R. J. R. (2004). The roles of orbital frontal cortex in the modulation of antisocial behavior. *Brain and Cognition*, 55, 198–208.

Blair, R. J. R. (2005). Applying a cognitive neuroscience perspective to the disorder of psychopath. *Developmental and Psychopathology*, 17, 865–891.

Blair, R. J. R., Colledge, E., Murray, L., & Mitchell, D. G. (2001). A selective impairment in the processing of sad and fearful expressions in children with psychopathic tendencies. *Journal of Abnormal Child Psychology*, 29, 491–498.

Blair, R. J. R., Jones, L., Clark, F., & Smith, M. (1997). The psychopathic individual: A lack of responsiveness to distress cues? *Psychophysiology*, 34, 192–198.

Blair, R. J. R., Peschardt, K. S., Budhani, S., Mitchell, D. G. V., & Pine, D. S. (2006). The development of psychopathy. *Journal of Child Psychology and Psychiatry*, 47(3/4), 262–275.

Blanchard, R. J. & Blanchard, D. C. (1990). Anti-predator defense as models of animal fear and anxiety. In Brain, P. F., Parmigiani, S., Blanchard, R. J., & Mainardi, D., (Eds.), *Fear and Defence*. (pp. 89-108). Chur.Harwood Acad.Pub.

Bowlby, J. (1973). *Attachment and Loss: Vol. II. Separation*. New York: Basic Books.

Bremmer, J. D., Randall, P., Vermetten, E., Staib, L., Bronen, R. A., Mazure, C., Capelli, S., McCarthy, G., Innis, R. B., & Charney, D. S. (1997). Magnetic resonance imaging-based measurement of hippocampal volume in posttraumatic stress disorder related to childhood physical and sexual abuse: A preliminary report. *Biological Psychiatry*, 41, 23–32.

Bremner, J. D. (2006). Traumatic stress: Effects on the brain. *Dialogues in Clinical Neuroscience*, 8(4), 445–61.

Campbell-Sills, L., Cohan, S. L., & Stein, M. B. (2006). Relationship of resilience to personality, coping, and psychiatric symptoms in young adults. *Behavior Research and Therapy*. 44(4), 585–599.

Carlson, V., Barnett, D., Cicchetti, D., & Braunwald, K. (1989). Disorganized/disoriented attachment relationships in maltreated infants. *Developmental Psychology*, 25(4), 525–531.

Caspi A., McClay, J., Moffitt, T. E., Mill, J., Martin, J., Craig, I. W. Taylor, A., & Poulton, R. (2002). Role of genotype in the cycle of violence in maltreated children. *Science*, 297, 851–854.

Conner, D. F. (2002). *Aggression and Antisocial Behavior in Children & Adolescents*. New York: Guilford Press.

Cook, A., Spinazzola, J., Ford, J., Lanktree, C., Blaustein, M., Cloitre M., DeRosa, R., Hubbard, R., Kagan, R., Liautaud, J., Mallah, K., Olafson, E., & van der Kolk, B. (2005). Complex trauma in children and adolescents. *Psychiatric Annals*, 35(5), 390–398.

Crittenden, P. (1992). Treatment of anxious attachment in infancy and early childhood. *Developmental Psychopathology*, 4, 575–602.

Crittenden, P. (1997). Truth, error, omission, distortion, and deception: The application of attachment theory to the assessment and treatment of psychological disorder. In: S. Dollinger & L. F. DiLalla (Eds.), *Assessment and Intervention Issues Across the Life Span* (pp. 35–76). Hillsdale, NJ: Erlbaum.

Crick, N. R. & Dodge K. A. (1996). Social information-processing mechanisms in reactive and proactive aggression. *Child Development*, 67(3), 993–1002.

Culp, R., Watkins, R., Lawrence, H., et al. (1991). Maltreated children's language and speech development: Abused, neglected, and abused and neglected. *First Language*, 11(33 Pt. 3), 377–389.

Damasio, A. R. (1994). *Descartes' Error: Emotion, Rationality and the Human Brain*. New York: Putnam (Grosset Books).

Daugherty, T. K., & Quay, H. C. (1991). Response perseveration and delayed responding in childhood behavior disorders. *Journal of Child Psychology and Psychiatry*, 32, 453–461.

Davies, D. (1999). *Child Development*. New York: Guilford Press.

de Leon, J., Susce, M. T., & Murray-Carmichael, E. (2006). The AmpliChip CYP450 genotyping test: Integrating a new clinical tool. *Molecular Diagnosis and Therapy*, 10, 135–351.

Dodge, K. A. & Coie, J. D. (1987). Social-information-processing factors in reactive and proactive aggression in children's peer groups. *Journal of Personality and Social Psychology*, 53(5), 1289–1309.

Dodge, K. A. (1991). The structure and function of reactive and proactive aggression. In: D. J. Pepler & K. H. Rubin (Eds.), *The Development and Treatment of Childhood Aggression* (pp. 210–218). Hillsdale, NJ: Lawrence Erlbaum.

Dodge, K., Lochman, J., Harnish, J., Bates, J., & Pettit, G. (1997). Reactive and proactive aggression in school children and psychiatrically impaired chronically assaultive youth. *Journal of Abnormal Psychology*, 106, 37–51.

Eichelman, B. (1987). Neurochemical and psychopharmacologic aspects of aggressive behavior. In: H. Y. Meltzer (Ed.), *Psychopharmacology: The Third Generation of Progress* (pp. 697–704). New York: Raven Press.

Fraiberg, S., Adelson, E., & Shapiro, V. (1987). Ghosts in the nursery: A psychoanalytic approach to the problems of impaired infant-mother relationships. *Selected writings of Selma Fraiberg* (pp. 101–136), Ohio State University Press.

Frick, P. J., Lilienfeld, S. O, Ellis, M., Loney, B., & Silverthorn, P. (1999). The association between anxiety and psychopathy dimensions in children. *Journal of Abnormal Child Psychology*, 27, 383–392.

Ford, J. D., Racusin, R., Ellis, C. G., Daviss, W. B., Reiser, J., Fleischer, A., & Thomas, J. (2000). Child maltreatment, other trauma exposure, and posttraumatic symptomatology among children with oppositional defiant and attention deficit hyperactivity disorders. *Child Maltreatment*, 5(3), 205–217.

Fox, J. A. (1995). Homicide offending patterns: A grim look ahead (abstract). In: *Scientific Proceedings of the Annual Meeting of the American Academy for the Advancement of Science*.

Foy, D, Guevara, M., Camilleri, A. (1996). Community violence. In D. J. Miller (Ed.), *Handbook of Posttraumatic Stress Disorders* (pp. 2–25). New York: Basic Books.

Gray, J. A. (1982). *The Neuropsychology of Anxiety: An Enquiry into the Functions of the Septo-hippocampal System*. Oxford: Oxford University Press.

Gray, J. A. (1987). *The Psychology of Fear and Stress*, 2nd edition. Cambridge, England: Cambridge University Press.

Gray, J. A. & McNaughton, N. (2000). *The Neuropsychology of Anxiety: An Enquiry into the Functions of the Septo-hippocampal System*, 2nd edition. Oxford: Oxford University Press.

Gregg, T. R. & Siegel, A. (2001). Brain structures and neurotransmitters regulating aggression in cats: Implications for human aggression. *Progress in Neuropsychopharmacology and Biological Psychiatry*, 25, 91–140.

Hare, R. D. (1995). Psychopaths: New trends in research. *The Harvard Mental Health Letter*, 12, 4–5, September.

Harvard Mental Health Letter. (2005). *The Biology of Child Maltreatment*, 21(12), 1–3.

Heim, C., Newport D. J., Miller, A. H., & Nemeroff, C. B. (2000). Long-term neuroendocrine effects of childhood maltreatment. *Journal of the American Medical Association*, 284(18), 2321.

House, T. H. & Milligan, W. L. (1976). Autonomic responses to modeled distress in prison psychopaths. *Journal of Personality and Social Psychology*, 34, 556–560.

Kagan, J. (1989). Temperamental contributions to social behavior. *American Psychologist*, 44, 668–674.

Kim-Cohen J., Caspi, A., Taylor, A., Williams, B., Newcombe, R., Craig, I. W., & Moffitt, T. E. (2006). MAOA, maltreatment, and gene-environment interaction predicting children's mental health: New evidence and a meta-analysis. *Molecular Psychiatry*, 10, 603–913.

Kramer, D. A. (2005). Commentary: Gene-environment interplay in the context of genetics, epigenetics, and gene expression. *Journal of American Child and Adolescent Pyschiatry*, 44:1, 19–27.

Lahey, B., Waldman, I., & McBurnett, K. (1999). Annotation: The development of antisocial behavior. *Journal of Child Psychology and Psychiatry*, 29, 669–682.

Lara, D. & Akiskal, H. S. (2006). Toward and integrative model of the spectrum of mood, behavioral, and personality disorders based on fear and anger traits: II. Implications for neurobiology, genetics, and psychopharmacological treatment. *Journal of Affective Disorders*, 94(1–3), 89–103.

LeDoux, J. (1999). *The Emotional Brain*. New York: Simon & Schuster.

LeDoux, J. (2002). *The Synaptic Self*. New York: Penguin Books.

Leibenluft, E., Blair, R. J. R., Charney, D. S., & Pine, D. S. (2003). Irritability in pediatric mania and other childhood psychopathology. *Annual New York Academy of Sciences*, 10008, 201–218.

Levenston, G. K., Patrick, C. J., Bradley, M. M., & Lang, P. J. (2000). The psychopath as observer: Emotion and attention in picture processing. *Journal of Abnormal Psychology*, 109, 373–386.

Levin, A. (2006). PTSD not sufficient to explain response to trauma. *Psychiatric News*, 41(16), 20.

Lykken, D. T. (1957). A study of anxiety in the sociopathic personality. *Journal of Abnormal and Social Psychology*, 55, 6–10.

Manuck, S. (2006). 6th International Congress of Neuroendocrinology (ICN 2006).

Mash, E. J. & Dozois, D. J. A. (1996). Child psychopathology: A developmental-systems perspective. In E. J. Mash & R. A. Barkley (Eds.), *Child Psychopathology* (pp. 3–60). New York: Guilford Press.

Mathews, V. P., Kronenberger, W. G., Wang, Y., Lurito, J. T., Lowe, M. J., & Dunn, D. W. (2005). Media violence exposure and frontal lobe activation measured by functional magnetic resonance imaging in aggressive and non-aggressive adolescents. *Journal of Computer Assisted Tomography*, 29(3), 287–92.

Matthys, W., Cuperus, J. M., & Van Engeland, H. (1999). Deficient social problem-solving in boys with ODD/CD, with ADHD, and with both disorders. *Journal of the American Academy of Child & Adolescent Psychiatry*, 38(3), 311–21.

Meyer-Lindenberg A., Buckholtz J., Kolachana B. S., Pezawas L., Blasi G., Wabnitz A., Honea R., Hariri A. R., Verchinski B., Callicott J., Egan M. F., Mattay V. S., & Weinberger D. R. (2006). Neural mechanisms of genetic risk f or impulsivity and violence in humans. *Proceedings of the National Academy of Sciences*, 103(16), 6269–6274.

Mezzacappa, E., Earls, A., & Kindlon, D. (1998). Executive and motivational control of performance task behavior, and autonomic heart-rate regulation in children: Physiologic validation of two-factor solution inhibitory control. *Journal of Child Psychology and Psychiatry*, 39, 525–531.

Miller, T. W. & Veltkamp, L. J. (1996). Trauma accommodation syndrome. In T.W. Miller, (Ed.), *Theory and Aassessment of Stressful Life Events* (pp. 95–98). Madison, Connecticut: International Universities Press.

Moyer, K. E. (1976). *The Psychobiology of Aggression*. New York: Harper & Row.

McFarlane, A. (1988). The phenomenology of posttraumatic stress disorders following a natural disaster. *Journal of Nervous and Mental Disorders*, 176, 22–29.

McNaughton, N. & Corr, P. J. (2004). A two-dimensional neuropsychology of defense: Fear/anxiety and defensive distance. *Neuroscience and Biobehavioral Reviews*. 28, 285–305.

Newman, J. P. & Kosson, D. S. (1986). Passive avoidance learning in psychopathic and nonpsychopathic offenders. *Journal of Abnormal Psychology*, 95, 252–256.

Niehoff, D. (1999). *The biology of violence*. New York: Free Press.

Ogden, P., Minton, K., & Pain, C. (2006). *Trauma and the Body*. New York: Norton series on interpersonal neurobiology.

Oxford, M., Cavell, T. A., & Hughes, J. N. (2003) Callous-unemotional traits moderate the relation between ineffective parenting and child externalizing problems: A partial replication and extension. *Journal of Clinical Child and Adolescent Psychology*, 32, 577–585.

Panksepp, J. (1998). *Affective Neuroscience: The Foundations of Human and Animal Emotions*. New York: Oxford University Press.

Parker, K. J., Buckmaster, C. L., Sundlass, K., Schatzber, A. F., & Lyons, D. M. (2006). Maternal mediation, stress inoculation, and the development of neuroendocrine stress resistance in primates. *Proceedings of the National Academy of Sciences*, 103(8), 3000–3005.

Pennington, B. & Ozonof, S. (1996). Executive functions and developmental pscychopathology. *Journal of Child Psychology and Psychiatry*, 37, 51–87.

Perry, B. & Pollard, R. (1998). Homeostasis, stress, trauma and adaptation. *Child and Adolescent Psychiatry Clinics of North America*, 7, 33–51.

Ploog, D. W. (2003). The place of the triune brain in psychiatry. *Physiology & Behavior*, 79, 487–493.

Pulkkinen, L. (1996). Proactive and reactive aggression in early adolescence as precursors to anti- and prosocial behaviors in young adults. *Aggressive Behavior*, 22, 241–257.

Rogeness, G. A., Javors, M. A., & Pliszka, S. R. (1997). Neurochemistry and child and adolescent psychiatry. *Journal of the American Academy of Child and Adolescent Psychiatry*, 31, 765–781.

Rutter, M., Dunn, J., Plomin, R., Simonoff, E., Pickles, A., Maughan, B., Ormel, J., Meyer, J., & Eaves, L. (1997). Integrating nature and nurture: Implications of person-environment correlations and interactions for developmental psychopathology. *Development and Psychopathology*, 9, 335–364.

Rutter, M., Moffitt, T. E., & Caspi, A. (2006). Gene-environment interplay and psychopathology: Multiple varieties but real effects. *Journal of Child Psychology and Psychiatry* 47(3/4), 226–261.

Ryan, G., Miyoshi, T., Metzner, J., Krugman, R., & Fryer, G. (1996). Trends in a national sample of sexually abusive youths. *Journal of the American Academy of Child & Adolescent Psychiatry*, 35, 17–54.

Shapiro, S. K., Quay, H. C., Hogan, A. E., & Schwarz, K. P. (1988). Response perseveration and delayed responding in undersocialized aggressive conduct disorder. *Journal of Abnormal Psychology*, 97, 371–373.

Shonk, S. M. & Cicchetti, D. (2001). Maltreatment, competency deficits, and risk for academic and behavioral maladjustment. *Developmental Psychology*, 37(1), 3–17.

Siegel, D. (2001). *The Developing Mind: How Relationships and the Brain Interact to Shape Who We Are*. New York: Guilford Press.

Soller, M. V., Karnik, N. S., & Steiner, H. (2006). Psychopharmacologic treatment in juvenile offenders. *Child and Adolescent Psychiatric Clinics of North America*, 15(2), 477–499.

Steiner, H., Garcia, I. G., & Matthews, Z. (1997). Posttraumatic stress disorder in incarcerated juvenile delinquents. *Journal of the American Academy of Child & Adolescent Psychiatry*, 36(3), 357–363.

Tiihonen, J., Hodgins, S., & Vaurio, O. (2000). Amygdaloid volume loss in psychopathy. *Society for Neuroscience Abstracts*, 2017.

van der Kolk, B. A. (2003). The neurobiology of childhood trauma and abuse. *Child and Adolescent Psychiatric Clinics of North America*, 12, 293–317.

van der Kolk, B. A. (2005). Developmental trauma disorder: Toward a rational diagnosis for children with complex trauma. *Psychiatric Annals*, 35(5), 401–408.

Vitiello, B., Behar, D., Hunt, J., Stoff, D., & Ricciuti, A. (1990). Subtyping aggression in children and adolescents. *Journal of Neuropsychiatry and Clinical Neuroscience*, Spring 2(2), 189–192.

Vitiello, B. & Stoff, D. M. (1997). Subtypes of aggression and their relevance to child psychiatry. *Journal of the American Academy of Child & Adolescent Psychiatry*, 36(3), 307–315.

Vitaro, F., Gendreau, P. L., Tremblay, R. E., & Oligny, P. (1998). Reactive and proactive aggression differentially predict later conduct problems. *Journal of Child Psychology and Psychiatry, and Allied Disciplines*, 39(3), 377–385.

Walker, J. L., Lahey, B. B., Russo, M. F., Frick, P. J., Christ, M. A. G., McBurnett, K., Loeber, R., Stouthamer-Loeber, M., & Green, S. M. (1991). Anxiety, inhibition, and conduct disorder in children: I. Relations to social impairment. *Journal of the American Academy of Child and Adolescent Psychiatry*, 30, 187–191.

Wootton, J. M., Frick, P. J., Shelton, K. K., & Silverthorn, P. (1997). Ineffective parenting and childhood conduct problems: The moderating role of callous-unemotional traits. *Journal of Consulting and Clinical Psychology*, 65, 292–300.

Chapter 4
Threat Assessment in School Violence

Connie Callahan

Every time a high profile act of violence occurs at school, attention turns to the prevention of school violence. School violence affected 37 communities across the United States between 1974 and June 2000. The Columbine incident that took place in Littleton, Colorado, on April 20, 1999, imprinted the most violent of school attacks on American minds when 14 students and a teacher lost their lives. According to the U.S. Department of Education & U.S. Department of Justice (1999), over 60 million students attend over 100,000 schools and most will not fall prey to serious violence in schools, but Americans would like to know if they could have known about any attack planning and if they could have done anything to prevent such school violence.

Coie and Jacobs (1993) and Elias and Tobias (1996) have documented that prevention and early intervention efforts can reduce violence and other troubling behaviors in schools. Cornell (1998) and Quinn et al. (1998) indicate that research-based practices can help school communities recognize the warning signs early and that promising prevention and intervention strategies that involve the entire educational community, administrators, teachers, families, students, support staff, and community members can make school safer. However, not all schools provide comprehensive violence prevention plans.

Some schools opt for solutions like installing metal detectors or hiring a security guard, while others recognize that violence prevention calls for a comprehensive approach that infuses every aspect of school life. Bus and playground safety, Internet use policies, gang prevention, classroom management, anti-bullying policies, and identification and early intervention with students who are struggling psychologically encompass important areas of school safety. Effective efforts both protect the physical safety of students and staff and promote positive learning and social development.

The proven fundamentals of violence prevention include strategies that are child focused and support learning. Schools must balance building security with efforts that foster student resiliency, connectedness, and social competency. Specifically schools should create welcoming, nurturing school climates; enforce positive behavior and discipline for all students; support student mental health and wellness; develop and regularly review crisis and threat assessment plans; train staff in crisis procedures and risk factors for violence; maintain appropriate building security; develop collaborative relationships with local law enforcement and community services providers; and strengthen home–school connections. School safe plans in which students, teachers, and administrators pay attention to students' social and emotional needs as well as academic needs will promote a climate of school safety.

Staying focused on student needs and outcomes also makes violence prevention efforts more effective at one extreme end of the violence spectrum: threat assessment. Threat assessment is perhaps one of the most difficult areas in violence prevention because there is no single profile of a student who may pose a real threat and no assured way to predict if a student will become violent. As noted in Columbine and Springfield, troubled students can commit an act of violence without making a direct threat. Those in school settings need to learn to do two things— assess threats and work with at-risk students.

Trained school mental health professionals can help assess the multiple factors that put a student at risk and work with other members of crisis teams and professionals in the community to provide appropriate interventions. A process that focuses solely on identification, without intervention, will neither help the potential offender nor necessarily improve safety. A major problem that schools face is that most counselors, psychologists, and administrators in schools are not trained specifically in threat assessment or in violence prevention. School personnel can be involved in a threat assessment inquiry while most threat assessment investigations are left to law enforcement officials. Threat assessment inquiries can help school personnel make critical decisions about responding to situations involving the threat of targeted school violence and the assessment of threats themselves can help establish the need for immediate intervention if a threat has been received by a school. Too many children come to school in pain, feeling lonely, and face desperation and despair.

When adults and students respect each other, when students have a positive connection to at least one adult, and when students feel free to help friends and openly share concerns about students who are in distress, a good school climate for safety is created. A key element is teaching students how to share concerns about others. The U.S. Department of Education published a booklet, *Early Warning, Timely Response: A Guide to Safe Schools*. This booklet lists signs of at-risk students. At-risk signs can be taught to teachers, staff members, parents, and school student bodies. Everyone, including students, should be encouraged to watch for students exhibiting those signs and report to adults. When these signs are reported, a counselor, psychologist, or social worker should investigate the child to determine if there are serious problems lurking that need attention. This document came with a strong warning that warning signs should not be used to label students, but the warning signs can be a talking point to help students realize when one of their classmates may need adult assistance. This is not intended to be a PROFILE for violent students. Rather it is an at-risk list that should prompt officials to provide counseling and other services to students who may be having problems. Table 4.1 lists many characteristics of at-risk students.

Table 4.1 Early warning signs

Early warning sign	Definition	Reference
Social withdrawal	In some situations, gradual and eventually complete withdrawal from social contacts can be an important indicator of a troubled child	McConaughy and Skiba (1993); Skiba (1997)
Excessive feelings of isolation and being alone	Research has shown that the majority of children who are isolated and appear to be friendless are not violent. These feelings are sometimes characteristic of children and youth who may be troubled, withdrawn, or have internal issues that hinder development of social affiliations	Doll (1996); Garber et al. (1991)
Excessive feelings of rejection	In the process of growing up, and in the course of adolescent development, many young people experience emotionally painful rejection. Children who are troubled are often isolated from their mentally healthy peers. Their responses to rejection will depend on many background factors. Without support, they may be at risk of expressing their emotional distress in negative ways—including violence	Coie et al. (1990)
Being a victim of violence	Children who are victims of violence—including physical or sexual abuse—in the community, at school, or at home are sometimes at risk of becoming violent toward themselves or others	Browne and Finkelhor (1986)
Feelings of being picked on and persecuted	The youth who feels constantly picked on, teased, bullied, singled out for ridicule, and humiliated at home or at school may initially withdraw socially. If not given adequate support in addressing these feelings, some children may vent them in inappropriate ways—including aggression or violence	Saarni (1990); Greenbaum (1988)
Low school interest and poor academic performance	Poor school achievement can be the result of many factors. It is important to consider whether there is a drastic change in performance and/or poor performance becomes a chronic condition that limits the child's capacity to learn. In some situations—such as when the low achiever feels frustrated, unworthy, chastised, and denigrated—acting out and aggressive behaviors may occur	Hinshaw (1992)
Expression of violence in writings and drawings	Children and youth often express their thoughts, feelings, desires, and intentions in their drawings and in stories, poetry, and other written expressive forms. Many children produce work about violent themes that for the most part is harmless when taken in context. However, an overrepresentation of violence in writings and drawings that is directed at specific individuals (family members, peers, other adults) consistently over time may signal emotional problems and the potential for violence	Berman and Jobes (1991)
Uncontrolled anger	Everyone gets angry; anger is a natural emotion. However, anger that is expressed frequently and intensely in response to minor irritants may signal potential violent behavior toward self or others	Rothbart et al. (1995)
Patterns of impulsive and chronic hitting, intimidating, and bullying behaviors	Children often engage in acts of shoving and mild aggression. However, some mildly aggressive behaviors such as constant hitting and bullying of others that occur early in children's lives, if left unattended, might later escalate into more serious behaviors	Batsche and Knoff (1994)

(continued)

Table 4.1 (continued)

Early warning sign	Definition	Reference
History of discipline problems	Chronic behavior and disciplinary problems both in school and at home may suggest that underlying emotional needs are not being met. These unmet needs may be manifested in acting out and aggressive behaviors. These problems may set the stage for the child to violate norms and rules, defy authority, disengage from school, and engage in aggressive behaviors with other children and adults	Loeber (1983, 1990)
History of violent and aggressive behavior	Unless provided with support and counseling, a youth who has a history of aggressive or violent behavior is likely to repeat those behaviors. Aggressive and violent acts may be directed toward other individuals, be expressed in cruelty to animals, or include fire setting. Youth who show an early pattern of antisocial behavior frequently and across multiple settings are particularly at risk for future aggressive and antisocial behavior	Gardner et al. (1996); Menzies and Webster (1995)
Intolerance for differences and prejudicial attitudes	All children have likes and dislikes. However, an intense prejudice toward others based on racial, ethnic, religious, language, gender, sexual orientation, ability, and physical appearance—when coupled with other factors—may lead to violent assaults against those who are perceived to be different	Prothrew-Stith (1987)
Drug use and alcohol use	Apart from being unhealthy behaviors, drug use and alcohol use reduce self-control and expose children and youth to violence, either as perpetrators or as victims or both	Cook (1991)
Affiliation with gangs	Gangs that support antisocial values and behaviors—including extortion, intimidation, and acts of violence toward other students—cause fear and stress among other students. Youth who are influenced by these groups—those who emulate and copy their behavior, as well as those who become affiliated with them—may adopt these values and act in violent or aggressive ways in certain situations	Arthur and Erickson (1992); National School Safety Center (1990)
Inappropriate access to, possession of, and use of firearms	Gangs that support antisocial values and behaviors—including extortion, intimidation, and acts of violence toward other students—cause fear and stress among other students. Youth who are influenced by these groups—those who emulate and copy their behavior, as well as those who become affiliated with them—may adopt these values and act in violent or aggressive ways in certain situations	Poland (1993)
Serious threats of violence	Idle threats are a common response to frustration. Alternatively, one of the most reliable indicators that a youth is likely to commit a dangerous act toward self or others is a detailed and specific threat to use violence	Keller and Tapasak (1997)
Serious physical fighting with peers or family members	Serious fighting indicates that there is poor impulse control	Lemerise and Dodge (1993); Lochman et al. (1997)

Severe destruction of property	This goes beyond little acts of vandalism	Harris et al. (1993)
Other self-injurious behaviors or threats of suicide	With suicide, the third leading cause of death, such threats must always be taken seriously	Hillbrand (1995)

Note: Teachers and administrators—and other school support staff—are not professionally trained to analyze children's feelings and motives, but they are on the front line when it comes to observing troublesome behavior and making referrals to appropriate professionals, such as school psychologists, social workers, counselors, and nurses. They also play a significant role in responding to diagnostic information provided by specialists. Educators and parents—and sometimes students—can recognize certain early warning signs. In some situations and for some youth, different combinations of events, behaviors, and emotions may lead to aggressive rage or violent behavior toward self or others. A good rule of thumb is to assume that these warning signs, especially when they are presented in combination, indicate a need for further analysis to determine an appropriate intervention.

This chart was devised from the booklet *Early Warning, Timely Response: A Guide to Safe Schools.*

The cornerstone of school violence prevention strategies should be to create cultures and climates of safety, respect, and emotional support within the school setting. Attending to warning signs should create a supportive environment where emotional intelligence is emphasized (Goleman, 1995). Resnick et al. (1997) indicate that students who experience a sense of emotional "fit" may be less likely to engage in or be victimized by harmful behavior. Schools that emphasize personal contact and connection between adults and students allow students to turn to adults for help when they see a student exhibiting at-risk behaviors. This breaks any code of silence that might inhibit any child from bringing concerns about a friend's behavior to the attention of responsible adults and sets the stage so that students are more likely to turn to a trusted adult for help in resolving problems. According to Pollack and Shuster (2000), in several cases of school shootings, lethal plans were shared with other students but no one told adults. This is in keeping with the finding of the Safe School Initiative.

According to Vossekuil et al. (2002), the Safe School Initiative was created and implemented through the Secret Service's National Threat Assessment Center and the Department of Education's Safe and Drug-Free Schools Program. These programs joined the Department of Education's expertise in helping schools facilitate learning through the creation of safe environments for students, faculty, and staff. The Secret Service has shared its experience in studying and preventing targeted violence. The Safe School Initiative began with a study of the thinking, planning, and other preattack behaviors engaged in by students who carried out school shootings.

The findings of the Safe School Initiative indicate that there are plans that educators, law enforcement officials, and others can pursue in response to the problem of school violence. Specifically, Initiative findings suggest that these officials may wish to consider focusing their efforts to formulate strategies for preventing these attacks in two principal areas:

- Developing the capacity to pick up on and evaluate available or knowable information that might indicate that there is a risk of a school attack.
- Employing the results of these risk evaluations, or "threat assessments," in developing strategies to prevent potential school attacks from occurring.

Support for these suggestions is found in the ten key findings of the Safe School Initiative study:

1. Incidents of targeted violence at school are rarely sudden, impulsive acts.
2. Prior to most incidents, other people knew about the attacker's idea and/or plan to attack.
3. Most attackers did not threaten their targets directly prior to advancing the attack.
4. There is no accurate or useful "profile" of students who engage in targeted school violence.

5. Most attackers engaged in some behavior, prior to the incident, that caused concern or indicated a need for help.
6. Most attackers were known to have difficulty coping with significant losses or personal failures. Many had considered or attempted suicide.
7. Many attackers felt bullied, persecuted, or injured by others prior to the attack.
8. Most attackers had access to and had used weapons prior to the attack.
9. In many cases, other students were involved in some capacity.
10. Despite prompt law enforcement responses, most shooting incidents were stopped by means other than law enforcement intervention.

Note that in most school shootings, the shooters did provide signs of their actions. One student had planned to shoot students in the lobby of his school prior to the beginning of classes. He told two friends exactly what he had planned and talked to three other students to keep them out of harm's way. Another student asked his friends to help him get ammunition for one of his weapons and he sawed off the end of a rifle to make it easier to conceal beneath his clothes. The students "leaked" information to others. If the leaked information had been reported to an adult, a threat assessment could have been conducted.

Educators and other adults can conduct a threat assessment inquiry to pick up on these signals and make appropriate referrals. By inquiring about any information that may have prompted some concern, an investigator may be able to develop a more comprehensive picture of the student's past and current behavior, and identify any indications that the student is intent on or planning to attack.

In developing a threat assessment protocol, the primary purpose would be to assess the actions, communications, and circumstances that indicate an individual intends to attack and is engaged in planning for that event. Appropriate authorities would need to gather information, evaluate facts, and determine if a student poses a threat of violence.

Individuals who have information about students that is cause for concern should know how to refer this information and to whom. The threat assessment team should designate a member of the team to serve as the initial point of contact for information of possible concern. The availability of this point of contact should be made known community-wide. An anonymous tip line may be of use if there is a process in place to carefully evaluate the information that is received by means of this approach. Threat assessment can be carried out by a team member who serves as the initial point of contact. This team member will screen information and determine whether to initiate a threat assessment inquiry or to consult other members of the team. School personnel can use the following forms to gather information about a student who may pose a threat to himself/herself or others in a school setting.

Threat Assessment Referral Form (Kentucky Department of Education, 2000)

If you become concerned that an individual may pose a risk for harming himself or others, complete this form by stating your concern, checking the Warning Signs of which you are aware, and explaining items checked. Turn it in directly to the school's principal or designee. In an *Imminent* safety threat, notify principal immediately and take immediate action to secure or isolate the individual, and move other students from harm's way.

Individual under concern_____ **Date of birth** _____

Person(s) completing this form_____ **Room/phone** _____

School_____ **Date of referral** _____

I. Reason for Referral (explain your concerns) _____

_____

_____

II. Imminent Warning Signs (when an individual displays Imminent Warning Signs, take immediate action to maintain safety, mobilize law enforcement, & appropriate school personnel).

- ☐ 1. Possession and/or use of firearm or other weapon
- ☐ 2. Suicide threats or statements
- ☐ 3. Detailed threats of lethal violence (time, place, method)
- ☐ 4. Severe rage for seemingly minor reasons
- ☐ 5. Severe destruction of property
- ☐ 6. Serious physical fighting with peers, family, others

III. Early Warning Signs (mark items, then elaborate below)

- ☐ 7. Social withdrawal or lacking interpersonal skills
- ☐ 8. Excessive feelings of isolation & being alone
- ☐ 9. Excessive feelings of rejection
- ☐ 10. Being a victim of violence, teasing, bullying
- ☐ 11. Feelings of being picked on
- ☐ 12. Low school interest, poor academic performance
- ☐ 13. Expressions of violence in writings & drawings
- ☐ 14. Uncontrolled anger
- ☐ 15. Patterns of impulsive & chronic hitting & bullying
- ☐ 16. History of discipline problems
- ☐ 17. History of violent, aggressive & antisocial behavior across settings (i.e., fighting, fire setting, cruelty to animals, vandalism, etc., especially begun before age 12)
- ☐ 18. Intolerance for differences, prejudicial attitudes
- ☐ 19. Drug & alcohol use
- ☐ 20. Affiliation with gangs
- ☐ 21. Inappropriate access, possession, use of firearms
- ☐ 22. Threats of violence (direct or indirect)
- ☐ 23. Talking about weapons or bombs
- ☐ 24. Ruminating over perceived injustices

☐ 25. Seeing self as victim of a particular individual

☐ 26. General statements of distorted, bizarre thoughts

☐ 27. Feelings of being persecuted

☐ 29. Depression

☐ 28. Obsession with particular person

☐ 30. Marked change in appearance

IV. Explain checked items; describe known Precipitating Events *(use back if needed)*

_____

_____

V. Turn in this form and any materials you may have which may be necessary to conduct a preliminary risk assessment (i.e., writings, notes, printed e-mail or Internet materials, books, drawings, confiscated items, etc.).

FOR OFFICE & EMERGENCY MANAGEMENT TEAM USE:

Date Received: _____ School Case Manager assigned to follow

referral: _____

Threat Assessment Worksheet (2 pages)

Coupled with the Referral Form (which addresses Warning Signs), this outline addresses Risk Factors, Precipitating Events, and Stabilizing Factors. The worksheet is designed to provide a concise way to organize known concerns when conducting a preliminary risk assessment and to list relevant school and agency involvement.

Individual under concern _____ Date of birth _____

Person(s) completing this form_____

Parent/legal guardian name_____ Phone _____

School _____ Date of referral _____

I. School & Agency Involvement (past or present) *To determine if safety concerns have been noted by others. List name, contact information & date of involvement if known*:

School Law Enforcement or Discipline Referrals _____

_____

Special Education, 504, or Under Consideration _____

_____

School-based Mental Health or Social Services _____

_____

Family Resource and Youth Services Center _____

_____

Community Social Services _____

_____

Police, Juvenile Court, Probation Services _____

_____

Community Mental Health Services _____

_____

Current or prior institutionalization or foster care placemen _____

_____

Other_____

_____

Comments/concerns expressed by any of the above _____

_____

II. Risk Factors *(indicate if Observed, Documented, or Suspected; circle O, D, S, respectively)*

In possession or has access to weapons (O, D, S) ⸺⸺⸺⸺⸺⸺

History of impulsive violent or other antisocial behavior (O, D, S) ⸺⸺⸺

⸺⸺⸺⸺⸺⸺⸺⸺⸺⸺⸺⸺⸺

Child abuse/neglect (O, D, S) ⸺⸺⸺⸺⸺⸺⸺⸺⸺

⸺⸺⸺⸺⸺⸺⸺⸺⸺⸺⸺⸺⸺

Isolation or social withdrawal (O, D, S) ⸺⸺⸺⸺⸺⸺⸺

⸺⸺⸺⸺⸺⸺⸺⸺⸺⸺⸺⸺⸺

Domestic violence or other family conflict (O, D, S) ⸺⸺⸺⸺⸺

⸺⸺⸺⸺⸺⸺⸺⸺⸺⸺⸺⸺⸺

Depression, mental illness, medical ailment (O, D, S) (list current medications)

⸺⸺⸺⸺⸺⸺⸺⸺⸺⸺⸺⸺⸺

⸺⸺⸺⸺⸺⸺⸺⸺⸺⸺⸺⸺⸺

Substance abuse or drug trafficking (O, D, S) ⸺⸺⸺⸺⸺⸺

⸺⸺⸺⸺⸺⸺⸺⸺⸺⸺⸺⸺⸺

Fire setting (O, D, S) ⸺⸺⸺⸺⸺⸺⸺⸺⸺⸺⸺

⸺⸺⸺⸺⸺⸺⸺⸺⸺⸺⸺⸺⸺

Threat Assessment Worksheet

II. Risk Factors *(cont.) (indicate Observed, Documented, or Suspected, O, D, S, respectively)*

Bed Wetting (O, D, S) _____

_____

Cruelty to animals (O, D, S) _____

_____

Preoccupation with real or fictional violence (O, D, S) _____

_____

Repeated exposure to violence (desensitization) (O, D, S) _____

_____

Gang involvement or affiliation (O, D, S) _____

_____

Other _____

_____

III. Precipitating Events *(recent triggers which may influence violence)*

Recent public humiliation/embarassment (whether instigated by adult or peer)

_____

_____

Boyfriend/girlfriend relationship difficulties _____

_____

Death, loss or other traumatic event _____

_____

Highly publicized violent act (such as a school shooting) _____

_____

Family fight or conflict _____

_____

Recent victim of teasing, bullying or abuse _____

_____

Other _____

_____

IV. Stabilizing Factors *(factors which may minimize or mitigate likelihood of violence)*

Effective parental involvement _____

_____

Involved with mental health; list provider or agency (if known) _____

_____

Social support networks (church, school, social organizations) _____

_____

Close alliance with a supportive adult (counselor, mentor, teacher, minister, etc.)

_____

Positive, constructive peer group _____

_____

Appropriate outlets for anger or other strong feelings _____

_____

Positive focus on the future or appropriate future events _____

_____

Other _____

_____

V. Category of Risk *(Determine a Risk for Harm Category based on available information)*

Imminent - High - Moderate - Minor - Low/No (date & time of determination _____)

NOTE: RFH Categories represent a distinct moment in time and may change from hour to hour, and day to day. Following an initial assessment, it is essential to monitor on-going status, to reassess level of risk according to new information, and to document significant changes.

Risk (or Threat) Assessment Concepts

I. **Warning Signs**: A sign or indicator that causes concern for safety.

    A. Imminent Warning Sign: A sign which indicates that an individual is very close to behaving in a way that is potentially dangerous to self or others. Imminent Warning Signs call for *immediate* action by school authorities and law enforcement.

    B. Early Warning Signs: Certain behavioral and emotional signs that, when viewed in a context, may signal a troubled individual. Early Warning Signs call for a referral to a school's Threat Assessment Team for assessment.

II. **Risk Factors**: Historical or background conditions which may influence the potential for violence. These factors may include family history of violence, prior antisocial behavior, mental health background, and various social factors.

III. **Precipitating Events**: Recent events or "triggers" which may increase potential for violence. These factors may include recent family conflict, rejection from a significant peer, serious conflict with a teacher, etc.

IV. **Stabilizing Factors**: Support systems or networks in place for an individual which may *decrease* the likelihood for violence. These factors may include effective parental relationships, positive peer groups, strong relationship with a teacher, counselor, or therapist, etc.

V. **Threat Assessment**: The process of reviewing Warning Signs, Risk Factors, Precipitating Events, and Stabilizing Factors, to determine the Risk for Harm category and develop an appropriate plan of action.

Risk for Harm Categories

Risk for Harm categories provide a way for schools to determine and assign a level of risk based on a review of Warning Signs, Risk Factors, Precipitating Events, and Stabilizing Factors. Based on level of risk, the Emergency Management Team develops action plans to maintain safety and to help an individual gain access to needed services or interventions. The descriptors following each category are not an exhaustive list, but are provided as a frame of reference.

Category 1: Imminent Risk for Harm

An individual is, or is very close to, behaving in a way that is potentially dangerous to self or others. Examples include detailed threats of lethal violence, suicide threats, possession and/or use of firearms or other weapons, and serious physical fighting. Most of these individuals will qualify for immediate hospitalization or arrest. Responses may include immediate action to secure individual, arrest or hospitalization, facility lock down, security response, parent notification, background or records check, "return to school plans," and ongoing case management.

Category 2: High Risk for Harm

An individual has displayed significant Early Warning Signs, has significant existing Risk Factors and/or Precipitating Events, and has few Stabilizing Factors. May not qualify for hospitalization or arrest at present, but requires referrals for needed services and active case management. Responses may include immediate action to secure individual, security response, parent notification, psychological consult/evaluation, and background check.

Category 3: Moderate Risk for Harm

An individual has displayed some Early Warning Signs and may have existing Risk Factors or recent Precipitating Events, but also may have some Stabilizing Factors. There may be evidence of internal emotional distress (depression, social withdrawal, etc.) or of intentional infliction of distress on others (bullying, intimidation, seeking to cause fear, etc.). Responses may include security response, parent notification, psychological consult/evaluation, background or records check, and ongoing case management.

Category 4: Minor Risk for Harm

An individual has displayed minor Early Warning Signs, but assessment reveals little history of serious Risk Factors or dangerous behavior. Stabilizing Factors appear to be reasonably well established. There may be evidence of the unintentional infliction of distress on others (insensitive remarks, "teasing" taken too far, etc.). Responses may include review of school records, parent notification, psychological consult, and security response.

Category 5: Low/No Risk for Harm

Upon assessment it appears that there is insufficient evidence for any risk for harm. Situations under this category can include misunderstandings, poor decision making, false accusations from peers (seeking to get other peers in trouble), etc. Responses may include investigation of the situation, notification and involvement of others as needed, etc.

Brief Interview Outline for Individual Under Concern

When interviewing an individual about safety concerns, one method is to ask questions which move from general introduction to fact finding, to recognition of concerns, to assessing support networks, to developing an outline for next steps. The following questions are not intended to be a scripted interview, but provide a sample structure for the kinds of questions which may need to be asked. Individuals using this outline are encouraged to use their professional judgment and experience, and to broaden or alter the questions. Note, in general it is good to avoid "yes or no" questions.

1. "Seems like you've been having a hard time lately, what's going on?" *(to establish rapport and trust and to open dialog in a nonthreatening way)*
2. "What is your understanding of why you've been asked to come to the office?" *(to review factual events)*
3. "What is your understanding of why school staff are concerned?" *(to determine if student is aware of effect behavior has on others)*
4. "What has been going on recently with you at school?" *(to look into possible precipitating events such as peer conflict, student–teacher interactions, and failing grades; follow appropriate leads)*
5. "How are things going with your family?" *(to look into events such as recent moves, divorce, deaths or losses, and conflict)*
6. "What else is going on with you?" *(to look into events outside of school such as community unrest, threats, police involvement, and medical issues)*
7. "Who do you have to talk to or assist you with this situation?" *(to determine what supports or stabilizing factors may be available or in place such as mental health professionals, peer groups, family supports, and church groups)*
8. "Given (whatever is going on), what are you planning to do?" or, "What are you thinking about doing?" *(follow up on appropriate leads, including the level of detail in stated plans, ability to carry out plans, etc.)* **(NOTE: If there is an IMMINENT RISK take immediate action to maintain safety by contacting school security and/or 911)**.
9. Close with a statement that describes short-term next steps (i.e., "I'll need to contact your parents to talk about…" or "You will be suspended for two days, then we'll…"). Try to determine student's affect or mood prior to his/her departure, and alert others if necessary.

Assessment Questions for Mental Health Professionals

Individual under concern _____ **Date of birth** _____

Parent/legal guardian name _____ **Phone** _____

Mental health professional's name _____ **Phone** _____

Person(s) requesting information _____ **Phone** _____

School name _____ **Date of referral** _____

The following outline is provided by schools to mental health professionals when referrals are made for "Risk for Harm" assessments. In order to serve students who may pose a safety risk to themselves or others, it is essential that the child's school has appropriate information about his/her potential for dangerous behavior.

Suggested use: School staff should complete this form and provide it (with accompanying materials as appropriate) to the mental health professional who will be conducting an evaluation. The mental health professional should then assess the concerns and address them in a report back to the school.

I. Brief description of reason for current referral, and a listing of any items which may accompany this referral (Threat Assessment Worksheet, student notes, printed e-mails, writing assignments, relevant documentation from other sources, etc.):

_____

_____

_____

_____

II. Requested information _(please address these questions in your report to the school)_:

1. What is this individual's understanding regarding the serious nature of their recent actions (behavior, oral or written communications, gestures, etc.)?
2. What is their understanding of the distress, harm, fear, etc., caused by their actions?
3. What is this individual's understanding of the inappropriateness of their actions?
4. What is your understanding of the causes of this individual's actions?
5. What, if anything, is planned to address these issues and prevent their recurrence?
6. At this time, what level of risk is this individual (low, moderate, high, or critical)?
7. If or when this individual returns to school, what may school staff, parents or others need to know to assist and support the student and take action when needed?
8. Other question(s):_____

_____

_____

Take Home Message

A major principle of threat assessment is that each investigation stands on its own. Inferences and conclusions about risk should be guided by an analysis of facts and behaviors specific to the concerned person and the given situation. Any student with the motive, intent, and ability potentially is capable of mounting a targeted attack at school. Judgments about a student's risk of violence should be based upon analysis of behaviorally relevant facts, not on "traits" or "characteristics" of a given individual or of a class of individuals.

References

Arthur, R. & Erickson, E. (1992). *Gangs and Schools*. Holmes Beach, FL: Learning Publications.

Batsche, G.M. & Knoff, H.M. (1994). Bullies and their victims: Understanding a pervasive problem in the schools. *School Psychology Review*, 23, 165–174.

Berman, A.L. & Jobes, D.A. (1991). *Adolescent Suicide: Assessment & Intervention*. Washington, DC: American Psychological Association.

Browne, A. & Finkelhor, D. (1986). Impact of child sexual abuse: A review of the research. *Psychological Bulletin*, 99, 66–77.

Coie, J.D. & Jacobs, M.R. (1993). The role of social context in the prevention of conduct disorder. *Development and Psychopathology*, 5, 263–275.

Coie, J.D., Dodge, K.A., & Kupersmidt, J. (1990). Peer group behavior and social status. In S.R. Asher & J.D. Coie (Eds.), *Peer Rejection in Childhood* (pp. 178–201). New York, NY: Cambridge University Press.

Cook, P.J. (1991). The technology of personal violence. In M. Toney (Ed.) *Crime & Justice: An Annual Review of Research*, Vol. 14, (pp. 235–280). Chicago, IL: Chicago University Press.

Cornell, D.G. (1998). *Designing Safer Schools for Virginia: A Guide to Keeping Students Safe from Violence*. Charlottesville, VA: University of Virginia, Thomas Jefferson Center for Educational Design.

Doll, B. (1996). Children without friends: Implications for practice and policy. *School Psychology Review*, 25, 165–183.

Elias, M.J. & Tobias, S.E. (1996). *Social Problem-Solving: Interventions in the Schools*. New York, NY: The Guilford Press.

Garber, J., Quiggle, N.L., Panak, W., & Dodge, K.A. (1991). Aggression and depression in children: Comorbidity, specificity, and social cognitive procession. In D. Cicchetti & S.L. Toth (Eds.), *Internalizing and Externalizing Expressions of Dysfunction: Rochester Symposium on Developmental Psychopathology*, Vol. II. Hillsdale, NJ: Erlbaum.

Gardner, W., Lidz, C.W., Mulvey, E.P., & Shaw, E.C. (1996). Clinical versus actuarial predictions of violence in patients with mental illnesses. *Journal of Consulting and Clinical Psychology*, 64, 602–609.

Goleman, D. (1995). *Emotional Intelligence*. New York: Bantam Books.

Greenbaum, S. (1988). *School Bullying & Victimization*. Malibu, CA: National School Safety Center.

Harris, G.T., Rice, M.E., & Quinsey, V.C. (1993). Violent recidivism of mentally disordered offenders: The development of a statistical prediction instrument. *Criminal Justice and Behavior*, 20, 315–335.

Hillbrand, M. (1995). Aggression against self and aggression against others in violent psychiatric patients. *Journal of Consulting and Clinical Psychology*, 63, 668–671.

Hinshaw, S.P. (1992). Externalizing behavior problems and academic underachievement in childhood and adolescence: Causal relationships and underlying mechanisms. *Psychological Bulletin*, 111, 127–155.

Keller, H.R. & Tapasak, R.C. (1997). Classroom management. In A. Goldstein & J.C. Conoley (Eds.), *School Violence Intervention: A Practical Handbook*. New York, NY: The Guilford Press.

Kentucky Department of Education. (2000). *School-centered emergency management and recovery guide*. Frankfort, KY: Kentucky Department of Education.

Lemerise, E.A. & Dodge, K.A. (1993). The development of anger and hostile interactions. In M. Lewis & J.M. Haviland (Eds.), *Handbook of Emotions* (pp. 537–546). New York, NY: Guilford.

Lochman, J.E., Dunn, S.E., & Wagner, E.E. (1997). Anger. In G.G. Bear, K.M. Minke, & A. Thomas (Eds.), *Children''s Needs: Development, Problems and Alternatives* (pp. 149–160). Bethesda, MD: National Association of School Psychologists.

Loeber, R. (1983). The stability of antisocial and delinquent child behavior: A review. *Child Development*, 53, 1431–1446.

Loeber, R. (1990). Development and risk factors of juvenile antisocial behavior and delinquency. *Clinical Psychology Review*, 10, 1–42.

McConaughy, S.H. & Skiba, R.J. (1993). Comorbidity of externalizing and internalizing problems. *School Psychology Review*, 22, 421–436.

Menzies, R. & Webster, C.D. (1995). Construction and validation of risk assessments in a six year follow-up of forensic patients: A tridimensional analysis. *Journal of Consulting and Clinical Psychology*, 63, 766–778.

National School Safety Center (1990). *Gangs in Schools: Breaking Up is Hard to Do*. Pepperdine, CA: Author.

Poland, S. (1993). *Crisis Manual for the Alaska Schools*. Juneau, AK: State Department of Education.

Pollack, W. & Shuster, T. (2000). *Real Boys' Voices*. New York: Random House.

Prothrew-Stith, D. (1987). *Violence Prevention Curriculum for Adolescents*. Newton, MA: Education Development Center.

Quinn, M.M., Osher, D., Hoffman, C.C., & Hanley, T.V. (1998). *Safe, Drug-Free, & Effective Schools for all Students: What Works*. Washington, DC: Center for Effective Collaboration & Practice. American Institutes for Research.

Resnick, M., Bearman, P.S., & Blum, R.W. (1997). Protecting adolescents from harm. *Journal of American Medicine Annuals*, 278(10), 823–832.

Rothbart, M.K., Posner, M.I., & Hershey, K.L. (1995). Temperament, attention, and developmental psychopathology. In D. Cicchetti & D. Cohen (Eds.), *Manual of developmental psychopathology* (pp. 315–340). New York: Wiley.

Saarni, C. (1990). Emotional competence: How emotions and relationships become integrated. In R.A. Thompson (Ed.), *Socio-emotional development* (pp. 115–182). Lincoln, NE: University of Nebraska Press.

Skiba, R. (1997). Conduct disorders. In G.G. Bear, K. Minke, & A. Thomas (Eds.), *Children''s Needs II: Development, Problems, & Alternatives*. Washington, DC: National Association of School Psychologists.

U.S. Department of Education & U.S. Department of Justice (1999). *1999 Annual Report on School Safety*. Washington, DC: Authors.

Vossekuil, B., Fein, R., Reddy, M., Borum, R., & Modzeleski, W. (May 2002). *The Final Report and Findings of the Safe School Initiative: Implications for the Prevention of School Attacks in the United States*. Washington, DC: U.S. Secret Service and U.S. Department of Education.

Chapter 5
Social Information Processing and Aggression in Understanding School Violence: An Application of Crick and Dodge's Model

Amy Nigoff

The current chapter will review a theory of how children interpret and process social situations and how these processes can be biased in a way that leads the child to aggression. Children are in school for 8 h of their day. Most of their social interactions occur there, when they are in classrooms or on the playground with other children. Mistakes and biases in the social information processing steps often manifest at school. By possessing an understanding of these steps, one would be in a better position to prevent aggression from happening. The current examination will consist of a review of a theory of social information processing and research connecting biases in processing to aggression. Finally, we will present a scenario exploring how social information processing theories can be used to treat and prevent school violence.

Mental health workers have benefited from theories of social psychologists and cognitive psychologists. Both of these areas are more recent additions to psychological thought but both have had tremendous influence on current thought and conceptualization. These areas have added to previous thinking consisting mainly of psychoanalytic theory and behaviorism. The current chapter will present a theory created from the marriage of social and cognitive psychologies.

From the beginning of the cognitive movement precipitated by a work by Ulric Neisser in 1967, information processing has held the place as a major tenet of cognitive psychology. Information processing model theorists assert that there is an ordered sequence of events that an individual will go through in order to make sense of his or her surroundings and social interactions. Broadbent (1958) created the first diagram that demonstrated the steps people use to process information. The model was created by comparing the human brain to a computer, a brand new invention that had the world's attention. It was hypothesized that there is a sequential order of steps and each step is influenced by the previous step. At each stage of processing, a conclusion is reached which will thus affect the next stage and all future stages. Information processing theorists use cognitive psychology processes such as memory, perception, decision making, and knowledge representation (Newell, 1990) as well as cognitive psychology constructs such as internal representations, scripts, schemas, and heuristics.

T. W. Miller (ed.), *School Violence and Primary Prevention.*
© Springer 2008

A question placed before theorists is what are these stages? The current chapter will review theories of these stages and how an understanding of these stages can lead to a better understanding of aggression in children and its alleviation and prevention. A model by Dodge and colleagues (Crick & Dodge, 1994; Dodge, 1986) will receive the most attention because of its presence in the literature as a leading model.

Before going further, the definition of aggression needs to be identified. *The American Heritage® Dictionary of the English Language*: Fourth Edition (2000) defines aggression as (1) the act of initiating hostilities or invasion; (2) the practice or habit of launching attacks; or (3) hostile or destructive behavior or actions. Violence is defined as physical force exerted for the purpose of violating, damaging, or abusing. Aggression is not the same as violence, which has an inclusion of some form of physical force applied to it. This distinction is necessary because aggression in schools is not limited to physical fighting. Most researchers divide aggression into three categories: physical aggression, verbal aggression, and social manipulation (e.g., Mynard & Joseph, 2000). Social manipulation typically uses the social network to inflict harm on the target (e.g., excluding someone from the group). Popular culture has minimized the effects of social manipulation by making light of the issue with movies (e.g., *Mean Girls*) and books (e.g., *Mean Chick, Cliques, and Dirty Tricks* by Erika V. Shearin Karres, 2004). We know from prevalence studies that the report of bullying decreases as children mature (DeVoe et al., 2002); however, this may be due to children learning more subtle ways to aggress. Children may be less likely to label this behavior as unacceptable due to the minimization in popular media.

Huesmann (1988) utilized theories of aggression and incorporated developments in cognitive psychology to create a model of information processing. He hypothesized that to understand aggressive responses, one must include the child's cognitive abilities and these information processing procedures. These areas, combined with learning from experience and observing others, will lead a child to exhibit aggressive behavior.

Huesmann (1988) describes "cognitive scripts" that are accessed by a child when confronted by a situation. A script is a guide for behavior. It is a step-by-step guide that specifies the steps in a situation that must be taken to reach the desired end. The script will assist the child in evaluating a situation leading to a decision on how to react. The process identified contains steps leading to a response. These steps are (1) encounter social problem; (2) evaluate environmental cues; (3) search memory for script to guide behavior; (4) evaluate generated script; and (5) behave according to script. During the evaluation step, if the child finds the evaluation unfavorable, the child will return to the search step to identify a different script that can be evaluated. Only the favorable script would thus be enacted.

Individual differences which will affect responses are readily observed in this model (Huesmann, 1988). At the beginning of the social interaction, each individual will have different cognitive abilities and behaviors that have been experienced. Every individual has different experiences.

Dodge (1986) formulated a model to explain how social cognitions are interwoven with social behaviors. Specifically, he hypothesized a model that could be applied to understand why someone would choose an aggressive response. He postulated that biases in social cue interpretation would lead to an aggressive act. In his model, a bias in thinking often belies the true intent of another's actions.

Dodge integrated and elaborated on previous models that focused on social skills deficits. Previous models were problematic because they often searched for a single factor that could predict aggression such as deficits in role-taking, problem solving, or low empathy. The models also ignored the fact that aggressive behaviors are situation specific. Finally, the models did not postulate a theory of why social cognitions lead to aggressive behaviors (Dodge, 1986).

Dodge's (1986) model describes how people respond to social cues using social cognitions. He posits that people begin with a body of biologically determined capabilities and storehouse of past experiences, socialized rules and knowledge, and schemas. A schema involves strict rules through which an individual will view situations. The storehouse contains memories and information gathered by the individual over time. These capabilities and memories are personalized to each individual. Social cues are received by the individual. In a series of steps, the individual processes the presented social information using the aforementioned biologically determined capabilities and memories of past experiences. The steps the individual takes to process social cues occur rapidly and sequentially. Every step is experienced although not necessarily at a conscious level. When a situation is novel or unfamiliar, the steps may be slower and at a conscious level. Dodge makes the assertion that either consciously or unconsciously, the individual invariably uses all social information processing steps.

Deviant responses to social cues are due to a failure to respond in a skillful or unbiased manner. Because individuals have different biological information and social experiences, their processing is individualized. The model provides a way to hypothesize how individuals understand and interpret social situations as a function of their past experiences and innate abilities (Dodge, 1986).

Crick and Dodge (1994) further developed the original model reflecting advances in conceptual and empirical innovations in psychology. This model differs from that developed by Dodge (1986) in that it provides more linkages between steps of processing. This is represented by the change in the model's shape, originally linear, to the circular shape of the newly formulated model. The change to a circular model also addresses concerns of researchers who believe that social information processing follows a simultaneous parallel path instead of the more rigid, sequential steps. The reformulated model accounts for this by presenting the model as circular and providing feedback loops in processing; the sequential steps are retained, however, in the belief that the model provides "heuristic value for understanding the processing of a single stimulus" (p. 77).

There are six steps in the reformulated model of social information processing. For a pictorial representation of the steps, see Fig. 5.1. The first step is the encoding process of the social cues received through the senses. Encoding the cues involve attending to appropriate cues and chunking information. Heuristics are often

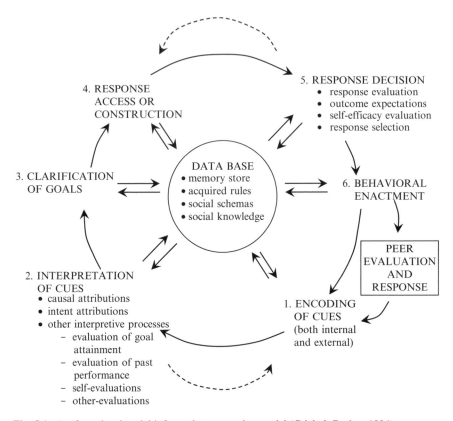

Fig. 5.1 A reformulated social information processing model (Crick & Dodge, 1994)

employed to economically encode information. Deficient or inaccurate encoding of social cues, such as not encoding all available cues, may lead to deviant responses. Cues may be selectively encoded to support future interpretations (Crick & Dodge, 1994; Dodge, 1986).

The second step in social information processing is the mental representation and interpretation process. Cues are integrated with past experiences producing a meaningful understanding of the social situation. This skill develops with age as the individual constructs and refines decision rules for understanding the social situation. Cognitive heuristics, schemas, scripts, and working models of relationships are used in order to guide processing at this step, making processing more efficient. As in the first step, deficiencies at this level will lead to cognitive biases while interpreting the cues. One example of this is the hostile attribution error, which will be discussed subsequently. Also, some individuals see aggression as normal and will acquire scripts and schemas that use aggression. Further, scripts may be malleable to deviant interpretations and thus encourage problematic behavioral responses. Interpretations made during this exchange will have an effect on future encoding and interpretation of social cues (Crick & Dodge, 1994; Dodge, 1986).

The third step is the only step added during the reformulation (Crick & Dodge, 1994); this is the step where the individual makes a clarification of goals for the social situation. Individuals begin with certain goals due to past experiences that may be revised in regard to the current social situation. Goals can be internal or external to the individual. An example of an internal goal is self-survival; examples of external goals are obtaining a reward and developing social relationships. Inappropriate goals are relationship damaging and will result in deviant behavior (cf., positively socially adjusted individuals who will choose goals that are relationship enhancing). This step was originally a part of the next stage; however, by separating this step out, more attention and research may be focused on it.

The fourth step involves the search for possible behavioral responses that are appropriate to how the social information was encoded, interpreted, and to what goal the individual is working toward. Available responses are constructed through the socialization process and are selected using a combination of past experiences, the ability to generate responses, rule structures, and the processes used in resolving the previous steps. When the situation is novel, new responses may be constructed to respond to social cues. If the previous steps have been conducted in an aberrant way, deviant responses will be generated. Deviant responses may occur at this step if the individual has inadequate search skills or has conducted a biased search (Crick & Dodge, 1994; Dodge, 1986).

Step 5 involves choosing a response to the social situation (Crick & Dodge, 1994; Dodge, 1986). Responses are chosen carefully as they may be situation specific (effective only in a specific situation) and involve specific behavioral capabilities concerning the individual's ability to carry out the decision. Further, an analysis of consequences must be performed. Estimations of consequences may be biased by the previous steps or due to past experiences. The response is decided upon by considering outcome expectations and self-efficacy evaluation. The individual may need to return to step 4 for additional response generation if there are no satisfactory response choices available. If, during step 2, the individual made a hostile attribution to the other person's intent, the response chosen will mirror this and will more likely be aggressive. The mistake of an overestimation of positive consequences may lead the individual to choose an aggressive response.

The sixth and final step of social information processing occurs when the response is enacted (Crick & Dodge, 1994; Dodge, 1986). This is the culmination of the process. Verbal and motor skills that have been developed through rehearsal, feedback, and practice are employed to act out the chosen response. An individual's previous experience with the chosen response will influence the response's effectiveness.

At the conclusion of step 6, the other(s) involved will react to the individual's chosen behavior, which constitutes a new social cue restarting the social information processing. The other person's response will be incorporated into the individual's memories of past experiences that will influence how the steps will be processed during future social situations (Crick & Dodge, 1994; Dodge, 1986).

Lemerise and Arsenio (2000) contend that the model created by Dodge and colleagues (Crick & Dodge, 1994; Dodge, 1986) leaves out a pivotal piece of the puzzle, namely, emotion. Lemerise and Arsenio assert, like some theorists before them, that emotion is distinctly different from cognition and that through adding emotion to the model, we can have a more complete understanding of how an individual identifies the response to a social situation. One such theorist is Albert Bandura (1994) who identified different definitions for affective processes ("process regulating emotional states and elicitation of emotional reactions") and cognitive processes ("thinking processes involved in the acquisition, organization, and use of information"; p. 71).

Lemerise and Arsenio (2000) suggest adding emotional considerations to the steps of social information processing already identified by Dodge and colleagues (Crick & Dodge, 1994; Dodge, 1986). These researchers identify that the emotions being displayed by the other actor(s) in the situation as well as the emotional tie the child has with the others will affect each step in the processing model. They also suggest more attention be paid to the child's own emotional state. In the database, a child may also have a predisposition for specific emotions or an "emotion style." Further, children may have different levels of ability to regulate emotions. Also, the child's current state of emotion, at the time of the social cue, should be taken into account. During the encoding step, Crick and Dodge identify internal as well as external cues. Lemerise and Arsenio assert that both the child's emotional state and the other actor's perceived emotional state will be encoded. Lemerise and Arsenio also state that the emotional attachment to the other person should be considered at this step. As in their example, children will react diametrically different when being teased by a friend and when being teased by the school bully.

During clarification of goals, Crick and Dodge (1994) identified an individual's current emotional state as having an effect on which type of goal will be endorsed. Lemerise and Arsenio (2000) suggest adding a consideration of the child's interpretation of the other individual's emotional cues. If the child has interpreted the other individual as being angry or aiming to be hurtful, then the child will clarify a goal based on this interpretation. If the child is attached to the other individual through friendship, this emotion may lead to a different goal being identified.

Steps 4 and 5, response access and response decision, can be affected by the intensity of emotion being experienced (Lemerise & Arsenio, 2000). If a youth is intensely experiencing a negative emotion, then negative responses will be accessed and generated. The concept of heuristics teaches us that the when angry feelings are activated, angry responses are more likely to occur. In step 5, a self-efficacy evaluation is made in regards to responses generated. Bandura (1994) states that the state of experiencing a positive mood will increase an individual's self-efficacy evaluation. Further, being in a "despondent" mood will decrease self-efficacy evaluation. Again, note that all steps in the social information processing model are affected by previous steps.

Once the child enacts the behavior (step 6), the child will observe the other's emotional response. This will be incorporated into the database. This information will be used by the child in future situations in order to guide the decision-making process.

Dodge's (1986) model and Crick and Dodge's (1994) reformulated model have been supported by empirical evidence. Most of the research presented is of data from Dodge's and colleagues' laboratories. However, the model has found support in the United States and in other countries by numerous other researchers including VanOostrum and Horvath (1997), Andreou and Metallidou (2004), and Orobio de Castro et al. (2003).

Results of social information processing studies support differences between aggressive and nonaggressive children in each step of social information processing model and data support that a combination of factors best predicts aggression. Also noted is that predictions of social behavior are situation specific. This indicates that the behavioral response in one domain does not significantly predict the behavioral response in another domain. There may, however, be a general processing pattern due to the marginal cross-domain predictability of aggression (Crick & Dodge, 1994; Dodge, 1986).

The research presented concerns the application of social information processing to aggressive individuals. However, social information processing has also been applied to other types of individuals including prosocial youth (Nelson & Crick, 1999). During stage two, unlike aggressive children, prosocial youth were less likely to make hostile attributional errors and more likely to make benign attributions; they were also less distressed concerning the provocation than were non-prosocial youth. Prosocial participants were more likely to make positive evaluations of prosocial behavior responses. Further, they were more likely to scorn instrumental goals and instead support relational goals (Nelson & Crick, 1999).

The social information processing model (Crick & Dodge, 1994; Dodge, 1986) can be used to distinguish youth who are proactively aggressive and those who are reactively aggressive. Proactive aggression is based on the model of social learning put forth by Bandura (1973). Bandura asserts that aggression is a socially acquired instrumental behavior motivated by reinforcement. With the social learning model, Bandura explained that aggression is instrumental in order to gain rewards. In the context of social learning, aggression is developed through learning and reinforcement; when rewards are acquired, the individual's use of aggression is validated and continued. Reactive aggression's roots are in the frustration–aggression model forwarded by Dollard et al. (1939) and refined by Berkowitz (1962). This theory identifies aggression as an angry reaction to a perceived frustration.

The distinction between proactive and reactive aggression is necessary for the current discussion as many studies of social information processing biases and deficits use this distinction. Bullying, by definition, is a form of proactive aggression (Dodge, 1991). Reactive aggression is seen as a retaliatory response or temper tantrums.

Crick and Dodge (1996) hypothesized that individuals who are reactively aggressive have a bias in step 2 (mental representation and interpretation) in that they attribute hostile intent to ambiguous situations and would thus react with a retaliatory response. Further, they hypothesized that individuals who are proactively aggressive have biases in steps 3 (goal selection), 4 (response search), and 5 (response decisions). Proactively aggressive individuals focus on goal attainment (i.e., the goal pulls for a behavior). These individuals choose goals that are instrumental in nature. Responses generated in step 4 will support the individual's outcome expectancies. During step 5, the response will be chosen that also supports their perceived positive outcome expectancies. Further, the individual will incorporate their feeling of self-efficacy in performing the behavior during the response decision. These specific social information processing variables will be discussed subsequently.

Berkowitz (1977) demonstrated that the individual's interpretation of the intention of the other person is related to their response choice. Milich and Dodge (1984) systematically studied how, when the provocateur's intent is unknown, aggressive children may attribute hostility to an ambiguous act. If the individual processes the provocateur as acting aggressively, a retaliatory response will be chosen, thus demonstrating reactive aggression. Dodge (1986, 1991) hypothesized that this is a bias in the second step of social information processing which leads people to make this type of aggressive interpretation. The bias is processed from past experiences and may result from an expectation of being the victim of aggression due to the individual being the victim of aggression previously. This is apparent in Dodge's (1986) and Crick and Dodge's (1994) model that identified a storehouse of previous experiences that is accessed in order to interpret the current social cue. Fittingly, this is characteristic of reactively aggressive individuals and thus of victims who are the repeated victim of aggression. Called hostile attributional bias, this is the probability of attributing hostile intent to another person when the situation does not warrant hostility. If the individual has been the victim of previous aggression, that heuristic would be activated easily, thus attributing hostility to the current social cue. Dodge and Newman (1981) found that a hostile attributional bias most likely occurred when the social cues were selectively encoded for hostility (step 1).

Hostile attributional bias has been demonstrated in research by Dodge and Coie (1987) who found that reactively aggressive boys (in first through third grades) were inaccurate in interpreting peers' cues. Specifically, they found that the reactively aggressive group of boys attributed hostile intention to ambiguous situations; the proactively aggressive group did not differ from nonaggressive children in the amount of hostile attributions. More recently, Orobio de Castro et al. (2005) found supporting results among aggressive boys aged 7–13. Partial correlations were computed to assess the unique relationship between type of aggression and hostile attributional bias. With the effects of proactive aggression partialed out, a significant correlation was found between reactive aggression and making hostile attributions. On the other side, children who were proactively aggressive were not significantly associated to hostile attribution scores after the effects of reactive aggression were controlled.

Research has shown that hostile attribution can be influenced by priming negative feelings. When alerted to possible hostile intent, children may access representations of hostile memories more easily and thus attribute hostility when the situation is ambiguous. Victims, who face, by definition, continuous physical, verbal, and emotional abuse have many representations in their thoughts ready to receive hostility and thus encourage them to make this attributional error (Berkowitz, 1990; Orobio de Castro et al., 2003).

Dodge (1991) reported that proactively aggressive individuals have expectations of a positive result for their aggressive behavior which causes them to have a positive attitude toward aggression. These positive expectations for aggressive behavior come from instrumental goals decided on in stage three and will result in the individual choosing an aggressive response in step 5 of social information processing. This is found among proactively aggressive children but not for reactively aggressive children. Crick and Dodge (1996) hypothesized that proactively aggressive individuals have a more positive attitude toward aggression because of what can be gained by the aggressive behavior.

More recently, Vernberg et al. (1999) gave a measure of attitude toward aggression, adapted from Slaby and Guerra (1988), to 1105 junior high students. The measure consists of three factors including Aggression is Legitimate and Warranted, Aggression Enhances Status and Power, and One Should Not Intervene in Fights. Only boys and girls who were identified as bullies scored high on all three of these factors ($r = .61$, $r = .30$, and $r = .28$, respectively; $p < 001$). Neither victims of bullying nor those who reported no involvement in bullying had high scores on the measure showing discriminate value for this variable in identifying the three bully groups.

Erdley and Asher (1996) found that children who were rated as aggressive by their peers were higher on choosing aggressive responses. Further, children who were rated as aggressive had fewer problem-solving responses when provided with a scenario where the intent of the "aggressor" was ambiguous. The researchers also found that aggressive children were more likely to choose a goal of revenge or to make themselves look better to their peers. Also discovered, in concordance with other literature, was that aggressive children had difficulty in identifying peaceful solutions to provocations.

Crick and Dodge (1996) tested a combination of biases to assess how they are related to proactive and reactive aggression. Participants included 624 children (9–12 years of age) in a large metropolitan area. Results supported the hypotheses indicating that there was a difference in how reactive and proactive children process social information. Specifically, the reactive aggressive group expressed more hostile attributions than the nonaggressive and the proactively aggressive group among 11- and 12-year-olds. Proactively aggressive children evaluated more positive outcome expectations for aggressive behavior than for non-proactive aggression. Further, proactively aggressive individuals also had a higher belief in their ability to carry out aggressive behaviors. In relation to social goals, proactively aggressive children exhibited more instrumental goals that were self-enhancing, supporting the hypothesis of a processing bias during step 3. Conclusions from Crick and Dodge indicate that social information processing theory can discriminate between proactively and reactively aggressive individuals.

One major advantage of Crick and Dodge's (1994) social information processing model is the ease of explanation to children. The model is easily described in computer terms, indeed, this is how the model was formulated in the first place.

Perception, problem solving, and memory are analogous to data reading, data processing, and storage capabilities. The action taken by the person can be compared to a computer's output. Although this comparison can be limiting, it is helpful in explaining to a society that is entrenched in computer usage.

One drawback of the social information processing model presented by Dodge and colleagues (Crick & Dodge, 1994; Dodge, 1986) is that the model may not be applicable to children with mild intellectual disabilities. This was demonstrated in a study by van Nieuwenhuijzen et al. (2006). The authors concluded that children with mild intellectual disabilities did not use steps of the social information processing model as did children without intellectual disabilities. Specifically, in step 5 (response decision), the children in the study did not use response evaluation, self-efficacy evaluation, response selection to choose the response that would be enacted in step 6. However, their data supported that the children in the study did encode cues, interpret them, and generate responses. Many children who are aggressive also have mild intellectual disabilities. The information provided by this study will allow us to better focus interventions on the other steps in the model.

Prevention and Treatment

School violence is extremely prevalent (DeVoe et al., 2002; Haynie et al., 2001; Nansel et al., 2001; National Children's Home, 2004). In its most severe form, 699,800 children were the victims of a violent act, including assault, rape, and robbery, on school grounds in the year 2000 (DeVoe et al., 2002). DeVoe et al. also found that, on school grounds, 8.9% of school age children had been threatened or injured with a weapon, 12.5% been involved in a physical fight, and 7.9% were victims of bullying. Research also indicates that aggression continues without intervention. Huesmann et al. (1984) found that participants who were aggressive as 8-year-old children were more aggressive as 30-year-olds. They were more likely to have served jail or prison sentences than their nonaggressive counterparts.

As discussed before, many of these acts of aggression can be connected to biases and mistakes children have in making sense of social situations. School violence can be decreased by those who work with children who have an understanding of why these acts of violence occur in the first place and by knowledge and practice of effective interventions. This is an opportunity that cannot be passed by. Children in schools are a "captive" audience and are easily accessed. Performing interventions that would help a child develop skills might save years of aggressive behaviors that will only lead to incarceration.

Skills training techniques have been established in both the literature and in practical application. Typically, the training consists of easy to understand steps and techniques to build a youth's repertoire. As identified above, skill deficits, deficiencies, biases, and mistakes lead to aggressive behaviors. Social information processing models can be used to assist clinicians in identifying which areas a youth may be having difficulty. The take home message, however, is that children who exhibit high levels of aggression have missing skills, have biases, and make mistakes at multiple stages in processing. From what has been previously discussed, it is a conglomeration of mistakes that result in aggression. The focus for working with aggressive youth should be on what steps the youth is having trouble. With that in mind, a number of interventions can be applied for the best possible outcome.

Finally, a situation is presented in which a youth might react aggressively. The steps of the model will be considered, including interventions that can be made at each step to help the child to decrease aggressive responses.

Harry is walking down the hall for his next class. Draco, a fellow classmate, bumps into him in passing. Draco comments to Harry and to Draco's friends, "I love your hair."

Harry is a 14-year-old boy who is in high school. Harry has had multiple experiences with aggression; his cousin and his uncle, with whom he lives, do not regard him as an important part of the family and are aggressive toward him. While his uncle is verbally aggressive, his cousin is physically assaultive. His aunt is a quiet bystander. Harry also has had a bad morning. He performed poorly in his class with his most disliked professor (database of information). Harry encodes the cue of Draco's statement with regards to his current bad mood (step 1). Harry also ignores the cues from Draco of genuineness positive regard. At this stage, Harry has made the mistake of selective encoding. He only encoded the cues that were negative. An intervention at this point can be to help Harry to identify the other cues that occurred that he had ignored. It would also be helpful to aid Harry in identifying the nonverbal cues of the situation. What did he miss because it was not verbal?

Harry next interprets the cue (step 2). He assumes that Draco is being mean. He believes that Draco is making fun of his hair, which is notoriously disheveled. Work can be done at this level to help Harry in clarifying the intent of ambiguous situations. He could be helped at this stage with questioning the automatic thought associated with the hostile attribution as well as generating alternative explanations that do not include hostility.

Teacher (T): Harry, he said that you had nice hair. Why is that a negative comment?

Harry (H): I know he was saying it to be mean. He always says mean things to me. He's never nice.

T: Is there a possibility that he wasn't being mean?

H: No! He never says anything nice. He always makes comments when his friends are around to make me look bad!

T: Maybe though, he wasn't being mean this time. Is it even possible that he was not being mean?

H: I guess there's a possibility but it's a really small chance.

Harry has begun to recognize that there may have been a chance that the other youth was not being negative. Harry's tendency was to automatically assume negativity. By encouraging Harry to realize, at least the possibility, that Draco was not being mean is a positive step in the right direction. Here is another way to help Harry to question his automatic assessment of hostility.

T: What would you have thought about the situation if it had been a friend who made the comment about your hair?

H: If it had been my friend Ron, I would have thought that he was being nice and that he noticed how I had used gel to try to get my hair to be tamer.

T: So why is it that you immediately assumed that Draco was being negative and mean?

This technique will decrease or change the emotional involvement by reframing the situation into something less hostile.

T: What do you believe Draco was meaning when he made the comment about your hair?

H: He was making fun of my hair. Why else would he have made a comment?

T: If you made the comment to one of your friends, what would you have meant by the statement?

H: I would have meant that the new style they were trying out was nice and that it looked good.

T: So why couldn't this have been what Draco was meaning? Is there another reason why Draco might have said this?

This is an example of perspective taking which is designed to help Harry to better understand Draco's motives and Draco's goals for his comment.

Harry will then identify the goal for his behavior (step 3). Because Harry may have already made the interpretation that Draco was being hostile, Harry may feel as if he needs to retaliate in order to save face. At this step, an intervention may include forced generation of other goals that are possible.

T: OK, Harry, take just a few seconds and let's talk about this. What are you trying to accomplish right now?

H: I want Draco to look stupid in front of his friends, just like he did to me!

T: But, isn't that the girl you like, there, by her locker? Do you want to look like a hot head to her?

H: Well, no. She got mad at me a couple of weeks ago when I tried to beat up that other kid who was making fun of me. She said I looked stupid with how red my face got.

T: So wouldn't it be better then to be the bigger person. Wouldn't that be more impressive to her and your friends?

Without an intervention, Harry will most likely pick a goal that he has used before due to easy access and familiarity.

Harry has chosen the goal of retaliation. He is angry and he feels slighted in front of his classmates. In order to achieve the goal of retaliation, Harry identifies a couple of ways in which he could respond. He could make fun of Draco because of his blonde hair, he could make a joke about Draco's own performance in class that morning, or he could be violent and physically attack Draco (step 4). All of these responses will result in the goal of retaliation. An intervention could be made here by guiding Harry through different responses that are possible. At this step, responses may be limited in order to reach the goal decided previously. Harry also considers walking away from Draco and not providing Draco with the satisfaction that he has hurt Harry's feelings.

Harry must evaluate the different responses that he has generated (step 5).

T: Harry, why don't you just walk away from Draco?

H: I can't. I'm so angry right now, I have to do something! I can't just walk away, that will make me look stupid to my friends!

T: I've seen you walk away from others before. Remember a couple of weeks ago when another student made fun of you because of how scared you got while watching a movie? You ignored him and walked away.

H: Yeah, I did. My friends were really proud of me.

T: So you've been successful at it before, I bet you could do it again!

The intervention involves increasing Harry's self-efficacy, his belief that he can walk away from the situation successfully.

In regard to the violent response, he does not believe that he can control his anger. Self-efficacy in his confidence to control his anger could be better developed. Self-efficacy can be increased by practicing a new skill by role-playing and in-vivo experiences. Harry would benefit from verbal skills training such as trainings on the different communication styles (assertive, aggressive, and passive). Assertive responding is calm and respectful. Assertiveness also incorporates "I" statements that reflect how Harry feels in the current situation. If Harry were more confident in his ability to successfully use assertive communication, he would be more likely to choose this response.

Finally, Harry decides to aggress against Draco and starts a physical fight with him (step 6). The response has been enacted. The bystanders are cheering for their particular friend. The fight is broken up but not before Harry has bloodied Draco's nose. He gets detention for the fight but his friends brag about his ability to better Draco. The results from this social interaction are incorporated into his database of information which he will use to process social information in the future.

Take Home Message

The steps of social information processing occur quickly. It is important to encourage Harry and other children to "think before acting" and to "do the right thing," both phrases that are used in skills trainings. The social information processes are not automatic but are quick and often without conscious decisions (Crick & Dodge, 1994). It is helpful to slow down in order to provide the opportunity to consider consequences of actions. As we can see in this example, the first mistake was very early in the processing procedure. Making an early intervention would help to decrease the likelihood of an aggressive response.

Knowledge of the social information processing model is helpful for anyone working with aggressive children. Having an increased understanding of the order of the steps will help by allowing us to identify interventions that can happen early. In the above case, if Harry had been able to generate different explanations for Draco's comment, all steps after that would have been affected. Social skills trainings are prevalent as empirically supported treatments and interventions. Applying these trainings with an understanding of social information processing will result in positive interventions that will decrease aggressive behaviors.

References

Andreou, E. & Metallidou, P. (2004). The relationship of academic and social cognition to behaviour in bullying situations among Greek primary school children. *Educational Psychology*, 24(1), 27–41.

Bandura, A. (1973). *Aggression: A Social Learning Analysis*. Englewood Cliffs, NJ: Prentice-Hall.

Bandura, A. (1994). Self-efficacy. In V. S. Ramachaudran (Ed.), *Encyclopedia of Human Behavior* (Vol. 4, pp. 71–81). New York: Academic Press.

Berkowitz, L. (1962). *Aggression: A Social Psychological Analysis*. New York: McGraw-Hill.

Berkowitz, L. (1977). Situational and personal conditions governing reaction to aggressive cues. In D. Magnusson & N. S. Endier (Eds.), *Personality at the Crossroads: Current Issues in Interactional Psychology*. Hillsdale, NJ: Erlbaum.

Berkowitz, L. (1990). On the formation and regulation of anger and aggression. *American Psychologist*, 45, 494–503.

Broadbent, D. E. (1958). *Perception and Communication*. New York: Pergamon Press.

Crick, N. R. & Dodge, K. A. (1994). A review and reformulation of social information-processing mechanisms in children's social adjustment. *Psychological Bulletin*, 115, 74–101.

Crick, N. R. & Dodge, K. A. (1996). Social information-processing mechanisms on reactive and proactive aggression. *Child Development*, 67, 993–1002.

DeVoe, J. F., Peter, K., Kaufman, P., Ruddy, S. A., Miller, A. K., Planty, M., Snyder, T. D., Duhart, D. T., & Rand, M. R. (2002). *Indicators of School Crime and Safety: 2002*. Washington, DC.: U.S. Departments of Education and Justice, NCES 2003–009/NCJ 196753.

Dodge, K. A. (1986). A social information processing model of social competence in children. *Minnesota Symposium in Child Psychology*, 18, 77–125.

Dodge, K. A. (1991). The structure and function of reactive and proactive aggression. In D. J. Pepler & K. H. Rubin (Eds.), *The development and treatment of childhood aggression* (pp. 201–218). Hillsdale, NJ: Lawrence Erlbaum Associates.

Dodge, K. A. & Coie, J. D. (1987). Social-information-processing factors in reactive and proactive aggression in children's peer groups. *Journal of Personality and Social Psychology*, 53, 1146–1158.

Dodge, K. A. & Newman, J. P. (1981). Biased decision-making processes in aggressive boys. *Journal of Abnormal Psychology*, 90, 375–379.

Dollard, J., Doob, L. W., Miller, N. E., Mowrer, O. H., & Sears, R. R. (1939). *Frustration and Aggression*. New Haven, Connecticut: Yale University Press.

Erdley, C. A. & Asher, S. R. (1996). Children's social goals and self-efficacy perceptions as influences on their responses to ambiguous provocation. *Child Development*, 67, 1329–1344.

Haynie, D. L., Nansel, T., Eitel, P., Crump, A. D., Saylor, K., Yu, K., & Simons-Morton, B. (2001). Bullies, victims, and bully/victims: Distinct groups of at-risk youth. *Journal of Early Adolescence*, 21, 29–49.

Huesmann, L. R. (1988). An information processing model for the development of aggression. *Aggressive Behavior*, 14, 13–24.

Huesmann, L. R., Eron, L. D., Lefkowitz, M. M., & Walder, L. O. (1984). Stability of aggression over time and generations. *Developmental Psychology*, 20, 1120–1134.

Lemerise, E. A. & Arsenio, W. F. (2000). An integrated model of emotion processes and cognition in social information processing. *Child Development*, 71, 107–118.

Milich, R. & Dodge, K. A. (1984). Social information processing in child psychiatric populations. *Journal of Abnormal Child Psychology*, 12, 471–490.

Mynard, H. & Joseph, S. (2000). Development of the multidimensional peer-victimization scale. *Aggressive Behavior*, 26, 169–178.

Nansel, T. R., Overpeck, M., Pilla, R. S., Ruan, W. J., Simons-Morton, B., & Scheidt, P. (2001). Bullying behaviors among US youth: Prevalence and association with psychosocial adjustment. *Journal of the American Medical Association*, 285, 2094–2100.

Nelson, D. A. & Crick, R. (1999). Rose-colored glasses: Examining the social information-processing of prosocial young adolescents. *Journal of Early Adolescence*, 19, 17–38.

Newell, A. (1990). *Unified theories of cognition*. Cambridge, MA: Harvard University Press.

National Children's Home (2004). Is it true that children can be bullied online and via mobiles? In *Internet safety FAQ*. Retrieved May 21, 2005, from http://www.nch.org.uk/information/index.php?i=134.

Orobio de Castro, B., Slot, N. W., Bosch, J. D., Koops, W., & Veerman, J. W. (2003). Negative feelings exacerbate hostile attributions of intent in highly aggressive boys. *Journal of Clinical Child and Adolescent Psychology*, 32, 56–65.

Orobio de Castro, B., Merk, W., Koops, W., Veerman, J. W., and Bosch, J. D. (2005). Emotions in social information processing and their relations with reactive and proactive aggression in referred aggressive boys. *Journal of Clinical Child and Adolescent Psychology*, 34, 105–116.

Slaby, R. G. & Guerra, N. G. (1988). Cognitive mediators of aggression in adolescent offenders: 1. Assessment. *Developmental Psychology*, 24, 580–588.

van Nieuwenhuijzen, M., de Castro, B. O., van der Valk, I., Wijnroks, L., Vermeer, A., & Matthys, W. (2006). Do social information-processing models explain aggressive behaviour by children with mild intellectual disabilities in residential care? *Journal of Intellectual Disability Research*, 50, 801–812.

VanOostrum, N. & Horvath, P. (1997). The effects of hostile attribution on adolescents' aggressive responses to social situations. *Canadian Journal of School Psychology*, 13, 48–59.

Vernberg, E. M., Jacobs, A. K., & Hershberger, S. L. (1999). Peer victimization and attitudes about violence during early adolescence. *Journal of Clinical Child Psychology*, 28, 386–395.

Chapter 6
The Roles of Morality Development and Personal Power in Mass School Shootings

Ken Kyle and Stephen Thompson*

Introduction

Much as many Americans today speak of a pre- and post-9/11 political world, some speak of a pre- and post-Columbine world of education. As a number of K-12 educators, academicians, and journalists suggest (e.g., McKenna & Haselkorn, 2005; cf. Martinson, 2000; Lawrence & Birkland, 2004), Columbine and the other well-publicized mass school shootings (and attempted school shootings) that occurred during the 1990s have coalesced in the public mind, becoming a watershed event. Media coverage was wide-ranging and intense, and as Hancock (2001) points out, much of it was presented out of context (for examples of media coverage, see links provided at CNN.com, 2001; cf. Moore, 2003). As one prominent example, the March 19, 2001, cover of *Time* magazine proclaimed, "The Columbine Effect" and offered stories on "Inside the Mind of the California Killer," "Confronting the Classroom Code of Silence," and "Why Some Kids Snap–and Others Don't" (cf. Gibbs, 2001). Indeed, Pam Riley, executive director of the Center for the Prevention of School Violence, publicly described Columbine as "the 'Pearl Harbor' of school violence" (see Dunne, 2000). This, despite the fact that statistically schools are safer than homes and neighborhoods in terms of likelihood of children experiencing violence.

Hancock writes: "National education statistics show that, at most, thirty-five children were murdered in school during the 1997–1998 academic year, while 2,752 were killed beyond campus" (Hancock, 2001, p. 77). As the Justice Policy Institute points out, during the 1998–1999 school year, the year of the Columbine mass school shootings, a child had about a one in two million chance of being killed in school. Indeed, of the 40 children (and adults) killed at schools during the 1997–1998 school year, 11 were killed in mass school shootings. Similarly, on average, 11 children died each day of that school year from family violence (Donohue et al., 1998). Leone et al. (2000) point out that most crimes in schools are thefts, and the majority of injuries to children at school are nonviolent. Evidence of the uncommon nature of such violence is found in the fact that "until the release of the 1998 federal

---

* Names appear in alphabetical order. Each author contributed equally to this chapter.

T. W. Miller (ed.), *School Violence and Primary Prevention.*
© Springer 2008

school crime and safety index…there was no national reporting mechanism for the shootings, homicides, or suicides that occurred on school campuses" (Furlong & Morrison, 2000, p. 77).

Nevertheless, in response to reports of an "epidemic" of mass school shootings, many school boards, school districts, state governments, as well as the federal government, took decisive action, enacting or strengthening a variety of security-related policies (Robelen, 1999; McCollum, 2004; cf. Austin 2003). Berger reports:

> A recent U.S. Department of Education survey of public schools found that 96% required guests to sign in before entering the school building, 80% had a closed campus policy that forbids students to leave campus for lunch, and 53% controlled access to their school buildings… A National School Board Association survey of over 700 school districts throughout the United States found that 39% of urban school districts use metal detectors, 75% use locker searches, and 65% use security personnel…. Schools have introduced stricter dress codes, put up barbed-wire security fences, banned book bags and pagers, and have added "lock down drills" and "SWAT team" rehearsals to their safety programs. (Berger, 2002, p. 119; cf.Fox & Harding, 2005; Brunner & Lewis, 2006).

Some of these measures are more provocative than others. As an example, consider a controversial policy recently adopted by The Independent School District of Burleson, Texas. The district now trains students to fight against school shooters, using their strength in numbers to overwhelm perpetrators, rather than to hide and passively await rescue in locked-down, secure classrooms. This approach is based upon the recommendations of some security experts who suggest that waiting for police to take control of a school shooting scenario is a deadly mistake. Rather, they suggest, students should take tactical control by overwhelming school shooters, literally throwing everything available at the shooters, including books, backpacks, chairs, etc. The idea is that an interrupted and possibly off-balance shooter can be tackled and held until authorities arrive. However, such recommendations are not without their detractors. One serious concern is, of course, for the safety of the student or students leading the charge, as they could potentially draw an immediate and deadly response from the shooter (Von Fremd, 2006).

Up until the spate of mass school shootings and attempted mass school shootings in the 1990s, many may have thought that school violence primarily affected large urban schools (cf. Cirillo et al., 1998), and some may have attached a socioeconomically (or even racially or ethnically) based significance to their understanding of school violence. As Sheley and Wright (1998) suggest,

> Recent shootings by students of peers and teachers in school settings, where such events were markedly unexpected, have provoked fear and outrage in America. For many, the "youth-gun problem" seems be spreading beyond inner cities to suburbs and small towns and from "bad boy" cultures (i.e., those characterized by relatively high poverty, crime, unemployment, and school dropout rates) to "good boy" cultures (characterized by fewer such social ills).

Commentator Tim Wise is even more direct:

> Two more white children are dead and thirteen are injured, and another "nice" community is scratching its blonde head, utterly perplexed at how a school shooting the likes of the one

yesterday in Santee, California could happen. After all, as the Mayor of the town said in an interview with CNN: "We're a solid town, a good town, with good kids, a good church-going town… an All-American town." Yeah, well maybe that's the problem.

I said this after Columbine and no one listened so I'll say it again: white people live in an utter state of self-delusion. We think danger is black, brown and poor, and if we can just move far enough away from "those people" in the cities we'll be safe. If we can just find an "all-American" town, life will be better, because "things like this just don't happen here."

Well, bullshit on that. In case you hadn't noticed, "here" is about the only place these kinds of things do happen. (Wise, 2001)

Still, no matter the source of impetus for change, we agree that informed consideration of school violence and appropriate policies are needed. And while we acknowledge that mass school shootings are relatively rare, we take this opportunity to consider mass school shootings specifically, and then to explore lessons learned that might apply to all school violence.

Therefore, following a demographic discussion of mass school shootings, we present an argument built around moral philosophy and other related factors that appear to contribute to the phenomenon of mass school shootings. The premises of this argument follow an intensifying progression, in that each newly presented premise builds upon the former premise resulting in a sequence of contributing factors potentially leading to school violence. In essence, when taken together, this sequence of factors may lead to acts of extraordinary violence. Out of this argument we develop a partial model of mass school shootings, a model that takes a number of *necessary*, but *not sufficient* variables into account in explaining mass school shootings. We contend that the greater the knowledge of necessary conditions, the greater the chance of developing effective preventative policies and interventions.

In presenting this argument and model, we develop the following premises. First, children whose primary socialization through family interactions does not effectively encourage development of a personal system of ethics may have difficulty accepting and living within socially accepted mores and ethical systems. Second, we consider the effects of peer associations on the moral development of children, and develop the premise that children deprived of positive peer group socialization may behave outside of socially accepted ethical systems. Third, we discuss the possible results of poor socialization. We hold that children from whom encouragement and esteem are consistently withheld suffer in their understanding of their own significance as persons. Therefore, such children may behave in increasingly deviant ways to achieve some form of esteem. Fourth, we suggest that school environments reflecting the intense social competition permeating larger society positively acknowledge and reward students who best demonstrate societal norms, and withhold esteem from students who do not reflect societal norms. Accordingly, such school environments exacerbate the isolation and insignificance that some poorly socialized students with underdeveloped moral philosophies feel. In essence, such highly charged competitive environments provide fertile ground for extraordinary manifestations of violence. Finally, we consider our model's potential to aid in understanding acts of extraordinary school violence, and suggest how our efforts may inform debate over acts of "ordinary" school violence.

Mass School Shootings, Perpetrators and Victims

Before discussing various means to address mass school shootings, placing such violent events in context is essential. Accordingly, we present our working definition of mass school shootings. We report the prevalence of mass school shootings in the United States of America (USA) and abroad, and present some characteristics of victims and perpetrators associated with mass school shootings in the USA since 1992. We briefly touch upon some of the more widely circulating reasons offered to explain mass school shootings, and we consider the useful commonalities that underlie mass school shootings.

Mass School Shootings Defined

There are various ways to define extraordinary acts of school violence like mass school shootings. For purposes of this chapter, a mass school shooting (1) takes place at a school, the grounds immediately adjacent to a school, or at a school-related event (e.g., a school dance or field trip) and (2) is a spree killing or attempted spree killing (i.e., murders that follow no discernible pattern and occur in a very short span of time). This is not to say, however, that mass school shootings are not or cannot be planned.

Further, to simplify matters, we only consider mass school shootings perpetrated by a student or students directed at students or school personnel. Finally, we further limit our focus to perpetrators 18 years of age and younger in the USA. Accordingly, gang-related killings, individual revenge killings, and murder or attempted murder of an individual spouse, lover, or girlfriend or boyfriend, whether successful or not, do not meet our definition of mass school shootings, even if the attack results in multiple victims (i.e., in carrying out an attack bystanders are accidently killed or wounded).

Characteristics of Mass School Shootings

Mass school shootings are neither an exclusively US phenomena nor a new phenomena. Based upon information presented in Infoplease's (Infoplease, 2006) "A Time Line of Recent Worldwide School Shootings" and in keeping with our definition and criteria for classifying an attack as a mass school shooting, over 20 mass school shootings took place in six different countries between January 1, 1996, and December 1, 2006. However, the lion's share of mass school shootings occurred in the USA. One mass school shooting occurred in each of the following countries over this ten-year period: Argentina, Bosnia-Herzegovina, Canada, and the Netherlands. Two mass school shootings occurred in Germany, and 19 occurred in the USA.

We have found documented accounts of mass school shootings that meet our criteria dating back to the 1974 Orlean High School attack in Orlean, New York; although it is likely that there were earlier mass school shootings. In that attack, an 18-year-old male honors student killed three and wounded 11 (see Hancock, 2001, for summaries of other "early" mass school shootings). Unfortunately, as suggested earlier, records of such attacks were not kept in a systematic fashion.

Nevertheless, some have attempted to compile records of mass school shootings and violent attacks on schools (http://www.columbine-angels.com/SV_Home.htm and its linked pages and The National School Safety Center are particularly good sources). On the basis of these and other sources, we have compiled our own list of mass school shootings in the USA (see Table 6.1).

Table 6.1 Mass school shootings in the USA, August 1992 through November 8, 2006—demographic background of perpetrators and victims[a]

	Location	Perpetrators	Victims[c]
Date	School, state, school/community setting[b]	Race/ethnicity-biological sex, age committed suicide	Number-biological sex-student/staff, killed (K); wounded (W)
12/14/1992	Simon's Rock College, MA Rural; <7,500; largely White	Asian American male, 18	1 Male student, K 1 Male professor, K 4 (N/A) Students, W
1/18/1993	East Carter Counter High School, KY Rural; <4,000; overwhelmingly White	White male, 17	1 Female teacher, K 1 Male custodian, K
10/12/1995	Blackville-Hilda High School, SC Rural; <5,500; largely African American	African American male, 16, committed suicide	1 Female teacher, K 1 Male teacher, W
11/15/1995	Richland High School, TN Rural; <350; primarily White[b]	White male, 17	1 Female student, K 1 Male student, W 1 Male teacher, W
2/2/1996	Frontier Middle School, WA Rural; <35,000; majority White	White male, 14	1 Female student, K 1 Female student, W 2 Male students, K
2/19/1996	Bethel Regional High School, AK Rural; <12,000; primarily Native American	Native American male, 16	1 Male principal, K 1 Male student, K 2 Female students, W
10/1/1997	Pearl High School, MS Rural; <31,500; largely White	White male, 16	2 Female students, K 3 Female students, W 4 Male students, W
12/1/1997	Heath High School, KY Rural; <4,000; primarily White	White male, 14	3 Female students, K 5 Female students, W

(continued)

Table 6.1 (continued)

Date	Location School, state, school/community setting[b]	Perpetrators Race/ethnicity- biological sex, age committed suicide	Victims[c] Number-biological sex-student/staff, killed (K); wounded (W)
12/15/1997	Stamps High School, AR Rural; <2,100; majority African American	White male, 14	1 Female student, W 1 Male student, W
3/24/1998	Westside Middle School, AR Rural; <18,000; overwhelmingly White	White male, 13 White male, 11	4 Female students, K 1 Female teacher, K 9 Female students, W 1 Male student, W
4/24/1998	James W. Parker Middle School, PA Rural; <13,500; overwhelmingly White	White male, 14	1 Female teacher, W 1 Male teacher, K 2 Male students, W
5/21/1998	Thurston High School, OR Rural; <33,500; primarily White	White male, 15	2 Male students, K 15 Female students, W 9 Male students, W
4/20/1999	Columbine High School, CO Suburban; <41,000; primarily White	White male, 18, committed suicide White male, 17, committed suicide	3 Female students, K 9 Female students, W 1 Female teacher, W 9 Male students, K 1 Male teacher, K 14 Male students, W
5/20/1999	Heritage High School, GA Suburban; <29,500; majority White	White male, 15	1 Female student, W 5 Male students, W
12/6/1999	Fort Gibson High School, OK Rural; <4,500; majority White	White male, 13	1 Female student, W 3 Male students, W
3/5/2001	Santana High School, CA Semirural; <55,500; primarily White	White male, 15	2 Male students, K 3 Female students, W 8 Male students, W 1 Male student- teacher, W 1 Male security guard, W
3/22/2001	Granite Hills High School, CA Suburban; <43,000; largely White	White male, 18	3 Female students, W 2 Female teachers, W 3 Male students, W
4/24/2003	Red Lion Area Jr. High School, PA Suburban; <19,000; overwhelmingly White	White Male, 14, committed suicide	1 Male principal, K
9/24/2003	Rocori Senior High School, MN Rural; <8,500; overwhelmingly White	White male, 15	2 Male students, K

(continued)

Table 6.1 (continued)

Date	Location — School, state, school/community setting[b]	Perpetrators — Race/ethnicity-biological sex, age committed suicide	Victims[c] — Number-biological sex-student/staff, killed (K); wounded (W)
3/21/2005	Red Lake High School, MN Rural (reservation); <1,500; 100% Native American	Native American male, 16, committed suicide	4 Female students, K 1 Female teacher, K 5 Male students, K 7 Male students, W
11/8/2005	Campbell County High School, TN Suburban; <9,500; overwhelmingly White[b]	White male, 15	1 Male assistant principal, K 1 Male principal, W 1 Male assistant principal, W
3/14/2006	Pine Middle School, NV Urban; <180,500; majority White[b]	White male, 14	1 Female student, W 1 Male student, W
9/29/2006	Weston High School, WI Rural; <350; overwhelmingly White	White male, 15	1 Male principal, K
Summary	23 Mass school shootings in the USA Smallest community (2) <350 inhabitants Largest community <180,500 inhabitants 1 Urban school district 5 Suburban school districts 17 Rural or semirural school districts	Perpetrators—25 (*all male*) Race/ethnicity: 21 White; 1 African American; 1 Asian American; 2 Native Americans Suicides—5 Race/ethnicity: 3 White; 1 African American; 1 Native American	Murdered victims—54 (22 Females; 32 males) (41 Students; 13 staff) Wounded victims—127 (58 Females; 65 males)[d] (117 Students; 10 staff)

N/A, not available.

[a]Does not include attacks planned but foiled by authorities. Sources for this compilation (in no particular order) include http://www.colleges.com/admissions/collegesearch/college_search.taf?_function = detail&page = 9&type = 4&school_id = 1100092;http://www.columbine-angels.com/Shootings-2000–2004.htm; http://wfrv.com/topstories/local_story_272173022.html; http://www.columbine-angels.com/Shootings-1980–2000.htm; http://columbine.free2host.net/victim/injured.html; http://www.epodunk.com/cgi-bin/mobilityInfo.php?locIndex = 12536; The National School Safety Center (2005); http://en.wikipedia.org/wiki/School_shooting; http://www.epodunk.com/cgi-bin/popInfo.php?locIndex = 226440; http://www.columbine-angels.com/Shootings-2005–2009.htm; http://www.mayhem.net/Crime/intermittent.html; http://ar.localschooldirectory.com/schools_info.php/school_id/4978; http://www.schoolfolks.com/community/; http://jeffcoweb.jeffco.k12.co.us/profiles/demographics/high/columbine.pdf; Infoplease (2006); http://www2.indystar.com/library/factfiles/crime/school_violence/school_shootings.html.

[b]Community type, community population, school racial/ethnic composition (overwhelmingly ≥ 95%, primarily ≥ 85%, largely ≥ 70%, majority ≥ 50%). The school racial/ethnic composition is unavailable for Richland High School and Campbell County High School. Instead the community's racial/ethnic composition is substituted. Similarly, the racial/ethnic composition of Pine Middle School is unavailable. The district's racial/ethnic composition is presented in its place.

[c]Victims reported here do not include others killed or wounded outside of the school attack.

[d]Female and male injured victims do not equal 127 because the biological sex of four injured victims is unknown.

Between the start of the 1992 school year and December 1, 2006, when this chapter was completed, we identified 23 school attacks that match our criteria for a mass school shooting, although a number of planned attacks were uncovered and prevented as well (as a specific example, see Sanchez, 2004). All of these attacks were carried out by individual male students except in two instances in which two male students carried out coordinated, joint attacks. Of the 25 assailants, 21 were White, two were Native American, one was African-American and one was Asian-American. Victims included male and female students, teachers, administrators, and school staff members. And in at least one case females were targeted exclusively.

Mass school shootings took place in every region of the country; however, they clustered in the Deep South where nine of the 23 incidents occurred (two in Arkansas, one in Georgia, two in Kentucky, one in Mississippi, one in South Carolina, and two in Tennessee). No other regional clustering occurred, although California, Minnesota, and Pennsylvania experienced two mass school shootings apiece, and California's two mass school shootings, although not directly connected, occurred in the same school district within three weeks of one another. Only one of the mass school shootings took place in an urban setting, and this did not occur until 2006. Moreover, this incident did not take place in an urban center where school violence is stereotypically said to occur (recall Tim Wise's comments presented earlier). Sixteen incidents took place in rural community settings, including one in a Native American Reservation. One took place in a semirural/suburban community setting, and five took place in suburban community settings. All but four of the mass school shootings took place in schools that had a majority of White students, some overwhelmingly so. Moreover, only one of the minority race/ethnicity perpetrators was a student in a majority White district while one of the White perpetrators was a student in a majority African-American district.

No mass school shootings took place during the 1993–1994, 1994–1995, and 2001–2002 school years. A single mass school shooting took place during each of the following school years: 1999–2000, 2002–2003, 2003–2004, 2004–2005, and 2006–2007 (up to December 1, 2006). Two mass school shootings took place during the 1992–1993, 1998–1999, 2000–2001, and 2005–2006 school years. Four took place during the 1995–1996 school year, and six mass school shootings occurred during the 1997–1998 school year. The shortest time between attacks was 2 weeks, while 17 days separated two different sets of mass school shootings.

Suggested Causes

Given these incidents, scholars, government agencies, civic leaders, and concerned individuals have offered a wide variety of possible causes for specific mass school shootings and for mass school shootings generally. Some look for psychological explanations; for example, a Federal Bureau of Investigation (FBI) team of psychologists and psychiatrists declared one of the Columbine killers to be a certifiable psychopath and the other a depressive with suicidal tendencies (see Cullen, 2004). More generally, Metcalf (2001) asks whether there is a connection between the use of psychotropic drugs and extraordinary acts of violence by today's youth, including mass school shootings. The US Secret Service and Department of Education consider bullying to be a contributing factor to mass school shootings and school violence generally (reported in Danitz, 2000). Kimmel and Mahler (2003) go further and suggest that bullying involving homosexual taunts may play a significant role in mass school shootings (cf. Plummer, 2001; Poteat & Espelage, 2005). Coleman (2004) points to the media's culpability in facilitating copycat incidents of violence and suicide, including mass school shootings. North (1999) and Jahnkow (2001) argue that our society's glorification of war and militarism are underlying factors. Moreover, Jahnkow (2001) also asks whether subliminal racism may be a factor in some of the mass school shootings. Similarly, Fraser (2001) suggests that severe alienation for any who do not conform to shallow community norms driven by a history of intolerance and racism were factors in the Columbine massacre (cf. Thomas & Smith, 2004).

A Profile of Mass School Shooters?

In light of the demographic information on school shooters presented earlier (see Table 6.1) and these suggested factors, it seems unlikely that a simple solution to mass school shootings will be found. Indeed, such observations are confirmed by law enforcement officials too. As Dedman reports: "The Secret Service studied the cases of 41 children involved in 37 shootings at their current or former school, from 1974 to 2000.... The Secret Service researchers read shooters' journals, letters and poetry. [And] they traveled to prisons to interview 10 of the shooters...." (Dedman, 2000, p. 4). The results of their research: there is no appropriate profile for mass school shooters.

They found mass school shooters are not typically "loners" and few were diagnosed as mentally ill or had histories of drug and alcohol abuse. However, more than half had histories of depression or of feeling desperate. About three fourths of the school shooters studied contemplated or attempted suicide before their attacks. Similarly, "in more than three-fourths of the incidents, the attackers had difficulty coping with a major change in a significant relationship or loss of status, such as a lost love or a humiliating failure" (Dedman, 2000, p. 3).

The Secret Service researchers found that although the most frequent motivation for attackers was revenge, many had more than a single motive. They report that more than three quarters of the shooters held a real or imagined grievance against the target of their attack and/or others, and in most of the cases considered, the mass school shooting was the first violent act directed at the person thought to have caused the slight or injury (see Dedman, 2000, p. 2). Indeed, the researchers report that many saw the attack as a way to solve a problem. Bullying was common. Two-thirds of the attackers described feeling persecuted, bullied or threatened—not teasing but torment. Other problems they were trying to solve: a lost love, an expulsion or suspension, even a parent planning to move the family. (Dedman, 2000, p. 3)

In terms of familial and educational background there were no discernable patterns. "Some lived with both parents in 'an ideal, All-American family.' Some were children of divorce, or lived in foster homes. A few were loners, but most had close friends" (Dedman, 2000, p. 5). A few had disciplinary records. And while some were taking Advanced Placement courses and kept honor roll grade point averages, some were failing. As Robert A. Fein, a forensic psychologist with the Secret Service confided, "What causes these shootings, I don't pretend to know, and I don't know if it's knowable" (reprinted in Dedman, 2000, p. 5).

Despite Fein's confession and the seeming improbability of finding the definitive cause or factors that prompt children to commit extraordinary acts of violence such as mass school shootings, we suggest that we can effectively work to prevent future mass school shootings. While almost all children in the USA must respond to pressure to conform to homogenized community standards of acceptability, negotiate life in a covertly (and sometimes overtly) misogynist, racist, militaristic, and homoprejudiced society, ferret through the all too frequently violent messages and maladaptive practices communicated by popular culture and the media, and respond to bullying at some time in their lives, very few commit mass school shootings. At least one appreciable difference between those who react to these stressors by engaging in extraordinary violence and those who do not is the possession of a sufficiently strong ethical sensibility.

Accordingly, we suggest that one of the key variables meriting detailed consideration is the presence or absence of a sufficiently developed moral or ethical sensibility. In the case of mass school shooters, their actions clearly indicate they had a deficient or inadequately developed ethical system. In essence, we argue that a well-developed moral system counters violent and maladaptive behaviors promoted by society. Accordingly, in the remainder of this chapter, we develop a model of mass school shootings centering on the development of an effective ethical system. In doing so, we are not suggesting that other factors, especially social and cultural factors like overt and covert racism and misogyny, militarism, economic disparities, and the like, can or should be dismissed. We hold that to adequately respond to mass school shootings, both individual-level and social-level factors must be addressed. Thus, our model should be seen as a partial response to mass school shootings.

Moral Philosophy and Mass School Shootings

Throughout this chapter, we hold that an acceptable ethical system entails possession of personal moral principles. Smetana (1999) defines morality as "an individual's prescriptive understanding of how individuals ought to behave towards each other"

(p. 312). We concur with Smetana and others who argue that a moral system, or moral philosophy, is based upon concepts of welfare, trust, justice, and rights (Smetana, 1995; Turiel, 1998; cf. Nucci, 2002). Smetana (1999) further suggests that moral judgments are "obligatory, universalisable, unalterable, impersonal, and determined by criteria other than agreement, consensus, or institutional convention" (p. 312).

Thus, the responses to behaviors considered immoral will be based upon the responder's concern for the welfare of the victim of the observed immoral behavior. Further, Tisak and Tisak (1996) suggest that morality and aggression are related in that behavioral responses to each include concern for the welfare and rights of the individuals victimized by aggression, as well as immoral behavior. This association between moral—or immoral—behavior and aggression will be developed further in this chapter as we discuss the possible behaviors of morally deficient adolescents working through issues of blocked personhood.

Differences between the behavior of adult mass murderers and juvenile mass murderers may offer evidence of the effects of an under- or undeveloped system of moral philosophy among juvenile mass school shooters. Nearly one-third of adult mass murderers die immediately after committing their crimes (Palermo, 1999). Of the 85 mass murders perpetrated by adults, studied by Palermo, 28 committed suicide at the scene, or were killed by police. In contrast to the behavior of adult mass murderers, juvenile mass murderers commit suicide after committing their crime much less frequently (Palermo, 1999).

One reasonable explanation for this difference is that no matter the motivation leading adults to commit mass murder, some sense of right and wrong may cause deeper feelings of remorse or resentment after the crime, leading some of them to commit suicide, or choose death at the hands of police, rather than continue with life. Still, if those adult mass murderers who committed suicide at the scene had possessed an adequately developed sense of personal ethics, they might not have committed mass murder in the first place. However, if the presence of some level of a moral philosophy may lead to suicide by a murderer, perhaps an understanding of the dynamic of ethics can help primary caregivers and social institutions lead children in developing a sufficient ethical system so that they do not engage in extraordinary acts of violence when confronted with personal and social injustices.

Family and Moral Development

While at first glance, the terms "family" and "parent" may seem straightforward, in fact, they are highly contested and the source of much political rancor (Kyle, 2001; Lakoff, 2002). Therefore, throughout the remainder of this chapter, family will be understood in broad terms, referring to familial units in which adults practice a primary socialization role in the life of a child, or in the lives of children, while living with them. Adult guardians in familial units, whether solo or coupled, are the primary caregivers of the child or children in their charge. They may include, but not be limited to, one or both natural parents, stepparents, adoptive parents, foster parents, grandparents, and other extended family members assuming the role of guardianship. Also, parents need not be heterosexual in their sexual orientation, and may or may not be in a domestic relationship. Thus, parent and parents are used synonymously with child guardian and child guardians. What is more important than who primary caregivers may be is the intent and capacity of primary caregivers.

Debate over the development of moral philosophy in adolescents is driven by Kohlbergian stage development theory (see Kohlberg, 1969, 1981). Accordingly, moral reasoning is said to develop in stages throughout individuals' lives:

- At Stage One people obey rules in order to avoid punishment.
- At Stage Two people change their behavior in order to receive rewards.
- At Stage Three people look beyond themselves and begin to concentrate on winning approval from their peers. Behavior may be changed to avoid disapproval.
- At Stage Four people become interested in doing their duty. People begin to respect authority and are willing to abide by the social order.
- At Stage Five duties are determined by contracts and respect for others' rights. There is an emphasis on equality, democratic rights, and order.
- At Stage Six people have respect for the rules of the social order, but are also able to make personal choices in which universal well-being is a priority.

Persons at ages 9–11 are generally characterized as being within Stages One and Two. These two stages together are known as the premoral level. Most adolescents and many adults function at Stages Three and Four. These two stages together are known as the conventional level. Stages Five and Six are described as principled reasoning (cf. Claypoole, Moody & Peace, 2000). For many stage development theorists, few adults are thought to function at Stage Five, and fewer still at Stage Six.

Researchers aligned with Kohlberg's theory suggest that prosocial behavior is age related. This suggests that the changes taking place in persons during puberty are not only physical and cognitive but also moral. Thus, age-related changes include underdevelopment or appropriate development of moral reasoning, empathy and related emotional responses, and perspective taking (Fabes, 1999). From this perspective, children need both a sense of belonging and a sense of autonomy. As they move through early adolescence, they are presented with new and ever widening social opportunities allowing them to develop their moral reasoning.

Some, however, contend that stage development theory overemphasizes the role of extra-familial factors in moral development. For example, Walker (1999), Hart et al. (1999), Pratt et al. (1999), Walker and Hennig (1999), and White (2000) contend that family socialization processes in general—and parenting styles in particular—are highly influential in the development of children's moral reasoning. For such critics, adolescents most likely to engage in deviant behaviors lack a close affective bond with their parents, may not be monitored or supervised effectively, and/or may not be disciplined in a consistent manner, thus hampering the development of reasoned behavior (Vazsonyi & Pickering, 2000). Indeed, this appears to be the case with some mass school shooters. Lanata contends that the vast majority of the school shooters came from broken and/or troubled families. Charles "Andy" Williams, the shooter at Santana High School in Santee, Calif., lived with his father; his parents had been divorced for 10 years… Barry Loukaitais from Moses Lake, Wash., lived under the same roof with feuding parents who reportedly were planning divorce. The father of Luke Woodham of Pearl, Miss., reportedly left home when Luke was five. Kip Kinkel from Springfield, Ore., was small in stature, reportedly suffered from a learning disability and perhaps did not measure up to the athletic, academic or social standards of an achievement-oriented family. (Lanata, 2003, p. 22)

Nevertheless, whether one is an adherent or detractor of stage development theory, all seem to agree that parents do influence the development of their children's pro- or antisocial behavior (cf. Goetting, 1994). This influence comes from guardians' role in informing children about desirable behavior. It comes from providing models of appropriate behavior, and from encouraging appropriate behavior. Further, it comes from punishing inappropriate behavior, and encouraging the development of empathy (Eisenberg & Murphy, 1995).

Peer Relationships

Many researchers hold that peer relationships are significantly associated with moral reasoning in early adolescence (e.g., Bukowski & Sippola, 1996; Schonert-Reichl, 1999; Simmons & Blythe, 1987; Singer, 1999). Around middle school age, adolescents begin to select their peers by interest, rather than by convenience (Carlo et al., 1999); thus, children's worlds expand beyond their families to include peer relationships. As Simmons and Blythe (1987) suggest, these new, self-selected relationships play an important part in the development of self-esteem in children.

Singer's work (Singer, 1999), consistent with Kohlberg's (Kohlberg, 1969) perspective that peer relationships drive the development of moral philosophy in adolescents, explores the effects of "scope of justice" and "moral intensity" on adolescents' moral judgments. To better appreciate Singer's perspective, a number of terms need clarification. "Scope of justice" refers to a person's extent of justice concerns for another person. "Justice" refers to judgments of fairness, which may be influenced by such factors as friendship and a sense of concern for other. "Moral intensity" refers to a collection of components including the magnitude of the consequence of a moral act, the social consensus around the ethicality of the moral act, the likelihood that the moral act will occur, and the effect of the moral act on its target (Jones, 1991).

Key to stage development theory is the idea that moral reasoning is a function of intellect and cognition. Also foundational is the idea that the ultimate principle of morality is justice. For Kohlberg, justice entails "the reciprocity and equality of human rights, and of the respect for the dignity of human beings as individuals" (Kohlberg, 1981, p. 19). However, we note that these ideas were challenged by Gilligan (1982), who asserted that there is an alternative affective perspective to morality, care for and relationships with others. This affective component of moral reasoning is congruent with the idea of scope of justice; that is, the ethicality of judgments made by adolescents is likely to be influenced by their relationships with, or sense of concern for, others (Singer, 1999).

Additionally, most models of moral reasoning focus on the moral agent, or on the moral climate in which an ethical decision is made. The term "moral climate" refers to the set of moral values held by the dominant group within the social environment of the moral agent. These may, or may not, reflect universal values. The idea of moral intensity instead considers the moral issue itself. Testing adolescents for both scope of justice and moral intensity components, Singer (1999) found a difference between the responses of female and male adolescents. On the one hand, female adolescents tended to respond according to their extent of care for the person(s) involved in a moral dilemma in moral issues of benign consequence. However, in moral issues of harmful consequence, female respondents tended to shift to a justice perspective (Singer, 1999).

On the other hand, male adolescents rarely considered affective components in their ethicality judgments. They tended to regard morally questionable decisions with benign consequences as unethical, and morally questionable decisions with harmful consequences as more unethical (Singer, 1999). These results seem to suggest that adolescents tend to use a justice perspective in their ethicality judgments. These results also seem to agree with Kohlberg' contention that ethicality judgments in adolescents are a function of intellect and cognition, and that justice is a foundational theme in moral reasoning.

These ideas about the importance of cognition and intellect in adolescents' ethical judgment making run counter to much of the literature already considered about the development of moral reasoning in children through their primary socialization. That literature tended either to expand Kohlberg's perspective to include affective components such as care for others and relationships with others (e.g., Walker, 1999) or to reject Kohlberg's perspective altogether (e.g., Gilligan, 1982). Those rejecting Kohlberg's arguments tended to focus primarily on components such as care for others and relationships with others. The work by Gilligan (1982) is an example, and this care perspective on morality contrasts with the justice perspective, with its emphasis on rights and autonomy (Singer, 1999).

Consideration of this care–justice distinction may prove useful in understanding the development of moral reasoning in children. Children begin by first being influenced by the affective relationships with their primary caregivers. That influence expands as children mature to include components of intellect and cognition. By adolescence, children face an environment that expands beyond their families to include growing networks of peer relationships. As adolescents interact with peers, their opportunities for learning prosocial behaviors arise through role taking within those peer relationships. For example, by interacting within a peer network of friends who earn good grades in school, participate in extracurricular activities, and are less likely to engage in problematic behavior, adolescents may learn prosocial behaviors through those interactions. As Bukowski and Sippola (1996) suggest, when demonstrated to peers, prosocial behaviors are often reinforced by peer responses, developing a cycle of prosocial behavior among them. Further, this cycle is more likely to develop in peer relationships than among relationships between children and adults, probably because the social associations among peers are more equal in terms of power and influence, and thus distinct from the relationships between children and adults (Bukowski & Sippola, 1996).

In view of Kohlberg's and Piaget's work, Schonert-Reichl (1999) developed the assumption that social interactions play a central role in the development of more complex moral reasoning. In such interactions individuals have the opportunity to consider perceptions different from their own, and possibly to integrate such perspectives as they work to resolve their moral conflicts. Working to systematically address the dearth of research on peer interactions associated with moral development, Schonert-Reichl (1999) investigated the relations between moral reasoning and six dimensions of peer relationships. These six dimensions of peer relationships are peer acceptance, leadership status, friendship participation, friendship quality, peer assessments of social behavior, and friendship activity participation.

Peer acceptance is an assessment of a child's level of acceptance by their peers. Leadership status is an assessment of a child's peers' affinity to having that child in charge. Friendship participation assesses the number of friendship relationships a child has and, of those, which are better, and best, friends. Friendship quality assesses qualitative components of friendship such as caring, conflict resolution, betrayal, help, companionship, and intimate exchange. Peer assessments of social behavior include such components as prosocial behaviors (cooperation, trust), antisocial behaviors (fighting, group disruption, backbiting), and withdrawn behavior (shyness, easily pushed around). Friendship activities assess what children do when spending time with their friends (Schonert-Reichl, 1999).

Colby and Kohlberg (1987) compared responses to these assessments with assessments of moral reasoning based upon Kohlberg's Moral Judgment Interview. Schonert-Reichl's findings lend support to Kohlberg's assertion that peer relationships and interactions are associated with moral development. Children with a greater number of close friends scored higher in moral reasoning than those with fewer close friends (Schonert-Reichl, 1999). Similarly, children who were considered leaders by their peers also tended to score higher in moral reasoning (Schonert-Reichl, 1999). The results of the study suggest that peer relationships in early adolescence are significantly associated with moral reasoning.

What may be of particular value to this study are Schonert-Reichl's findings regarding the association between friendship quality and moral reasoning. Prosocial behaviors were associated significantly and positively with moral reasoning in the girls studied. However, both prosocial and antisocial behaviors were associated positively and significantly with moral reasoning in the boys studied. That antisocial behavior would be associated with moral reasoning is inconsistent with many previous studies that suggest a negative association between moral reasoning and antisocial behaviors (Schonert-Reichl, 1999). While previous studies used teacher assessments of antisocial behavior, Schonert-Reichl used peer nominations to gather data about antisocial behaviors. Further, it is possible that boys sometimes place a positive value on antisocial behavior. It could be that some boys view aggression as a way of obtaining social goals (Crick & Dodge, 1996; cf. Phoenix et al., 2003). Dodge and Coie (1987) suggest that there are two forms of aggressive behavior. One form, proactive aggression, is viewed by children as more positive than the second form, reactive aggression. The other form, reactive aggression, is hostile, and viewed more negatively by children.

Also noteworthy, of the children studied by Schonert-Reichl (1999), those perceived by peers to be socially withdrawn tended to measure lower in moral reasoning. In essence, children who are socially unassertive, who do not participate in high levels of social interaction, and who avoid confrontation may not acquire the necessary peer interaction that leads to moral growth. For Kohlberg (1969), "cognitive disequilibria" are those challenges that children experience as they interact with peers. Moreover, they serve as important components in the development of moral reasoning. Children who are rejected by the social hierarchy have fewer social interactions. Thus, they experience fewer opportunities for cognitive disequilibria (Schonert-Reichl, 1999). Hence, children withdrawn from, or rejected by, their peers have fewer opportunities for cognitive disequilibria, and as a result develop their moral reasoning faculties more slowly. This has important implications because those deprived of positive peer group socialization may rebel against or even reject socially accepted mores, values, and ethical systems. This was the case with the majority of the mass school shooters of the past two decades. As Lanata (2003) explains,

> Too often, the shooters were either "loners" or were involved in "outcast groups." Kroth, the group with which Luke Woodham was reportedly associated, immersed itself in a fantasy game very similar to "Dungeons and Dragons." A member of the group reportedly encouraged Woodham to torture and murder his family dog. Klebold and Harris [the Columbine shooters] had a negative impact on one another. ... They threatened classmates, criticized other groups, wore "Serial Killer" T-shirts and spent more than a year together planning the deadly assault at Columbine. (Lanata, 2003, p. 23; cf. Cullen, 2004)

In essence, as adolescents interact with peers, their opportunities for learning prosocial behaviors arise through role taking within those peer relationships. And as suggested earlier, prosocial behaviors, when demonstrated to peers, are often reinforced by peer responses, developing a cycle of prosocial behavior among them (cf. Bukowski & Sippola, 1996; Carlo et al., 1999).

Moreover, Schonert-Reichl (1999) reports that children with greater numbers of close friends exhibit a more developed sense of moral reasoning than do those with fewer close friends. Of the children in this study, those perceived by peers to be socially withdrawn tended to measure lower in moral reasoning. Children who are socially unassertive, who do not participate in high levels of social interaction, and who avoid confrontation may not acquire the necessary peer interaction that leads to moral growth. Children who are rejected by the social hierarchy often have fewer social interactions, resulting in fewer opportunities for cognitive disequilibria (Schonert-Reichl, 1999), that is, challenges that children encounter as they interact with peers, and are important components in the development of moral reasoning (see Kohlberg, 1969). Thus, children withdrawn from or rejected by peers have fewer opportunities for cognitive disequilibria, and as a result they seem likely to develop moral reasoning more slowly.

Personhood, Power, and Violent Behavior

At about four years of age, children begin to understand themselves as beings with extended selves. However, it is not until adolescence that human beings begin to think abstractly about their lives. Indeed, during adolescence, humans begin to construct narrative interpretations of their lives, only to continually revise and extend those narratives (McAdams, 1990). Similarly, it is during this time that humans begin to align themselves with the social identities available within their culture (Barresi, 1999). So long as the self-narratives adolescents devise are congruent with their society's predominant narratives, they are likely to receive positive social recognition. If self-constructed narratives are not congruent with the predominant narratives in their society, social identity, and even personhood, may not be recognized (Barresi, 1999).

For May (1972), however, personhood exists in relationship with personal power, so the issue of the exercise of personal power must be considered as well. May (1972) argues that there are five levels of power present as potentialities in every person's life: the power to be, self-affirmation, self-assertion, aggression, and violence. The power to be is given in the act of birth. This power is neither good nor evil. Neither is it neutral; it must be lived out. That is, power is active; for power to be neutral is for power to not exist. According to May (1972), for a person to exist is for that person to have power at some level. At the level of self-affirmation, the person's state of being must be affirmed. Questions of significance emerge from the quest for affirmation. Self-esteem or substitutes for it must be sought. Self-assertion occurs when self-affirmation meets resistance. This is a more overt form of self-affirmation, which demands attention. Aggression is yet a stronger form of self-assertion, which occurs when self-assertion has been blocked for a long time. Aggression moves beyond the person's own assertion or affirmation and enters the territory of others and demands power for the self. Violence occurs when aggressive efforts toward self-assertion are ineffective (May, 1972). If the other phases of behavior are blocked, then explosion into violence may be the only way that individuals or groups can find release from unbearable tension and achieve a sense of significance (May, 1972).

In cases where individuals are not afforded "normal" personhood by means of outside affirmation on a regular basis, it follows that their behavior may deviate from that considered normal by others. When individuals are placed in situations where a sense of personal significance is almost impossible to achieve, or worse, where open ridicule and humiliation are their "norm," their only release from the tension of continually blocked behavior and their need to achieve that sense of significance may lead to violence (see Klein, 1991; May, 1972; cf. Newman, et al., 2004).

In social groups, "when individuals find themselves participating in inequitable relationships, they become distressed. The more inequitable the relationship, the more distress individuals feel" (Deutsch, 1985, p. 15). Consequently, a person who perceives himself/herself to be a victim of injustice because of some deprivation will likely experience some degree of anger and express that anger toward others who caused or profited from the injustice.

The views and actions of Harris and Klebold, the Columbine High School shooters, support this principle. One of their classmates described the social climate at Columbine High School: "Columbine is a clean and good place except for those rejects [referring to Harris and Klebold and their friends]. Most students didn't want them there" (quoted in Gibbs & Roche, 1999, p. 50). Stancato (2003) suggests that this social estrangement left these young men alone in a quest to find meaning in a world that had rejected them. They turned to the "Trench coat Mafia" for that meaning, and the cult of Nazi values that group embraced. In so doing, they found further estrangement from their larger social world.

Gibbs and Roche (1999), in a *Time* magazine article, quoted Harris and Klebold from actual tapes reportedly made shortly before the massacre. They are reported to have said, "Isn't it going to be fun to get the respect we are going to deserve?" (Gibbs & Roche, 1999, p. 44). That they reportedly expected that violence and death would bring them respect illustrates the point here that a loss of personhood through social estrangement may lead to a violent attempt to find it.

At this point the issue of bullying must be addressed. School violence literature is replete with studies about bullying and its effect on the bullies and the bullied (e.g., Bullock, 2002; Galloway, 1994; Olweus, 1991, 1993). Clearly, bullying is a significant issue in the study of everyday school violence and is well documented. Nevertheless, we challenge the notion that school shootings occur as a direct result of bullying. We suggest that bullying certainly leads to hurt feelings, and sometimes violent responses, but mass school shootings are much more complex. We contend that the loss of personhood and the search for power that contribute to heinous violence and death are separate issues from bullying. Indeed, the experts at the FBI's Behavioral Science Unit acknowledge that bullying appeared to play a role in the lives of some, but not all, mass school shooters (Lanata, 2003). Accordingly, bullying may be a factor in mass school shootings, but it is neither necessary nor sufficient to explain them.

Competition, Cliques, and the School Environment

School environments and school curricula may facilitate higher incidences of violence if insufficient attention is paid to the zero-sum logic—and its corresponding dog-eat-dog worldview—communicated by many aspects of the school environment in the USA today and to the development of personal moral philosophy and interpersonal relationships learning (Stephens, 1995). Messerschmidt

(1993) contends that today's school environment emphasizes sports and academic success. Too often this environment encourages competition and fosters a sense of shame in losing. Similarly, this emphasis on the culture of sport success in US schools subordinates other interests that many not athletically inclined gravitate toward, for example, band, chorus, debate, and intellectual achievement (Kessler et al., 1985).

As a specific example, consider institutions as innocuous as junior high school and high school team sports such as football, basketball, and baseball (Johnson et al., 2001). Many contend that increasing competition, to the point of parents fighting among themselves at games, undercuts values such as cooperation (Riesman, 1954; cf. Sage, 1978; Staffo, 2001); and others have gone further, pointing to the connections between the sports and war metaphors (Shapiro, 1989).

Keep in mind that social interactions are self-perpetuating, Deutsch (1985) argues that modes of interaction breed themselves. Moreover, he suggests that competition is not natural, but learned. Persons are socialized to compete, and too often, the result is considered evidence of the inevitability of competition (Kohn, 1986). Likewise, cooperation, too, is learned. Competition will induce a vicious spiral of intensifying competition while cooperation will induce a spiral of increasing cooperation (Kohn, 1986). We contend that people have the capacity to be competitive and/or cooperative, but that these qualities are shaped by environmental and social factors. Further, we hold that learning to be more cooperative is a greater benefit to society than is learning to be more competitive or more individualistic (cf. Kohn, 1986).

Moreover, Kohn argues that competition generalizes. What is learned in one context is not confined there. As competition spreads to other contexts and assumes other forms, so too does aggression (Kohn, 1986). There is good evidence of a causal link between competition and aggression. Theorists propose that competition generates a high level of arousal; hence individuals are predisposed to respond with aggression if frustrated by some action or behavior. If this theory is correct, it would go a long way toward explaining why many individuals who lose may become aggressive (Kohn, 1986).

As children grow and interact they learn from their interactions. School curricula can include components that assist children with their understanding of the consequences of their interactions and relationships, leading to occurrences of peace, rather than violence. Indeed, as Klein (1992) explains, our schools are

> age-graded educational systems in which children and teachers have little choice of whether or not they work with one another and where the vast majority of students—those who aren't smart enough or adequately prepared—must live with the humiliating possibility of being treated as... failures. These systems are put together in such a way as to ensure the humiliation of repeated failure on the part of so-called disadvantaged children. (p. 265)

Accordingly, we argue that a school's internal environment, especially its dominant culture and subculture dynamics, is among the factors to consider in unraveling mass school shootings. Indeed, Garrick-Duhaney (2000) suggests that cultural factors are not given their due by persons responsible for formulating violence prevention programs. More specifically, she recommends that schools should focus on the cultural diversity of their students since heterogeneity is often a source of conflict, and sometimes a contributing factor to violence.

We contend that Garrick-Duhaney's (Garrick-Duhaney 2000) insights are applicable to the predominantly White suburban and rural schools where mass school shootings have historically occurred even though her work specifically addresses heterogeneous school environments. We do so because cultures, subcultures, and cliques that develop in such schools may be as real and as divisive for students as those relationships across race and ethnicity in the larger society. When larger ethnic issues such as skin color or national origin are absent, issues of subcultural identification may become more important (cf. Eckert, 1989). In such situations, diversity may include socioeconomic factors such as social class and family prestige, and include subcultural identities based on gender, religion, philosophy, academics, sports, avocation, or fashion. To the students interacting in such environments, the diversities present are their ecological reality. For example, consider the preliminary responses to a nationwide survey of students and teachers conducted by Teaching Tolerance. Early responses revealed that

- Of the first 1,000 students, 53% described their schools as quick to put people in categories;
- According to the students, the top three factors that create group boundaries at school are style (60 percent), athletic achievement (53 percent) and appearance (52 percent); the students cited race and ethnicity at 25 percent and 18 percent respectively;
- When asked about crossing boundaries, students rated those of appearance (17 percent) and style (16 percent) as the most difficult to get over. (Carnes, 2003, p. 3)

Implications and Recommendations

We suggest that what may begin as a deficiency in ethical development during primary socialization by parents and guardians may later be exacerbated by peers. Further, children who do not assert themselves socially, who do not participate in many social interactions, and who avoid confrontation may compound this early deficiency by failing to acquire the necessary peer interaction that leads to moral growth. Moreover, recall that cognitive disequilibria (see Kohlberg, 1969) are the challenges that children encounter as they interact with peers and are important components in the development of moral reasoning. Children who are rejected by the social hierarchy have fewer social interactions, resulting in fewer opportunities for cognitive disequilibria (Schonert-Reichl, 1999). In such instances, children with ethical deficiencies will make interpretations about their interactions with peers based on less complete data than their peers. That is, such children may not have developed the breadth of knowledge available to children with greater experience. Their behavioral responses will likely reveal their deficiencies to their peers, resulting in inequities in their relationships, thus eliciting ecological reactions (Walker, 2000). These ecological reactions may be interpreted as fair, or unfair, resulting in either mild tendencies towards conformity or further deviant behavior and marginalization. This process may spiral into power inequities and the marginalization of the less powerful; for example, they may be bullied and/or ostracized. Children on the unfortunate end of this spiral eventually find themselves ethically deficient, relatively powerless, and transitioning to secondary school, a place and time of great anxiety (Elias et al., 1985) where esteem and significance, too often, are awarded to those who best demonstrate the normal values of society—recall the comments of the Columbine shooters and their classmate reported earlier. Hence, such children are ill prepared to deal with the stress and potential humiliation of secondary school; and they may lash out in horrific ways like mass school shootings. This series of events/circumstances may be presented in the form of a partial model of mass school shootings (see Fig. 6.1).

Given this possibility, a more holistic, and hence, a possibly more effective, approach to school shootings would entail addressing the variables outlined above. Specifically, this approach would involve a constellation of interventions directed at the family, at peer relationships, at improving self-esteem, at bullying, and at reducing conflict and competition in schools. Specifically, we highlight the need for further research, and we consider some general approaches and specific primary prevention efforts related to family and parenting skills, and to competition and conflict reduction in schools.

Further Research

As presented here, the premises of our argument have followed an intensifying progression, describing a number of contributing factors that, when occurring in sequence, may result in mass school shootings. Our review of information on mass school shooters (see Gibbs & Roche, 1999; Lanata, 2003; Nicoletti et al., 1999; Stancato, 2003; Zinna, 1999) suggests that our model is accurate. Nevertheless, our review focused primarily on others' analyses of primary data. Thus, we believe that further review of our model in light of primary data seems appropriate. For example, as transcripts of interviews with surviving shooters (or would-be shooters), parents, teachers, counselors, and classmates of school shooters, personal diaries, and video recordings become available, these might be reviewed with an eye toward evaluating the contributing factors we emphasize, their sequence, etc.

Still, on the basis of our analysis and review of the literature, we are confident that programs designed to promote parenting styles and approaches conducive to the development of a sound moral philosophy among children would lessen the chance of future acts of extraordinary school violence. We are also confident that promoting parenting styles that improve the development of a sound moral philosophy in children would lessen incidents of more common forms of school violence such as bullying, theft, and vandalism. In other words, children whose behavior is informed by a sense of concern for others will extend that concern to their interpersonal relationships at all levels, reducing their likelihood of behaving in domineering, oppressive, or vengeful ways.

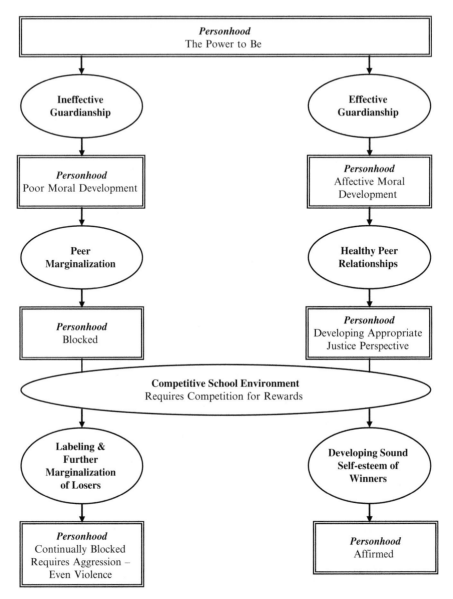

Fig. 6.1 A partial model of moral development. The purpose of this model is to contrast ideal types of the extremes of moral development. Most children develop somewhere in between these extremes, with varying degrees of result—some whose personhood is more or less affirmed, and some whose personhood is more or less blocked, requiring personal assertiveness in pursuit of esteem. We contend that children who become school shooters progress along a path closer to the ideal type on the left of our model, where personhood is continually blocked and the opportunities to develop the ability to deal with real relationships continually withheld until violent aggression is the last perceived recourse

Similarly, our work suggests that programs designed to lessen the competitive nature of schools generally have potential to preempt further acts of extraordinary school violence. Just as, we suspect, the patterns of behavior leading to violence may be changed by raising children's concern for the welfare of others, we are confident that the potential for violence at school, ordinary and extraordinary, could be further reduced by lowering levels of competition in schools. While the competition one might engage in as a personal challenge to perform better does not perpetuate a winner versus loser mentality, there is good evidence of a causal link between competition and aggression (May, 1937). Theorists such as Deutsch (1985) and May (1972) propose that competition generates a high level of arousal, and that an emphasis on competition may predispose participants to respond with aggression if frustrated by some action or behavior, such as losing (for more detailed discussion, see Thompson & Kyle, 2005).

Conclusion

Extraordinary incidents of mass murder and mass murder-suicide at school require extraordinary understanding and intervention. National news media attention on these incidents has blurred the issue, resulting in programs and policies that too often attempt only to further insulate schools from their environments. Lacking is consideration of those ideas that may reveal and resolve the reasons for mass murder committed by students. Those ideas lie in behavioral sciences literature about the development of a personal moral philosophy, and prosocial behavior in adolescents, and the struggle for power and significance in highly competitive suburban and some rural school environments.

Each of the premises of the argument presented here centers around a psychological or social issue that, when taken together with the others, may be understood as a contributing factor to incidents of extraordinary violence. Each of the psychological and social issues presented as premises of this argument, when taken alone, may simply lead to maladjusted adolescents, and probably not to school shootings. More simply, many children are raised in home environments that are not conducive to the development of a sound, personal moral philosophy; however, most of these children do not become school shooters. Likewise, many children are rejected and/ or bullied by their peers, but their marginalization alone probably does not lead to school shootings. Nevertheless, we have developed an argument exploring possible contributing factors to the phenomenon of school shootings. The premises of this argument follow an intensifying progression, in that each newly presented premise builds upon the former premise resulting in a sequence of contributing factors that, when taken together, may lead to extraordinarily violent behavior.

The essence of the argument is that children will develop at different rates and to different levels depending upon the particular influences of their developmental processes. Among the population of adolescents may be children who have developed a propensity for violence. That propensity for violence may result in the manifestation of violence as the opportunities for it occur. The best opportunity for controlling violence, then, may be to control the environments where the propensity for violence might be brought to fruition. Among such environments is the school environment. Zero tolerance policies and fortifications are attempts by schools to control the school environment for actual outbreaks of violence. The distinction proposed here is to control the school environment in such a way that the predilection for violence is abated.

This review further suggests that children who are not enabled to develop a strong personal system of ethics at home and who fail to develop significant relationships among their peers enter secondary school in need of a low-intensity, cooperative environment where they might work on building relationships conducive to moral development. If, instead, these students are subjected to a highly competitive school environment in which esteem is awarded to those most in compliance with societal expectations, and withheld from those least compliant, they may seek aggressive, and perhaps violent, means to achieve recognition and a sense of significance.

An important point must be reinforced here, that most children do not become school shooters. Table 6.1 demonstrates that despite the heinousness of these acts and the resulting attention because of it, they remain relatively few in number. Is the value of this discussion, then, limited to policies and procedures designed to address extraordinarily rare potentialities? We think not. We would suggest that while most children may not become mass murderers, many suffer at the hands of negligent parenting and are ill prepared for the labeling and marginalization that may come at the hands of their peers as they approach and enter adolescence. The very steps taken to abate the development of school shooters in extreme cases may also be quite useful for abating the suffering of many more children that would be otherwise marginalized.

References

Austin, V. L. (2003). Fear and loathing in the classroom: A candid look at school violence and the policies and practices that address it. *Journal of Disability Policy Studies*, 14, 17–22.

Barresi, J. (1999). On becoming a person. *Philosophical Psychology*, 12(1), 79–98.

Berger, R. R. (2002). Expansion of police power in public schools and the vanishing rights of students. *Social Justice*, 29, 119–130.

Brunner, J. & Lewis, D. (2006). Safety tips for principals: How to assess and respond to student threats. *Principal Leadership*, 7(2), 65–66.

Bukowski, W. M. & Sippola, L. K. (1996). Friendship and morality. In W. M. Bukowski & A. F. Newcomb (Eds.), *The Company They Keep: Friendship in Childhood and Adolescence* (pp. 238–261). Cambridge: Cambridge University Press.

Bullock, J. R. (2002). Bullying among children. *Childhood Education*, 78(3), 130–133.

Carlo, G., Fabes, R. A., Laible, D., & Kupanoff, K. (1999). Early adolescence and prosocial/moral behavior II: The role of social and contextual influences. *The Journal of Early Adolescence*, 19(2), 133–147.

Carnes, J. (2003). Editor's note: What if? *Teaching Tolerance*, 23(Spring), 3.

Cirillo, K. J., Pruitt, B. E., Colwell, B., Kingery, P. M., Hurley, R. S., & Ballard, D. (1998). School violence: Prevalence and intervention strategies for at-risk adolescents. *Adolescence*, 33, 319–330.

Claypoole, S. D., Moody, E. E., Jr., & Peace, S. D. (2000). Moral dilemma discussions: An effective group intervention for juvenile offenders. *Journal for Specialists in Group Work*, 25(4), 394–411.

CNN.com (2001). Are U.S. schools safe? In-depth Specials. Available online: *http://www.cnn.com/SPECIALS/1998/schools/* Downloaded December 2, 2006.

Colby, A. & Kohlberg, L. (1987). *The Measurement of Moral Judgment, Vol: Theoretical Foundations and Research Validation.* New York: Cambridge University Press.

Coleman, L. (2004). *The Copycat Effect: How the Media and Popular Culture Trigger the Mayhem in Tomorrow's Headlines.* New York: Paraview Pocket Books.

Crick, N. R. & Dodge, K. A. (1996). Social information-processing mechanisms in reactive and proactive aggression. *Child Development*, 67, 993–1002.

Cullen, D. (2004). The depressive and the psychotic: At last we know why the Columbine killers did it. Slate. Available online: *http://www.slate.com/id/2099203/* Downloaded December 2, 2006.

Danitz, T. (2000). Bullying contributes to school shootings, report says. Stateline.org. Available online: http://www.stateline.org/live/ViewPage.action?siteNodeId=136&languageID=1& content Id=14154 Downloaded December 5, 2006.

Dedman, B. (2000). Deadly lessons—school shooters: Secret Service findings. Chicago Sun-Times. Available online: *http://www.knowgangs.com/school_resources/deadlylessons.pdf* Downloaded December 2, 2006.

Deutsch, M. (1985). *Distributive Justice: A Social-Psychological Perspective.* New Haven: Yale University Press.

Dodge, K. A. & Coie, J. D. (1987). Social information-processing factors in reactive and proactive aggression in children's playgroups. *Journal of Personality and Social Psychology*, 53, 1146–1158.

Donohue, E., Schiraldi, V., & Zeidenberg, J. (1998). *Schoolhouse Hype: School Shootings, and the Real Risks Kids Face in America.* Washington, DC: Justice Policy Institute. Available online: *http://www.cjcj.org/pubs/shooting/shootings.html* Downloaded December 2, 2006.

Dunne, D. W. (2000). Are our children safe in school? Education World (March 6, 2000). Available online: *http://www.education-world.com/a_issues/issues071.shtml* Downloaded December 2, 2006.

Eckert, P. (1989). *Jocks and Burnouts: Social Categories and Identity in the High School.* New York: Teacher College Press.

Ehrlich, H. J. (1999). The Columbine high school shootings: The lessons learned. *Social Anarchism*, 27. Available online: *http://library.nothingness.org/articles/SA/en/display/336* Downloaded December 2, 2006.

Eisenberg, N. & Murphy, B. (1995). Parenting and children's moral development. In M. H. Bernstein (Ed.), *Handbook of Parenting: Applied and Practical Parenting* Vol. 4 (pp. 227–257). Mahwah, NJ: Lawrence Erlbaum.

Elias, M. J., Gara, M., & Ubriaco, M. (1985). Sources of stress and support in children's transition to middle school: An empirical analysis. *Journal of Clinical Child Psychology*, 14, 112–118.

Fabes, R. A. (1999). Early adolescence and prosocial/moral behavior I: The role of individual processes. *The Journal of Early Adolescence*, 19, 5–16.

Fox, C. & Harding, D. J. (2005). School shootings as organizational deviance. *Sociology of Education*, 78(1), 69–97.

Furlong, M. & Morrison, G. (2000). The school in school violence: Definitions and facts. *Journal of Emotional and Behavioral Disorders*, 8(2), 71–82.

Galloway, D. (1994). Bullying: The importance of a whole school approach. *Therapeutic Care and Education*, 3, 315–329.

Garrick-Duhaney, L. M. (2000). Culturally sensitive strategies for violence prevention. *Multicultural Education*, 7(4), 10–17.

Gibbs, N. & Roche, T. (1999). The Columbine tapes. *Time*, 154, 40–51.

Gibbs, N. (2001). It's only me. *Time*, 157. Available online http://www.time.com/time/magazine/ article/0,9171,1101010319-102025,00.html Downloaded January 2, 2008.

Gilligan, C. (1982). *In a Different Voice. Psychological Theory and Women's Development.* Cambridge, MA: Harvard University Press.

Goetting, A. (1994). The parent-crime connection. *The Journal of Primary Prevention*, 14, 169–186.

Hancock, L. (2001). The school shootings: Why context counts. *Columbia Journalism Review*, 40, 76–77.

Hart, D., Atkins, R., & Ford, D. (1999). Family influences on the formation of moral identity in adolescence: Longitudinal analyses. *Journal of Moral Education*, 28, 375–386.

Infoplease. (2006). A time line of recent worldwide school shootings. © 2000–2006 Pearson Education, publishing as Infoplease. 02, December 2006.<http://www.infoplease.com/ipa/ A0777958.html>.

Jahnkow, R. (2001). School violence: A result of 'bad parenting' or militarism. *San Diego Independent Media Center.* Available online: http://www.sandiego.indymedia.org/en/2002/01/336.shtml Downloaded January 2, 2008.

Jones, T.M. (1991). Ethical decision making by indviduals in organizations: An issue-contingent model. *Academy of Management Review,* 16, 366–395.

Johnson, D. A., Giler, J. I., Kneeland, W., & Crawford, S. A. (2001). In the hope of reducing violence, should schools require spectator silence at interscholastic sport competitions? *Journal of Physical Education, Recreation & Dance*, 72(3), 16–17.

Kessler, S., Ashenden, D. J., Connell, R. W., & Dowsett, G. W. (1985). Gender relations in secondary schooling. *Sociology of Education*, 58(1), 34–48.

Kimmel, M. S. & Mahler, M. (2003). Adolescent masculinity, homophobia, and violence. *American Behavioral Scientist*, 46, 1439–1458.

Klein, D. C. (1991). The humiliation dynamic: An overview. *The Journal of Primary Prevention*, 12, 93–121.

Klein, D. C. (1992). Managing humiliation. *The Journal of Primary Prevention*, 12, 255–268.

Kohlberg, L. (1969). Stage and sequence: The cognitive-developmental approach to socialization. In D. Goslin (Ed.), *Handbook of Socialization Theory and Research* (pp. 347–480). Chicago: Rand McNally.

Kohlberg, L. (1981). *The Philosophy of Moral Development: Moral Stages and the Idea of Justice.* San Francisco: Harper and Row.

Kohn, A. (1986). *No contest: The Case Against Competition.* Boston: Houghton Mifflin Company.

Kyle, K. (2001). The use and 'abuse' of family in policy matters. *Sociological Practice: A Journal of Clinical and Applied Sociology*, 3, 205–219.

Lakoff, G. (2002). *Moral Politics: How Liberals and Conservatives Think*, 2nd edition. Chicago: University of Chicago Press.

Lanata, J. C. (2003). Behind the scenes: A closer look at the school shooters. *Sheriff*, 55(Mar/Apr), 22–26.

Lawrence, R. G. & Birkland, T. A. (2004). Guns, Hollywood, and school safety: Defining the school-shooting problem across public arenas. *Social Science Quarterly*, 85, 1193–1207.

Leone, P. E., Mayer, M. J., Malmgren, K.,& Meisel, S. M. (2000). School violence and disruption: Rhetoric, reality, and reasonable balance. *Focus On Exceptional Children*, 33, 1–23.

Martinson, D. L. (2000). A school responds to controversial student speech: Serious questions in light of Columbine. *The Clearing House*, 73, 145–149.

Metcalf, G. (2001). The dope made me do it. Worldnetdaily.com. Available online: http:www. worldnet.com/news/articles.asp?ARTICLE_ID=21250 Downloaded December 9, 2006.

May, M. (1937). A research note on cooperative and competitive behavior. *American Journal of Sociology*, 42, 887–891.

May, R. (1972). *Power and Innocence: A Search for the Sources of Violence*. New York: W.W. Norton and Company, Inc.

McAdams, D. P. (1990). Unity and purpose in human lives: The emergence of identity as a life story. In A. I. Rabin, R. A. Zucker, R. A. Emmons, & S. Frank (Eds.), *Studying Persons and Lives* (pp. 148–200). New York: Springer.

McCollum, S. (2004). Zero tolerance: Safer schools or unfair rules? *Literary Cavalcade*, 57, 20–21.

McKenna, M. & Haselkorn, D. (2005). NCLB and the lessons of Columbine. *USA Today*, 133(May 2005), 20–22.

Messerschmidt, J. W. (1993). *Masculinities and Crime: Critique and Reconceptualization of Theory*. Lanham, MD: Rowman & Littlefield Publishers, Inc.

Moore, M. (2003). Bowling for Columbine. Metro? Goldwyn? Mayer studio. *The National School Safety Center*. *http://www.nsscl.org* Downloaded April 4, 2004.

National School Safety Center. (2004). *National School Safety Center^{TM}*, Available online: http://www.nsscl.org Downloaded January 2, 2008.

Newman, K. S., Fox, C., Harding, D., Mehta, J., & Roth, W. (2004). *Rampage: The Social Roots of School Shootings*. New York: Basic Books.

Nicoletti, J., Zinna, K., & Spencer-Thomas, S. (1999). *Violence goes to School: Lessons Learned from Columbine*. Lakewood, CO: Nicoletti-Flater Associates.

North, D. (1999). The Columbine High School massacre: American pastoral… American beserk. World Socialist Web Site. Available online: http://www.wsws.org/articles/1999/apr1999/colo-a27.shtml. Downloaded January 2, 2008.

North, D. (1999). The Columbine High School massacre: American pastoral... American beserk. *World Socialist Web Site*. Available online: http://www.wsws.org/articles/1999/apr1999/colo-a27.shtml.Downloaded January 2, 2008.

Nucci, L. (2002). Because it is the right thing to do. *Human Development*, 45(2), 125–129.

Olweus, D. (1991). Bully/victim problems among school children: Basic facts and effects of a school-based intervention program. In K. Rubin & D. Pepler (Eds.), *The Development and Treatment of Childhood Aggression* (pp. 411–488). Hillsdale, NJ: Lawrence Erlbaum.

Olweus, D. (1993). *Bullying at School: What we Know and What we Can Do*. Cambridge: Blackwell.

Palermo, G. B. (1999). Mass murder, suicide, and moral development: Can we separate the adults from the juveniles? *International Journal of Offender Therapy and Comparative Criminology*, 43(1), 8–20.

Phoenix, A., Frosh, S., & Pattman, R. (2003). Producing contradictory masculine subject positions: Narratives of threat, homophobia, and bullying in 11–14 year old boys. *Journal of Social Issues*, 59, 179–195.

Plummer, D. (2001). Policing manhood: New theories about social significance of homophobia. In C. Wood (Ed.), Sexual Positions, An Australian View (pp. 60–75). Melbourne: Hill of Content.

Poteat, V. P. & Espelage, D. L. (2005). Exploring the relation between bullying and homophobic verbal content: The homophobic content agent target (HCAT) scale. *Violence and Victims*, 20(5), 513–528.

Pratt, M. W., Arnold, M. L., Pratt, A. T., & Diessner, R. (1999). Predicting adolescent moral reasoning from family climate: A longitudinal study. *The Journal of Early Adolescence*, 19, 148–175.

Riesman, D. (1954). Football in America: A study in cultural diffusion. In D. Riesman (Ed.), *Individualism Reconsidered and Other Essays* (pp. 242–257). Glencoe, IL: Free Press.

Robelen, E. W. (1999). National policymakers trying range of measures to stem school violence. *Educator Week*, 18, 19–20.

Sage, G. H. (1978). American values and sport: Formation of a bureaucratic personality. *Journal of Physical Education and Recreation* 49, 42–44.

Sanchez, C. (2004). Profile: School in Virginia prepared when 12-year-old student brought weapons to school. National Public Radio: Weekend edition (July 11, 2004).

Schonert-Reichl, K. A. (1999). Relations of peer acceptance, friendship adjustment, and social behavior to moral reasoning during early adolescence. *The Journal of Early Adolescence*, 19, 249–279.

Shapiro, M. J. (1989). Representing world politics: The sport/war intertext. In J. Derian & M. J. Shapiro (Eds.), *International/Intertextual Relations* (pp. 69–96). Lexington, MA: Lexington Books.

Sheley, J. F. & Wright, J. D. (1998). High school youths, weapons, and violence: A national survey. *National Institute of Justice*. Available online: http://72.14.203.104/search?q = cache:9ij4LhhYxrOJ:www.ncjrs.gov/pdffiles/172857.pdf + perception + school + violence + inner + city&hl = en&gl = us&ct = clnk&cd = 1 Downloaded December 2, 2006.

Simmons, R. G. & Blythe, D. A. (1987). *Moving into Adolescence: The Impact of Pubertal Change and School Context*. Hawthorn, NY: Aldine.

Singer, M. S. (1999). The role of concern for others and moral intensity in adolescent's ethicality judgments. *The Journal of Genetic Psychology*, 160, 155–166.

Smetana, J. G. (1995). Parenting styles and conceptions of parental authority during adolescence. *Child Development*, 66, 299–317.

Smetana, J. G. (1999). The role of parents in moral development: A social domain analysis. *Journal of Moral Education*, 28, 311–320.

Staffo, D. F. (2001). Strategies for reducing criminal violence among athletes. *Journal of Physical Education, Recreation & Dance*, 72(6), 38–42.

Stancato, F. (2003). The Columbine tragedy: Adolescent identity and future recommendations. *The Clearing House*, 77(1), 19.

Stephens, R. D. (1995). *Safe Schools: A Handbook for Violence Prevention*. Bloomington, IN: National Education Service.

Thomas, S. P. & Smith, H. (2004). School connectedness, anger behaviors, and relationships of violent and nonviolent American youth. *Perspectives in Psychiatric Care*, 40(4), 135–148.

Thompson, C., Barresi, J., & Moore, C. (1997). The development of future-oriented prudence and altruism in preschoolers. *Cognitive Development*, 12, 199–212.

Thompson, S. (2002). Perspectives on school shootings: Morality, competition, and the power to be. Unpublished Masters Thesis. Pennsylvania State Harrisburg.

Thompson, S. & Kyle, K. (2005). Understanding mass school shootings: Links between personhood and power in the competitive school environment. *Journal of Primary Prevention*, 26(5), 419–439.

Tisak, M. & Tisak, J. (1996). My sibling's but not my friend's keeper: Reasoning about responses to aggressive acts. *The Journal of Early Adolescence*, 16, 324–340.

Turiel, E. (1998). The development of morality. In W. Damon (Series Ed.) & N. Eisenberg (Vol. Ed.), *Handbook of Child Psychology: Social, Emotional, and Personality Development* Vol. 3 (5th edition, pp. 863–932). New York: John W. Wiley & Sons, Inc.

Vazsonyi, A. T. & Pickering, L. E. (2000). Family processes and deviance: A comparison of apprentices and nonapprentices. *Journal of Adolescent Research*, 15(3), 368–391.

Von Fremd, M. (2006). Students trained to fight school shooters. ABC News.com. Available online: http://articles.news.aol.com/news/_a/students-trained-to-fight-school/20061018103309990004?ncid = NWS00010000000001 Downloaded December 2, 2006.

Walker, L. J. (1999). The family context for moral development. *Journal of Moral Education*, 28, 261–264.

Walker, L. J. & Hennig, K. H. (1999). Parenting style and the development of moral reasoning. *Journal of Moral Education*, 28, 359–374.

Walker, J. S. (2000). Choosing biases, using power and practicing resistance: Moral development in a world without certainty. *Human Development*, 43, 135–156.

White, F. A. (2000). Relationship of family socialization processes to adolescent moral thought. *Journal of Social Psychology*, 140, 75–91.

Wise, T. (2001). School shootings and white denial. Alter.net. Available online: *http://www.alternet. org/story/10560/* Downloaded December 2, 2006.

Zinna, K. (1999). *After Columbine: A Schoolplace Violence Prevention Manual*. Silverhorne, CO: Spectra Publishing Co., Inc.

Chapter 7
Multiple Contextual Levels of Risk for Peer Victimization: A Review with Implications for Prevention and Intervention Efforts

Noel A. Card, Jenny Isaacs, and Ernest V. E. Hodges

Overview In this chapter we will discuss the importance of considering risk—and alternatively, protective—factors for peer victimization that occur at multiple levels of children's ecological context, with the goal that this review will be useful for both basic research and prevention and intervention efforts. We will begin by defining peer victimization and identifying several well-established personal characteristics that place children at greater or lesser risk for being the targets of their peers' aggression. However, the majority of our review of risk and protective factors will focus on features of the child's context, and we will separate these contextual influences into those occurring across five levels of Bronfenbrenner's ecological taxonomy. We will then discuss the implications of these ecological risk and protective factors for prevention and intervention efforts and review prior prevention and intervention studies that have considered multiple contextual levels. We will conclude that studies that have failed to consider higher levels of contextual risk factors have been less effective than is desired and will offer suggestions for considering these ecological factors in future empirical and applied work.

Introduction and Background

Defining Peer Victimization

Peer victimization refers to being the target of aggression by peers. Two aspect of this definition merit attention. First, aggressive behavior refers to acts that are intended to hurt another person (Parke & Slaby, 1983) and includes behaviors that are either direct (physical aggression such as hitting, verbal aggression such as taunting) or indirect (social or relational aggression such as excluding from groups or spreading gossip; see Archer & Coyne, 2005), as well as those whose primary goal is to obtain rewards (instrumental aggression) or those enacted in response to a perceived threat (reactive aggression; see Card & Little, 2006a). These behaviors also subsume behaviors defined as bullying (Olweus, 1978), a topic that has recently witnessed considerable popularization (e.g., Espelage & Swearer, 2004). Thus, aggressive behaviors consist of a fairly wide range of acts. However, individual differences in these behaviors tend to be highly correlated (for a meta-analytic review of intercorrelations between overt and relational forms, see Card et al., 2007; for a meta-analytic review of intercorrelations between instrumental and reactive forms, see Card & Little, 2006a), as are individual differences in tendencies to be victimized by these various forms (e.g., Crick & Bigbee, 1998; Crick & Grotpeter, 1996; Prinstein et al., 2001). Given the high overlap among these different aspects of aggression and victimization, we will generally consider peer victimization undifferentiated by form or function in this chapter.

A second aspect of our definition of peer victimization that merits mention is that it is directed toward the child by peers. Typically, this means youths of similar age to the victim (often in same grade) and, as typically measured in a closed setting (e.g., schools), usually implies others who are in a similar or overlapping ecological context as the child. The implication of this latter observation for the present review is that many of the same ecological factors that have been found to promote aggressive behavior will in turn also promote youths being victimized by their peers. Although important areas for research and prevention in their own right, we will not consider in this chapter victimization that children receive from parents or other adults, siblings, or from unspecified others in the community (e.g., neighborhood violence); several other overviews of these broader aspects of victimization are available (e.g., Finkelhor & Dziuba-Leatherman, 1994; Finkelhor et al., 2005).

Victims of peer aggression have only recently been a focus of attention relative to research on aggressors (see Ladd, 2005; Olweus, 2001; for an early, overlooked exception, see Burk, 1897). Empirical attention to peer victimization emerged with the work of Dan Olweus in Norway and Sweden during the 1970s (Olweus, 1978, 2001) but did not receive much attention in the United States until the work of David Perry and colleagues in the late 1980s (Perry et al., 1988). Since this time research on peer victimization has increased exponentially, and there now exist hundreds of studies on the topic (see Card, 2003). Importantly, research has also been conducted across a range of countries, and results converge to indicate that peer victimization is a common problem predictive of maladjustment across all countries studied (see Smith et al., 1999).

Individual Characteristics and Peer Victimization

Considerable attention has been devoted to understanding the individual characteristics that are associated with being victimized by peers. Because we have reviewed these individual characteristics associated with peer victimization elsewhere (Card, 2003; Card et al., 2007), we will only briefly review these findings. Specifically, we will briefly review evidence regarding relations of peer victimization with demographic characteristics, internalizing and externalizing problems, socially competent behavior, academic characteristics, and self-concept.

The results of numerous studies converge to suggest that boys are more victimized by peers than are girls, though this may differ somewhat by form, with this gender difference being higher when considering overt victimization and negligible when considering relational victimization (e.g., Crick & Grotpeter, 1996; Prinstein et al., 2001). Somewhat surprisingly, ethnic minorities appear to be no more or less victimized, on average, than ethnic nonminorities (e.g., Boulton, 1995; Olweus, 1978; Siann et al., 1994); however, there is evidence to suggest that the content of this victimization may differ (e.g., racist name calling; Verkuyten & Thijs, 2002). Consideration of other physical characteristics (e.g., wearing glasses and being short) has yielded inconsistent findings, but research has consistently indicated that physical weakness places children at increased risk for being victimized by peers (e.g., Lagerspetz et al., 1982; Olweus, 1978).

Internalizing problems, such as depression, anxiety, loneliness, and socially withdrawn behaviors, have consistently been found to be strongly associated with peer victimization. Importantly, there is also evidence from longitudinal studies so as to make conclusions about directions of effects. As might be expected, there is evidence to suggest that peer victimization predicts increases in internalizing problems over time (e.g., Boivin et al., 1995; Hodges et al., 1999a; Hodges & Perry, 1999; Kochenderfer & Ladd, 1996; Ladd & Troop-Gordon, 2003). This is not surprising, and intuitive evidence would suggest this to be the case. What might be less obvious, however, is that internalizing problems also predict increases in peer victimization over time (e.g., Boivin et al., 1995; Egan & Perry, 1998; Hodges et al., 1999; Hodges & Perry, 1999). This may be because children with internalizing problems are seen as easy targets by potential aggressors, reward aggressors with signs of suffering, and have less support from peers (see below). Because internalizing problems are both antecedents and consequences of peer victimization, it may be the case that the emergence of either can lead to a vicious cycle of maladjustment and abuse (Hodges & Perry, 1999).

Externalizing problems include such behaviors as aggression, argumentativeness, delinquency, emotional dysregulation, and attention deficit/hyperactivity disorder (ADHD)-type symptoms. Broadly considered, these problems are associated with peer victimization, though it is necessary to consider more specific behaviors in order to gain a complete picture. Aggression and peer victimization tend to be essentially unrelated (e.g., Olweus, 1978; Perry et al., 1988; Pope & Bierman, 1999); the implication of this is that there exists a substantial portion of victims who are also aggressive against peers (i.e., aggressive-victims; Olweus, 1978; Pellegrini et al., 1999; Schwartz et al., 1997). In contrast, peer victimization is related to higher delinquency and, perhaps especially strongly, with emotional dysregulation (Pope & Bierman, 1999). The longitudinal evidence relating externalizing behaviors to peer victimization is mixed, but there is evidence that hyperactivity and emotional dysregulation leads to increases in victimization (Pope & Bierman, 1999; Shields & Cicchetti, 2001), perhaps because such behaviors are likely to annoy peers and provoke potential aggressors.

As might be expected, prosocial behaviors tend to relate to lower levels of peer victimization (e.g., Boulton & Smith, 1994; cf., Olweus, 1978). In a longitudinal study, Egan and Perry (1998) found that prosocial behavior predicted decreases in peer victimization, which suggests that it serves as a protective factor against victimization. Related socially competent behaviors, such as adaptive conflict management and assertiveness, may also be related to lower victimization (e.g., Schwartz et al., 1993), though these have not been as extensively studied as other behaviors.

Although not widely studied, there is some evidence that indicates that peer victimization is related to poor academic ability (e.g., on standardized tests; Buhs & Ladd, 2001) and school grades (Juvonen et al., 2000; Olweus, 1978). Unfortunately, there has not been adequate longitudinal research on these associations (and longitudinal studies that exist are inconclusive; e.g., Kochenderfer & Ladd, 1996), so we do not know the extent to which academic characteristics are antecedents or consequences of peer victimization. Either direction of effect seems plausible: extremely high or low (perhaps depending on context) academic ability may place children at risk for victimization, and it is also reasonable to assume that children who are victimized may be less focused on school work and academic performance. Clearer evidence is available that indicates that peer victimization predicts increases in school avoidance (Kochenderfer & Ladd, 1996), which might be expected to further impact school achievement.

Finally, peer victimization is related to various aspects of self-concept, including self-worth, perceptions of social competence, and perceptions of competence in a variety of domains (e.g., Egan & Perry, 1998; Graham & Juvonen, 1998; Neary & Joseph, 1994; Salmivalli & Isaacs, 2005). As for internalizing problems (see above), there appears to be a reciprocal relation between victimization and low self-concept: peer victimization, perhaps because it signals to children that they are devalued by (at least some) peers, predicts decreasing self-concept over time; and low self-concept, perhaps because it translates into submissive behaviors, predicts increases in victimization over time (Egan & Perry, 1998).

Ecological Risk Factors for Peer Victimization

Bronfenbrenner's Ecological Taxonomy

Context can be defined and conceptualized in many ways. However, Bronfenbrenner's (Bronfenbrenner, 1977; Bronfenbrenner & Crouter, 1983; Bronfenbrenner & Morris, 1998; for a review see Card et al., 2007) definition and taxonomy have been widely used and will serve useful in guiding our review of prior literature. Bronfenbrenner and Morris (1983) defined environment as "any event or condition outside the organism that is presumed to influence, or be influenced by, the person's development" (p. 359). Two points about this definition merit mention. First, this definition is broad, as it needs to be to encompass the numerous aspects of children's environment that may relate to their victimization. Second, this definition recognizes the bidirectional influence that exists between children and their environments. In other words, it considers not only the impact that context may have on the individual, which is likely intuitive, but also the fact that individuals both directly change the context they are in and seek out contexts with certain characteristics.

Bronfenbrenner (1977) originally proposed four increasingly distal-nested levels into which to divide aspects of children's contexts. The first of these is the *microsystem*, which consists of individuals' immediate contextual settings that are presumed to most directly affect (and be affected by) the individual. Examples of microsystems relevant to children's development include the peer group, school, and family. These microsystems likely have the most direct contextual impact on children's day-to-day functioning and exert the most direct influence on children's development. Moreover, the child is most capable of impacting these microsystems, more so than distal contextual levels (described below). For some microsystemic contexts, children may also be able to select some contexts over others (e.g., which peers they choose to affiliate with), an autonomy that generally increases with age.

Children develop within numerous microsystems that can overlap, such as when parents are involved in their children's school. This overlap among different microsystems occurs within what Bronfenbrenner's termed the *mesosystem*, which is the next distal level of context that encompasses multiple microsystems. An important feature of the mesosystem is the relationships it fosters between different microsystems, and the degree and quality of this overlap may be a potentially important aspect of mesosystemic variability. For example, some mesosystemic contexts may foster active, cooperative alliances between parents and teachers, whereas others may impede relationships or set up adversarial relationships. Another example of variability within the mesosystem is evident if some children's peer group consist primarily of peers from school, whereas others' consist primarily of children from other contexts.

The next level of context in Bronfenbrenner's taxonomy is the *exosystem*. This level consists of the larger formal or informal settings that encompass the mesosystems and microsystems. School systems and neighborhoods are two examples of exosystemic contexts, with the former being a more formal structure and the latter often being a more informal context. Continuing with the examples of the previous paragraph, it seems apparent that school systems may vary in the degree to which they facilitate positive interactions (vs. infrequent or negative interactions) between parents and school personnel; and the structures of school (e.g., the geographic area from which they draw students) and neighborhoods (the degree to which they provide ease and safety in traveling; opportunities for children to interact in playgrounds or formal activities) could influence both the qualities of children's peer group (affiliation with prosocial vs. deviant peers; a microsystemic characteristic) and the overlap between children's peer group and school (affiliation with peers inside vs. outside of school; a mesosystemic characteristic).

The most distal level of ecological context originally proposed by Bronfenbrenner (see 1977) is the *macrosystem*. This level includes the broader cultural, political, and economic patterns that exist within larger organizational bodies (e.g., cities and countries). The macrosystem impacts more proximal levels of context, though typically acting most directly on the exosystems. For example, economic neglect of education at the governmental level (as well as increased emphasis on academic test scores) can result in situations in which school districts must hire fewer, often less qualified school personnel and reduce or eliminate extracurricular activities for students. These influences of the macrosystem on the exosystem will in turn impact the more proximal contexts in which children develop, such as by making it more difficult for parents to develop relationships with teachers (a mesosystemic effect) and leaving students with more unsupervised time during which they are more likely to affiliate with delinquent peers (a microsystemic effect). Of course, the opposite directions of contextual influence can also occur. For example, if many youths affiliate within delinquent peer groups and crime increases, the exosystem (i.e., public opinion, government action) is likely to be impacted (unfortunately, the response is too often aimed at responding to this crime at the expense of education, thus creating a vicious macrosystemic cycle). Although this outwardly traveling influence is more likely to be due to the aggregation of multiple individuals, microsystems, etc., singular incidents can also affect the macrosystem. For example, the shootings that occurred at Columbine High School in 1999 (by two individuals who were heavily influenced by their microsystems of rejection and mutual deviant influence; see McCabe & Martin, 2005) greatly impacted public perceptions of youth violence and were followed by sweeping reforms of school policies toward weapons (e.g., through zero-tolerance policies).

Time can be an important component of context, though not one that is often considered (but see Bronfenbrenner, 1986; Card et al., 2007; Elder, 1997). This *chronosystem* refers to the historical context in which individuals and their ecological contexts (ranging from microsystems to macrosystems) are embedded. This can refer to either short- (e.g., highly publicized acts of violence) or long-term (e.g., depression era) historic periods. Moreover, this chronosystem intersects with all of the previously reviewed aspects of children's ecologies; for example, acts of violence can affect the history of a particular peer group (a microsystem), schools and communities (exosystems or mesosystems), and/or nations (macrosystems).

Microsystemic Risk Factors for Peer Victimization

Three microsystems that have been studied in relation to peer victimization are the peer group, the classroom or school climate, and the family. We will selectively review this research next.

The Peer Group

There is considerable research to suggest that children's relations with peers are strongly related to their experience of victimization (for reviews, see Card et al., 2007; Rodkin & Hodges, 2003). Children who are victimized are often rejected by peers (i.e., many peers dislike them) and are low in peer acceptance (i.e., few peers like them). There is sufficient evidence to conclude that this poor peer group status (i.e., high rejection and low acceptance) predicts increases in victimization over time (e.g., Boulton, 1999; Hanish & Guerra, 2000; Hodges & Perry, 1999; Ladd & Troop-Gordon, 2003). The reason for this may be because children who are rejected (and not well liked) by their peers may be seen as easy targets by aggressors, and aggressors may expect, and perhaps receive, reinforcement (e.g., peers laughing or cheering on attacks), or at least little punishment, for targeting these low-status children. Longitudinal studies also indicate that this poor social status is a consequence of peer victimization (Boivin et al., 1995; Boulton, 1999; Hodges & Perry, 1999; Ladd & Troop-Gordon, 2003; Pellegrini, 1995); thus victimization and social status may operate in a mutually reinforcing cycle, much like internalizing problems and low self-concept as reviewed above.

In addition to acceptance and rejection, an important aspect of the peer group is the extent to which it supports aggression toward victims. Consideration of social cognitions that peers hold toward victimized children indicate that all peers—not just aggressors—hold cognitions that support aggressive behavior toward these targets (Williard & Perry, 1990). In other words, both aggressive and nonaggressive children expect that aggressive behavior would result in more tangible rewards, more victim suffering, and be less likely to result in retaliation when directed toward peers viewed as highly victimized relative to those viewed as not victimized. Evidence also indicates that most children play some role in acts of aggression; in addition to aggressors and victims, children may function as assistants or reinforcers to aggressors or, conversely, as defenders of victims (Salmivalli et al., 1996; for a review, see Salmivalli, 2001). In other words, nearly all children play some role in aggressive incidents, even if not directly as aggressors. Furthermore, nearly all incidents of victimization involve additional peers, besides the aggressor and victim, playing a supporting role for the aggressor or a defending role for the victim (85% in an observational study by Craig & Pepler, 1995). The peer group, then, appears to represent a powerful microsystemic contextual influence on the occurrence of aggressive behavior toward certain victims.

Children's dyadic relationships may also place them at greater or lesser risk for peer victimization. The type of childhood relationship that has been most studied has been friendships. Research has consistently indicated that children who have friends, or who have more friends, are less victimized than children who do not have friends or who have fewer friends (e.g., Boulton et al., 1999; Hodges et al., 1999a, 1997; Hodges & Perry, 1999; Pellegrini et al., 1999; Salmivalli et al., 1997). As with group-level status, having few or no friends is both a risk factor (Boulton et al., 1999; Hodges et al., 1999a; cf., Hodges & Perry, 1999) and a consequence (Ladd et al., 1997; cf., Hodges & Perry, 1999) of peer victimization.

Friendships may reduce victimization because friends may protect the child from potential aggressors. Victimization may also lead to a lack of friendships because peers may distance themselves from the targeted child. Not all friends are equal, however, and the characteristics of friends and friendships are related to peer victimization. Having friends with certain characteristics (e.g., physical strength and peer acceptance) can protect children from victimization, but unfortunately the friends of victimized children tend to also be victimized, have personal and interpersonal risk factors themselves, and be unwilling or unable to offer protection (Haselager et al., 1998; Hodges et al., 1997, 1999a; La Greca & Harrison, 2005; Salmivalli et al., 1997).

Children who have antipathetic relationships (relationships in which both members dislike one another) also tend to be more victimized than those who do not (Abecassis et al., 2002; Card & Hodges, 2007; Parker & Gamm, 2003; Schwartz et al., 2003). Although having mutual antipathies and being rejected by peers are correlated, and there is little evidence that having mutual antipathies constitutes a unique risk factor (i.e., after controlling for rejection), there is evidence indicating that the characteristics of children's antipathies is uniquely related to peer victimization. Specifically, children are more likely to be victimized when their mutual antipathies are aggressive, are physically strong, do not suffer internalizing problems, and are not themselves victimized than when their antipathies do not have these characteristics (Card & Hodges, 2007). Moreover, consideration of specific aggressor–victim relationships indicates that victimization is disproportionately likely to occur within antipathetic relationships, especially when the antipathies possess the characteristics listed above, and this victimization within antipathetic relationships is more strongly related to maladjustment than is victimization within other relationships (Card & Hodges, 2007). Unfortunately, all studies of victimization and antipathies conducted thus far are concurrent, so we cannot be sure of the directions of effects.

This latter finding regarding victimization within specific relationships points to an important direction for future research: studying specific aggressor–victim relationships. There is evidence indicating that specific dyads account for much of the occurrence of aggression (as opposed to being due to some aggressors indiscriminately attacking others or some victims be targeted by all peers; Coie et al., 1999; Dodge et al., 1990), so consideration of these dyadic contexts seems important (see Pierce & Cohen, 1995). This does not imply that incidents of aggression necessarily occur with only one aggressor and one victim present; it is possible that two friends may share common targets for aggression (i.e., be engaged in aggressor–victim relationships with the same victim; see Card & Hodges, 2006) or that specific aggressors attack specific victims in settings in which others are present (e.g., in the presence of reinforcers; see above). There is evidence to indicate that dyad-specific social cognitions that the aggressor holds toward the victim is related to (and presumably underlies) this dyad-specific aggression (Hubbard et al., 2001). There is also preliminary evidence that the characteristics of the aggressor–victim relationships are related to the consequences of victimization—victimization from aggressors who are more powerful than the victim (e.g., greater physical strength and more accepted by peers) predicts maladjustment more strongly than does victimization within relationship with smaller power differentials (Card & Hodges, 2005). However, we generally know little about how aggressor–victim relationships form, are maintained, change over time, and terminate; we also have little information about how the characteristics of these relationships affect the outcomes of aggressors or victims in these relationships.

The School

The peer group and school are highly overlapping microsystems, especially for children whose peer group is located primarily within the school context. Moreover, relatively few studies have focused on identifying aspects of the school that serve as risk or protective factors for peer victimization, likely because of the necessary scale of such projects (i.e., it is necessary to sample numerous schools in order to identify how variability in their features are related to students' victimization). Nevertheless, several aspects of the school have been examined as distinct microsystemic risk factors for peer victimization, including staff approachability and training, physical structure of the school, and school size and location.

Several studies have examined whether and to whom victimized children report their abuse. These results indicate that only a fraction of victims report their abuse to teachers or staff members. Specifically, about half of elementary school-age children report victimization to teachers (O'Moore et al., 1997), with numbers falling to about one-third in middle school (Fekkes et al., 2005; Mellor; 1990; Smith & Shu, 2000) and to as low as 15% among adolescents (O'Moore et al., 1997). Thus, it appears that youths generally do not report their victimization to school professionals, often because they believe that such action will fail to improve, and may even worsen, their situation (Fekkes et al., 2005; Newman & Murray, 2005; Smith & Shu, 2000). In one survey, 69% of students thought that school professionals handled victimization problems poorly, whereas only 2% thought that these problems were handled "very well" (Hazler et al., 1991). When students do report their victimization to teachers, this tends to end or diminish the victimization about half the time, but fails to change or even makes the situation worse about half the time (Fekkes et al., 2005; Smith & Shu, 2000). Although these results are not quite as pessimistic as those suggested by the survey by Hazler and colleagues (1991), they certainly indicate that the responses could be improved. Teachers' perceptions confirm the need for improvement; in one survey, only 5% of teachers felt they had adequate training to deal with bullying situations (Byrne, 1994). However, schools in which teachers are aware of school policies on peer victimization and have received training to deal with bullying tend to have students who view teachers as more approachable and willing to take action against bullies and, more importantly, lower rates of peer victimization (Hazler, 1996; Siann et al., 1993; Smith & Shu, 2000).

Youths' reports of where they are victimized vary greatly across studies, with various samples each reporting classrooms, hallways, lunchrooms, playgrounds, and areas near the school (e.g., behind building, parking lots) as the most common sites for victimization (Astor et al., 1999; Baldry & Farrington, 1999; Borg, 1999; Fekkes et al., 2005; Mellor, 1990; O'Moore et al., 1997; Slee, 1995; Smith & Shu, 2000; Whitney & Smith, 1993). Congestion has been cited as a correlate of victimization (e.g., Siann et al., 1993), but the most extensive survey of locations of school violence suggests that an absence of adult presence in certain areas during certain times is most strongly related to victimization (Astor et al., 1999). It is likely the case that the location affects not only the occurrence of victimization but also the form and severity of victimization. Observational research indicates that overt victimization occurs disproportionately frequently on the playground, whereas relational victimization (which is more likely to escape adults' attention) more frequently occurs in classrooms (Craig et al., 2000). It may also be the case that victimization episodes may last longer and be less likely to end when victims show signs of suffering (e.g., crying) in unsupervised areas such as playgrounds than in classrooms—however, we are not aware of any studies that have evaluated this claim. Clearly, more research is needed to explain the variability across studies of where victimization occurs, the characteristics of schools that predict the variability, and the features of victimization experiences (and the impact these have on victims) occurring in different locations.

Neither school nor class size has consistently been found to be related to school differences in victimization (Lagerspetz et al., 1982; Ma, 2002; O'Moore et al., 1997; Olweus, 1978; Whitney & Smith, 1993; Wolke et al., 2001), although one study found a trend for larger schools and classrooms to contain higher rates of victimization (see Stephenson & Smith, 2002).

The Family

Familial factors that have been examined in relation to victimization include parenting behaviors, attachment styles, family dysfunction, family composition, and socioeconomic status.

Several components of parenting behaviors have been explored in association with peer victimization. Parents' provision of support (Abecassis et al., 2002; Haynie et al., 2001), involvement (Haynie et al., 2001; Nansel et al., 2001), and responsiveness (Ladd & Kochenderfer-Ladd, 1998) are all negatively associated with victimization. Other correlates may vary depending on the gender of the child. For example, there is mixed evidence that overprotectiveness and intense closeness are positively associated with victimization among boys, but not among girls (Finnegan et al., 1998; Ladd & Kochenderfer-Ladd, 1998; cf., Lagerpetz et al., 1982), whereas intrusive demandingness, coercion, and threat of rejection are positively associated to victimization among girls, but not among boys (Finnegan et al., 1998; Ladd & Kochenderfer-Ladd, 1998). Child abuse, a more extreme form of coercive parenting behavior, has also been connected to peer victimization (Duncan, 1999; Shields & Cicchetti, 2001). This relation has been accounted for by elevated emotional dysregulation by abused youths (Shields & Cicchetti, 2001), suggesting the process by which many of these familial correlates may antecede victimization—through the fostering of personal factors that may be expressed in the peer group that increase risk of victimization by peers.

Several aspects of parenting behaviors converge to influence attachment styles, suggesting that attachment styles may be associated with victimization as well. The empirical evidence of this association is mixed, however. Troy and Sroufe (1987) found that preschoolers with an insecure anxious–ambivalent attachment were more likely to be victimized in dyadic laboratory play situations. Similarly, Jacobson and Wille (1986) found that this anxious–ambivalent style assessed at 18 months predicted victimization in dyadic laboratory play among 3-year-olds, but not 2-year-olds. Among school-age children, Bowers et al. (1994) failed to find a significant correlation between victimization and attachment security, but these authors did not differentiate between avoidant and preoccupied (anxious–ambivalent) forms of insecurity. Indeed, when such distinctions are made in middle childhood, preoccupied, but not avoidant, attachment is related to greater victimization, at least for boys (Finnegan et al., 1996). Together, these results suggest a small to moderate association between victimization and attachment, specifically with anxious–ambivalent (or preoccupied) attachment. No study has yet examined this association longitudinally. Thus, preoccupied attachment may lead to victimization (perhaps through the manifestation of personal risk factors such as internalizing behaviors; Finnegan et al., 1996; Hodges et al., 1999b), but victimization might also affect attachment quality.

Two components of family structure that have been examined in association with victimization are family size and intactness (e.g., presence vs. absence of father). In several studies, these components have not been found to be significantly related to victimization (Berdondini & Smith, 1996; Bowers et al., 1994; Rigby, 1993), though some have found a small association between victimization and father absence (Bond et al., 2001; Flouri & Buchanon, 2002; Mellor, 1990). The mechanisms by which nonintact family structure leads to victimization may include higher risk of maladaptive parenting behavior brought on by parental distress, and lost opportunities for the child to develop social skills through interaction with a second parent. Across several studies, little evidence supports an association between family socioeconomic status and victimization (e.g., Borg, 1999; Olweus, 1978; Wolke et al., 2001; cf., Ma, 2002).

Mesosystemic Risk Factors for Peer Victimization

As we continue our review into more distal contextual levels, we find that the empirical basis for drawing conclusions becomes limited. Potential mesosystemic risk/protective factors for victimization might involve the quality of teacher–parent relations, the extent to which children's friends or antipathies are among schoolmates, or the presence of sibling or other family members among peers, to suggest just a few examples. Unfortunately, the majority of studies investigating these microsystemic risk factors do so in isolation, ignoring the critical interplay between these microsystems, or mesosystems. To provide just one example of this practice (noting that many studies are guilty of this, without meaning to single out this particular study): Perren and Hornung (2005) found that victimization was associated with low peer acceptance and low family support (two microsystemic variables), but did not evaluate whether the interaction (which would capture mesosystemic risk or protection) between peer acceptance and family support was associated with victimization.

The absence of empirical evidence regarding mesosystemic factors and victimization has not prevented recommendations for intervention. Various intervention programs involve educators becoming involved in children's peer relations (e.g., "befriending" interventions; see Boulton et al., 1999). Similarly, Besag (2002), for example, recommended that parents and teachers work together to intervene and prevent victimization (see also Sheridan et al., 2004). While we do not disagree with such recommendations—in fact, common sense suggests that these efforts might prove effective—we are concerned that such recommendations are made without a supporting empirical basis for doing so. Such an empirical basis exists supporting the importance of one mesosystemic characteristic, parent–school collaboration, for various aspects of academic development (see Sheridan et al., 2004), but it is not clear that similar effects exist for peer victimization. More attention to mesosystemic risk and protective factors for peer victimization is sorely needed.

Exosystemic Risk Factors for Peer Victimization

Consideration of exosystemic risk factors for peer victimization has primarily been limited to two features: rural versus urban school settings and neighborhood characteristics.

In terms of school location, there may be a small tendency for urban schools to have more victimization than rural schools (Lagerspetz et al., 1982). However, Nansel et al. (2001) failed to find associations between school location and rates of victimization in a nationally representative sample of over 15,000 youths in the United States, and several other studies have also failed to detect a difference between urban and rural schools (e.g., Hewitt, 1995). In total, it appears that there may exist a tendency for greater victimization in urban than in rural schools, but this difference appears to be fairly small in magnitude.

Studies of the aspects of neighborhoods that are related to incidences of peer victimization have considered primarily the poverty versus affluence of neighborhoods. In a convincing quasi-experimental study, Fauth et al. (2005) examined outcomes for youths whose families moved from economically disadvantaged, primarily minority neighborhoods to middle-class, primarily White neighborhoods (comparing these outcomes to those of youths who remained in disadvantaged neighborhoods). Results indicated lower neighborhood victimization for those youths who moved; unfortunately the authors of this study did not also assess in-school victimization. However, other evidence suggests that being the victim of neighborhood violence is associated with in-school victimization (Schwartz & Proctor, 2000), and that schools serving economically disadvantaged student bodies have higher rates of peer victimization (Dhami et al., 2005; cf., Ma, 2002). Together, this research suggests a substantial association between neighborhood poverty and peer victimization in schools.

Qualitative research of neighborhood geographies (Percy-Smith & Matthews, 2001) and social support (Spilsbury, 2005) supports the importance of other aspects of neighborhood contexts. However, these aspects have not been the focus of quantitative investigation, so it is difficult to make conclusions regarding the magnitude or association these other exosystemic factors have with peer victimization.

Macrosystemic Risk Factors for Peer Victimization

As mentioned, macrosystemic influences include broader cultural, political, and economic patterns that exist within larger organizational bodies such as cities or countries. In considering potential risk or protective factors at this level, it is reasonable to first consider evidence for *any* potential impact. For instance, it is natural to ask whether there is evidence that some cities or countries (i.e., macrosystemic entities) vary substantially in levels of peer victimization. The evidence thus far is unconvincing, or at least inconsistent—cross-national comparisons have generally indicated more similarities than differences in rates of victimization, and when differences are found, they are often not replicated across studies (see Eslea et al., 2004; Menesini et al., 1997; Österman et al., 1994; Smith et al., 1999). Although we would hesitate to conclude that cross-national differences do not exist, we believe that there is not yet adequate evidence to conclude the presence, directions, and magnitudes of such effects. Several factors make the detection of such effects challenging. First, the scope of such projects makes these data difficult to collect— researchers wishing to make cross-national comparisons must measure peer victimization among a representative sample of children from numerous countries, at obviously great cost in time and effort. Second, attention needs to be placed on ensuring comparable measurement across countries, which requires attention to the cultural and linguistic interpretation of items (see Smith et al., 2002) and the use of advanced statistical procedures (see Card & Little, 2006b). Finally, factors that may affect victimization at the national level (i.e., macrosystemic factors) overlap with historic factors, a consideration that should qualify interpretation of such differences (these two sources of differences could be partly separated by consideration of the shared and unique chronosytemic risk and protective factors across countries, as well as through extensive longitudinal research, though this adds to the aforementioned scope of cross-national comparisons).

Despite the challenges of studying macrosystemic risk factors for victimization, as well as the ambiguity of extant research in even identifying cross-national variability in victimization, we consider attention to this contextual level critically important. Intuition certainly supports the importance of school funding and attention to victimization—if schools and teachers do not receive adequate funding, training, and encouragement to prevent and intervene in victimization, it seems improbable that the problem will simply go away by itself.

One salient macrosystemic policy change that has occurred in the United States, largely in reaction to highly publicized school shootings, is the adoption of so-called "zero-tolerance" policies. These policies are primarily aimed toward weapon carrying but have also been extended to aggressive behavior more generally. Although it is encouraging that such macrosystemic efforts have been directed toward reducing school violence, these policies have been critiqued; specifically, there is concern that such policies are ineffective, change actual reporting practices regarding aggression and victimization as much as the actual occurrence, and artificially reduce violence statistics by removing problematic students rather than helping them (see Chesney-Lind & Belknap, 2004; Peebles-Wilkins, 2005).

Chronosystemic Risk Factors for Peer Victimization

Given the relatively short history of research on peer victimization, it is not possible to draw strong conclusions regarding chronosystemic risk. The little evidence available suggests that peer victimization has been a longstanding problem: it was described in an 1857 novel by Thomas Hughes, *Tom Brown's Schooldays* (see Rigby, 2001); it was first recognized as a topic for scientific study in the late nineteenth century (Burk, 1897) and became the focus of modern quantitative research in the 1970s in Scandinavia (see Olweus, 1991) and in the 1980s in the United States (Perry et al., 1988). Nevertheless, two aspects of the chronosystem merit consideration.

First, there is the possibility that incidents of violence lead to further incidents of violence. McCabe and Martin (2005) presented evidence that school shootings often happen in close succession to one another and argued that subsequent school shootings may be at least partially in response to the media coverage (which some individuals may view as rewarding for the violent behavior). Considering more normative forms of aggression, it is plausible that children who witness aggressors being rewarded (e.g., by peers cheering the aggression, perceiving aggressive individuals as popular or "cool") would be motivated to themselves enact aggression toward peers. Alternatively, it would be expected that witnessing aggression that is punished by peers or adults might decrease further aggression. These processes would suggest that the local (i.e., short-term) chronosystem plays a role in aggression and victimization.

More typical considerations of chronosystemic influence on development focus on long-term, historic phenomena (e.g., Elder, 1997). In this respect, there is simply insufficient empirical research on chronosystemic risk factors for peer victimization. Consideration of historic changes in schools within the United States over the last several centuries provides some interesting possibilities (see McCabe & Martin, 2005): during the colonial period (i.e., prior to 1776) there was considerable variability in the amount and source (e.g., apprenticeships, church) of education, and corporal punishment by these "teachers" was common; from 1776 through the mid-1800s, schooling was more structured but was still heavily reliant on both religion and corporal punishment; from mid-1800s to mid-1900s was a period of reform in which religious control of schools diminished while government control increased, and corporal punishment became less common; and the mid-1900s through the present witnessed both an increasing accountability for schools and an increasing presence of organized gangs in schools. Although these chronosystemic factors have not been sufficiently studied to link them to aggressive behavior across time, intuition suggests that several of these features (e.g., modeling of aggression by adults, the amount and content of moral teaching) could influence the incidence of children's victimization by peers. We suspect that a combination of historical research, systematic integration of the accumulating research base, and very long-term prospective studies will be needed to understand these chronosystemic influences.

Prevention and Intervention

Prevention programs vary in terms of the target group they select and their intended impact. Currently they can be classified into three categories: universal, selective, and indicated (Mrazek & Haggerty, 1994). Universal preventive programs are designed to be delivered to entire populations. Many school-based interventions include all of the student body and fall into this category. Selective preventive programs focus on at-risk individuals or groups. For example, early intervention programs designed to reduce entry in criminal activities for children living in extremely impoverished, high-crime neighborhoods can be viewed as a form of selective prevention. Indicated prevention programs are usually more intense and costly and are used to target high-risk individuals who demonstrate early signs of problematic outcomes. For example, young children who display early indicators of academic or behavioral problems may be selected to receive special services in hopes of preventing the evolution of more complex and impairing problems.

Victimization prevention programs within the school have represented all of these categories. In addition, direct treatment for those who have already emerged as chronic victims or aggressors can be used in isolation, or in conjunction, with preventive programs. Regardless of the taxonomy used, the overarching focus for many programs devised to prevent in-school victimization share the ultimate goal of creating a safe school environment that is free of peer harassment and hostility.

Ecological Systems Theory, as described above, provides a rich way to conceptualize and devise programs aimed at preventing victimization from developing and intervening once it has emerged. Viewing social problems such as victimization as a multilevel phenomenon can help to guide the development of effective prevention programs (Choi, 2003). Indeed, many prevention efforts have utilized our growing knowledge base regarding the impact of multiple contextual levels on child development. One of the first large-scale, multifaceted, and contextually informed bully/victimization intervention programs to be implemented and systematically evaluated was Olweus' (Olweus, 1993) Bullying Prevention Program. The goal of the program is to provide a school (and preferably also a home) environment characterized by warmth and prosocial interactions. Positive adult involvement from both parents and school personnel is coupled with clear, firm limits for unacceptable behavior and consistent nonaggressive, nonhostile consequences for rule violations. In addition, both school personnel and parents receive educational material describing bullying and suggestions for counteracting it. The core features of the program are implemented at the school level, class level, and the level of individual students. School-level efforts include the formation of a coordinating committee to oversee the program, a school-wide awareness and involvement in anti-bullying efforts, increased monitoring of students, and regular meetings between parents and school staff. In the classroom, clear rules against bullying and regularly scheduled class discussions about bullying are provided. For students involved in bullying, both bullies and victims are required to participate in serious talks about bullying, and parents of both parties are included in discussions.

Olweus' program was first implemented with ~2,500 students in Bergen, Norway, in conjunction with a Norwegian, nationwide anti-bully campaign. Results from this program (Olweus, 1991, 1993) revealed substantial reductions in bully–victim problems (around 50%) as well as reductions in other types of antisocial behaviors (e.g., vandalism) and reports of positive changes in the social climate of the classrooms. This program was also implemented in Rogaland, Norway (Roland, 2000); however, the results were markedly different from the Bergen project. Three years after the implementation of the anti-bullying program in Rogaland, overall rates of bullying had actually increased. The differences in program outcomes have been attributed to poor implementation of the program and lack of external support in Rogaland (Roland, 2000; Smith et al., 2003). For example, packages of information were merely sent to Rogaland schools and periodic monitoring and visits from a research team were not provided, whereas the schools in Bergen had received this additional monitoring and support. In a meta-analysis of 14 whole-school anti-bullying interventions, the effect sizes for bullying and victimization were all small, negligible, or negative (Smith et al., 2003). The one exception was for Olweus' (Olweus, 1993) intervention; the effects for both bullying and victimization were medium. More recent whole-school anti-bullying prevention programs have also demonstrated small to negligible reductions in victimization and aggression (e.g., Frey et al., 2005). The variability in efficacy of these multilevel interventions points to the need to more systematically evaluate factors that differentiate outcomes among programs that share the common goal of alleviating victimization utilizing a whole-school approach with multilevel methods of intervention.

As suggested by the disparate outcomes of the Bully Prevention Program in Bergen and Rogaland, an important factor that may influence efficacy may be the level of program implementation. There is accumulating evidence that high-quality implementation is associated with greater intervention effects (Aber et al., 1998; Eslea & Smith, 1998; Kallestad & Olweus, 2003; Roland, 2000; Salmivalli et al.,

2005). Certain teacher- and school-level factors are associated with greater program implementation, including teachers' ability to communicate openly with one another, thoroughly reading the prevention program material, believing it is important to counteract bullying in school, and their emotional responsiveness and empathic understanding of victims, as well as the school's overall interest and attention to bullying problems (Kallestad & Olweus, 2003). This suggests that ongoing program monitoring, a strong commitment and genuine interest by school personnel, adequate training and knowledge about victimization and ways to intervene, and continued staff support may be central to the proper implementation, and the ultimate efficacy, of these comprehensive programs. Further study is needed to account for variability in program outcomes, especially those that were attempted replications of Olweus' Bullying Prevention Program, in order to evaluate factors that contribute to more rigorous victimization prevention program implementation (Forgatch, 2003). In addition, the idea of sufficient dosage may relate not only to the quality of implementation but also to the length and intensity of implementation. There is a growing *consensus* regarding the need to examine whether the targets of preventive efforts are exposed to enough of the intervention to allow for desired and enduring effects (see Nation et al., 2003).

It is possible that the multicomponent nature of a whole school, contextually informed approach to preventing victimization, may overburden educators, especially those who have limited resources. It may be important to streamline interventions to increase adherence. In order to do this effectively, it is important that the researchers thoroughly analyze the effects of each program component, in isolation and in conjunction with others. Although there has yet to be systematic evaluations teasing apart the effects of each component of multilevel, whole-school victimization prevention programs, there is some evidence that different types and levels of interventions have varying effects on the reduction of aggression and victimization. For example, Fraser et al. (2005) found some increased effects in lowering aggression and social cognitions supporting aggression by adding a teacher and parent component to a social problem solving skills training intervention, but these additional benefits were modest. When comparing the effects of four types of interventions for externalizing behaviors among high-risk adolescents, it was found that the parent-focused intervention showed short-term superiority to peer focused, combined parent and peer focused, and adolescent self-directed intervention conditions (Dishion & Andrews, 1995). In fact, adolescents in the small peer training groups intervention condition appeared to show a worsening of delinquent and aggressive behaviors, suggesting iatrogenic effects of congregating groups of high-risk adolescents. A similar effect was found when comparing a classroom-based aggression prevention program to one that also included a small peer group training component for high-risk early adolescents, with the latter group showing a worsening in aggressive behavior (Metropolitan Area Child Study Research Group, 2002). These results demonstrate that certain program components meant to improve student behavior may actually exacerbate aggressive behavior. Similarly, some more intensive programs have failed to show incremental effects on reducing aggressive behavior, compared to less intensive interventions (e.g., Cavell & Hughes, 2000).

A developmental–ecological framework (Tolan et al., 1995) not only acknowledges the importance of considering multiple social contextual influences when conceptualizing models of child adjustment and when devising prevention programs but also recognizes the centrality of viewing processes as woven within a developmental context. Effects of different types of victimization and aggression interventions have varied depending on the age of the child, with some demonstrating somewhat more positive effects with younger children (e.g., Orpinas et al., 2003; Stevens et al., 2000; Salmivalli et al., 2005; Smith et al., 2004) and others favoring the older children in their sample (e.g., Flannery et al., 2003). Although it would be ideal to implement prevention programs very early on (Cummings et al., 2000), well before serious victimization problems emerge, it is central that interventions be timed for when they can have the greatest impact (Nation et al., 2003).

Evaluation of the timing of interventions, as well as differentiating the impact of varying program components, can also be complicated by important contextual factors. The complex interplay between program components, developmental factors, and larger contextual factors was demonstrated by the work of Metropolitan Area Child Study Research Group (2002) on aggression prevention. It examined the effects of three aggression prevention programs, delivered at various stages of development, among two different urban communities. They examined the relative efficacy of targeting increasing levels of the child's social ecology, comparing no treatment, classroom training, classroom training plus small group peer group training, and a combined classroom-, peer-, and family-focused intervention. Second, they compared children receiving the different programs during early elementary school, those receiving it in late elementary school, and those who received both the early and the late interventions. Finally, they compared results from two different urban communities, Chicago and Aurora Illinois. Both communities were largely economically disadvantaged, but Chicago residents had greater mean levels of adversity (e.g., poorer, overall lower functioning, and fewer resources). For the late-intervention students, there were no positive intervention effects on levels of aggressive behavior; however, those in the classroom plus peer condition actually became more aggressive than children receiving no intervention. For the early intervention students, those children in the class, peer, and family condition differed from children receiving no intervention, but the results were qualified by their community context. Those from the lower-adversity area (i.e., Aurora) decreased in aggression but those from the higher-adversity area (i.e., Chicago) increased in aggression. The same pattern of results was evident for children receiving both early and late intervention. Thus, not only was the developmental timing and type of intervention associated with differential changes in aggression, the community context also played a pivotal role in altering the nature of outcomes.

Other studies have also demonstrated the importance of considering context when evaluating interventions designed to reduce aggression, victimization, and the attitudes that promote these behaviors. For example, context effects were explored in a study comparing Prime Time, a program focused on building child competencies for aggressive children through working with the children and their teachers and parents, with Lunch Buddies, a program focused on changing aggressive children's peer ecologies through the use of a student mentor during lunchtime (Hughes et al., 2005). Although initial outcome evaluations demonstrated no differences between these two interventions in changing levels of aggression, additional analyses revealed that Lunch Buddies was more effective than Prime Time in high-adversity schools (i.e., high aggression, number of students eligible for free or reduced priced lunch, and mobility) but Prime Time was more effective in reducing aggression in low-adversity schools (Hughes et al., 2005). These results suggest that bolstering child competencies is most effective in reducing aggression in higher-functioning environments but altering the peer ecology is more central in more adverse school environments. This pattern suggests the importance of examining the larger context that students are embedded in to fully appreciate what types of aggression prevention programs work most effectively.

Another example of contextually differentiated efficacy was evident in a study examining the Resolving Conflict Creatively Program, a program that trains teachers and peer mediators to help children make good choices when faced with conflict (Aber et al., 1998). Efficacy was greatest for classes that demonstrated a high level of program implementation, but these effects were minimized for children in high-risk classes (i.e., classes with norms that favored aggression) and high-risk neighborhoods (i.e., high in poverty and homicide).

Other studies have found a somewhat different pattern of results for their aggression prevention programs. For example, the classroom-based behavior management prevention program called the Good Behavior Game (Dolan et al., 1989) has been shown to produce the greatest reductions in rates of aggressive, disruptive behavior for highly aggressive boys in highly aggressive classes (Kellam et al., 1998). In addition, the family-focused prevention program, SAFEChildren, promoted decreases in aggressive behavior only for high-risk children and children from high-risk families (Tolan et al., 2004). When examining general intervention effects, the whole sample demonstrated no changes in aggression. Only by looking at specific types of children, those deemed high risk or from high-risk families, could effects be found.

Our review of the outcomes of aggression and victimization prevention programs highlights the need to examine both individual factors, such as age and level of aggression, and contextual factors, such as family/community functioning and class norms, to better understand factors that contribute to program fit. The question of proper program fit is the cornerstone to understanding what works under what conditions. The evolution of successful victimization prevention programs relies on our ability to further develop, integrate, and apply our growing understanding of the multiple contextual risks for victimization. By systematically evaluating how individual, peer, class, school, family, and larger community and societal factors relate to variability in victimization prevention program efficacy we may be able to better account for differential levels of efficacy across samples and the lack of efficacy of conceptually sound interventions and provide more tailor-made prevention programs given the characteristics of target individuals and groups. In order to do this effectively, we may need to expand our conceptualization of appropriate levels of contexts to target for intervention.

Although it is recognized that more efficient victimization prevention programs may decrease cost, increase program adherence, and allow for more widespread implementation, it is clear that risk and protective factors for victimization exist in multiple levels of children's ecological contexts. Despite efforts to systematically include several levels of the child's ecology, many multilevel interventions fail to include the family in their intervention efforts. Strong evidence has accumulated that in parent–child relations parents are involved in the development and mainte-nance of aggressive behavior; parent–child relations have also been implicated in differentiating victims from nonvictims (for reviews, see Hodges et al., 2003; Perry et al., 2001). Thus, parental involvement in intervention efforts may prove to be a valuable, yet largely untapped resource. Furthermore, as children progress through their education they experience changes in teachers, classes, peer groups, and often schools. The home environment is one of the few environments that can endure throughout a child's development. Although some interventions incorporate ongo-ing parent involvement and/or training, some that espouse a "parent component" to their intervention may grossly underutilize parents in their efforts. For example, programs that involve parents by simply mailing overviews of the programs to their homes (e.g., O'Moore & Minton, 2005) may not, in fact, elicit any additional parental involvement.

Another potentially instrumental context that is rarely tapped in bully/victim prevention programs is the larger community outside the school. Community-level interventions have been largely used to combat health risk behaviors such as smok-ing, pregnancy, and drug abuse. The results of these prevention programs have yielded many positive effects, although some have failed to produce the desired outcomes (Wandersman & Florin, 2003). Like the family environment, once children leave the confines of the school they are subject to being immersed in the culture of their community. The community works as an exosystemic context that frames and shapes the contexts embedded within; thus it may have a distal, or even proxi-mal, influence on them. Therefore, community efforts may not only shape children's experiences in the community but also positively predispose the microsystems that are often directly targeted for intervention (e.g., school, peer group).

In summary, a significant limitation of much of the prior work evaluating victimization prevention programs is the lack of systematic evaluation of both treat-ment components and contextual moderators of intervention efficacy. In addition to expanding our exploration of ecologically relevant variables, we may need to evaluate them contemporaneously in both additive and complex moderational models.

Challenges and Future Directions

Although research in the last few decades has done much to improve our under-standing of the personal risk factors for peer victimization, relatively little research has considered the contextual risk factors for victimization. The research reviewed in this chapter represents some exceptions, but considerably more work is needed to provide a complete understanding of contextual risk and how these can inform prevention and intervention efforts.

Challenges to conducting basic research on contextual risk factors for victimization include difficulties in both design and analysis. In terms of design, studies that adequately sample multiple contexts must be quite large and therefore require substantial investments of effort and time. This investment is compounded when conducting longitudinal research, which is necessary to establish temporal relations among individual characteristics, various levels of contextual influence, and victimization experiences. Even when researchers are able to collect such data, the complexity of analyzing these data might be daunting. Special consideration is needed to account for the nesting of individuals within contexts, which themselves may be partially overlapping; the complexity of these analyses increases when one is trying to model longitudinal change (see Little et al., 2007).

Prevention and intervention efforts face even greater challenges. Not only must research evaluating the effectiveness of these efforts deal with the same design and analysis challenges as basic research, but there is the added challenge of manipulating contextual factors. Two aspects of this challenge merit consideration. First, there is the very real challenge that many contextual features may be difficult or impossible to change. Changes to microsystemic contextual factors such as school or family characteristics are themselves challenging, changes to more distal contextual factors (neighborhood features and funding for schools) may be outside of the researcher's or practitioner's power, and changes to chronosystemic features are impossible (unless one has access to a time machine). A second challenge is that even if one can affect change in a contextual risk factor, the specificity of such a manipulation is questionable. For example, a researcher's efforts to change an exosystemic feature (e.g., increasing contact between teachers and parents) might actually change a microsystemic feature (e.g., teachers feeling more responsible for responding to victimization), so conclusions from this study might attribute the benefit of the prevention or intervention effort to the wrong aspect of context. Although this might seem to be of little concern if one is interested only in the effectiveness of the study, it substantially undermines our understanding of which contextual risk factors should be targeted and ultimately results in inefficient returns on our prevention and intervention efforts.

Conclusions

Our understanding of contextual risk factors for peer victimization, and their implications for prevention and intervention, is far from complete. Nevertheless, the existing research demonstrates the importance of considering such contextual risk factors, and we hope that our organization of these findings in terms of Brofenbrenner's models (see Bronfenbrenner & Morris, 1998; Card et al., in press) will provide a useful framework for considering these risk factors. Further basic and applied research on these risk factors, although challenging, is needed if we are to improve the effectiveness of current efforts to prevent or intervene in children's victimization by peers.

References

Abecassis, M., Hartup, W. W., Haselager, G. J. T., Scholte, R. H. J., & Van Lieshout, C. F. M. (2002). Mutual antipathies and their developmental significance. *Child Development*, 73, 1543–1556.

Aber, J. L., Jones, S. M., Brown, J. L., Chaundry, N., & Samples, F. (1998). Resolving conflict creatively: Evaluating the developmental effects of a school-based violence prevention program in neighborhood and classroom context. *Development and Psychopathology*, 10, 187–213.

Archer, J. & Coyne, S. M. (2005). An integrated review of indirect, relational, and social aggression. *Personality and Social Psychology Review*, 9, 212–230.

Astor, R. A., Meyer, H. A., & Behre, W. J. (1999). Unowned places and times: Maps and interviews about violence in high schools. *American Educational Research Journal*, 36, 3–42.

Baldry, A. C. & Farrington, D. P. (1999). Types of bullying among Italian school children. *Journal of Adolescence*, 22, 423–426.

Berdondini, L. & Smith, P. K. (1996). Cohesion and power in the families of children involved in bully/victim problems at school: An Italian replication. *Journal of Family Therapy*, 18, 99–102.

Besag, V. (2002). Parents and teachers working together. In M. Elliot (Ed.), *Bullying: A Practical Guide to Coping for Schools* (pp. 114–125). London: Pearson Education.

Boivin, M., Hymel, S., & Bukowski, W. M. (1995). The roles of social withdrawal, peer rejection, and victimization by peers in predicting loneliness and depressed mood in childhood. *Development and Psychopathology*, 7, 765–786.

Bond, L., Carlin, J. B., Thomas, L., Rubin, K., & Patton, G. (2001). Does bullying cause emotional problems: A prospective study of young teenagers. *British Medical Journal*, 323, 480–484.

Borg, M. G. (1999). The extent and nature of bullying among primary and secondary school children. *Educational Research*, 40, 137–153.

Boulton, M. J. (1995). Patterns of bully/victim problems in mixed race groups of children. *Social Development*, 4, 277–293.

Boulton, M. J. (1999). Concurrent and longitudinal relations between children's playground behavior and social preference, victimization, and bullying. *Child Development*, 70, 944–954.

Boulton, M. J. & Smith, P. K. (1994). Bully/victim problems in middle-school children: Stability, self-perceived competence, peer perceptions, and peer acceptance. *British Journal of Developmental Psychology*, 12, 315–329.

Boulton, M. J., Trueman, M., Chau, C., Whitehand, C., & Amatya, K. (1999). Concurrent and longitudinal links between friendships and peer victimization: Implications for befriending interventions. *Journal of Adolescence*, 22, 461–466.

Bowers, L., Smith, P. K., & Binney, V. (1994). Perceived family relationships of bullies, victims, and bully/victims in middle school. *Journal of Social and Personal Relationships*, 11, 215–232.

Bronfenbrenner, U. (1977). Toward an experimental ecology of human development. *American Psychologist*, 32, 513–531.

Bronfenbrenner, U. (1986). Ecology of the family as a context for human development: Research perspectives. *Developmental Psychology*, 22, 723–742.

Bronfenbrenner, U. & Crouter, A. C. (1983). The evolution of environmental models in developmental research. In P. H. Mussen (Series Ed.) & W. Kessen (Volume Ed.), *Handbook of Child Psychology: History, Theory, and Methods*, Vol. 1 (pp. 357–414). New York: Wiley.

Bronfenbrenner, U. & Morris, P. A. (1998). The ecology of developmental processes. In W. Damon (series ed.) & R. M. Lerner (volume ed.), *Handbook of Child Psychology: Theoretical Models of Human Development*, Vol. 1 (pp. 993–1028). New York: Wiley.

Buhs, E. S. & Ladd, G. W. (2001). Peer rejection as an antecedent of young children's social adjustment: An examination of mediating processes. *Developmental Psychology*, 37, 550–560.

Burk, F. L. (1897). Teasing and bullying. *Pedagogical Seminary*, 4, 336–371.

Byrne, B. (1994). Bullies and victims in a school setting with specific reference to some Dublin schools. *Irish Journal of Psychology*, 15, 73–87.

Card, N. A. (2003). Victims of peer aggression: A meta-analytic review. Poster presented at the biennial meeting of the Society for Research in Child Development, Tampa, FL.

Card, N. A. & Hodges, E. V. E. (2005). Power differential in aggressor-victim relationships. In N. A. Card & E. V. E. Hodges (Chairs), *Aggressor-Victim Relationships: Toward a Dyadic Perspective*. Paper Presented at the Biennial Meeting of the Society for Research in Child Development, Atlanta, GA.

Card, N. A. & Hodges, E. V. E. (2006). Shared targets for aggression by early adolescent friends. *Developmental Psychology*, 42, 1327–1338.

Card, N. A. & Hodges, E. V. E. (2007). Victimization within mutually antipathetic peer relationships. *Social Development*, 16, 479–496.

Card, N. A. & Little, T. D. (2006a). Proactive and reactive aggression in childhood and adolescence: A meta-analysis of differential relations with psychosocial adjustment. *International Journal of Behavioral Development*, 30, 466–480.

Card, N. A. & Little, T. D. (2006b). Analytic considerations in cross-cultural research on peer relations. In X. Chen, D. C. French, & B. Schneider (Eds.), *Peer Relations in Cultural Context* (pp. 75–95). New York: Cambridge University Press.

Card, N. A., Isaacs, J., & Hodges, E. V. E. (2007). Correlates of school victimization: Recommendations for prevention and intervention. In J. E. Zins, M. J. Elias, & C. A. Maher (Eds.), *Bullying, Victimization, and Peer Harassment: A Handbook of Prevention and Intervention* (pp. 339–368). New York: Haworth Press.

Card, N. A., Little, T. D., & Bovaird, J. A. (2007). Modeling ecological and contextual effects in longitudinal studies of human development. To appear In T. D. Little, J. A. Bovaird, & N. A. Card (2007). *Modeling Ecological and Contextual Effects in Longitudinal Studies of Human Development* (pp. 1–11). Mahwah, NJ: Lawrence Erlbaum.

Card, N. A., Stucky, B. D., Sawalani, G. M., & Little, T. D. (2007). Direct and Indirect Aggression During Childhood and Adolescence: *A Meta-Analytic Review of Gender Differences, Intercorrelations, and Relations to Maladjustment*. Manuscript submitted for publication.

Cavell, T. A. & Hughes, J. N. (2000). Secondary prevention as context for assessing change processes in aggressive children. *Journal of School Psychology*, 38, 199–235.

Chesney-Lind, M. & Belknap, J. (2004). Trends in delinquent girls' aggression and violent behavior: A review of the evidence. In M. Putallaz & K. L. Bierman (Eds.), *Aggression, Antisocial Behavior, and Violence Among Girls: A Developmental Perspective* (pp. 203–220). New York: Guilford.

Choi, J. N. (2003). How does context influence individual behavior? Multilevel assessment of the implementation of social innovations. *Prevention & Treatment*, 6, No Pagination Specified. (DOI: 10.1037/1522–3736.6.1.623c).

Coie, J. D., Cillessen, A. H. N., Dodge, K. A., Hubbard, J. A., Schwartz, D., Lemerise, E. A., & Bateman, H. (1999). It takes two to fight: A test of relational factors and a method for assessing aggressive dyads. *Developmental Psychology*, 35, 1179–1188.

Craig, W. M. & Pepler, D. J. (1995). Peer processes in bullying and victimization: An observational study. *Exceptionality Education Canada*, 5, 81–95.

Craig, W. M., Pepler, D., & Atlas, R. (2000). Observations of bullying in the playground and in the classroom. *School Psychology International*, 21, 22–36.

Crick, N. R. & Bigbee, M. A. (1998). Relational and overt forms of peer victimization: A multiinformant approach. *Journal of Consulting and Clinical Psychology*, 66, 337–347.

Crick, N. R. & Grotpeter, J. K. (1996). Children's treatment by peers: Victims of relational and overt aggression. *Development and Psychopathology*, 8, 367–380.

Cummings, E. M., Davies, P. T., & Campbell, S. B. (2000). *Developmental Psychopathology and Family Process: Theory, Research, and Clinical Implications*. New York: Guilford Press.

Dhami, M. K., Hoglund, W. L., Leadbeater, B. J., & Boone, E. M. (2005). Gender-linked risks for peer physical victimization in the context of school-level poverty in first grade. *Social Development*, 14, 532–549.

Dishion, T. J. & Andrews, D. W. (1995). Preventing escalation in problem behaviors with high-risk young adolescents: Immediate and 1-year outcomes. *Journal of Consulting and Clinical Psychology*, 63, 538–548.

Dodge, K. A., Price, J. M., Coie, J. D., & Christopoulos, C. (1990). On the development of aggressive dyadic relationships in boys' peer groups. *Human Development*, 33, 260–270.

Dolan, L., Turkkan, J., Werthamer-Larrson, L., & Kellam, S. G. (1989). *The Good Behavior Game Training Manual*. Baltimore, MD: The John Hopkins Prevention Research Center.

Duncan, R. D. (1999). Maltreatment by parents and peers. The relationship between child abuse, bully-victimization, and psychological distress. *Child Maltreatment*, 4, 45–55.

Egan, S. K. & Perry, D. G. (1998). Does low self-regard invite victimization? *Developmental Psychology*, 34, 299–309.

Elder, G. H., Jr. (1997). The life course and human development. In W. Damon (Series Ed.) & R. M. Lerner (Volume Ed.), *Handbook of Child Psychology* (5th edition, Vol. 1, pp. 939–992). New York: Wiley.

Eslea, M. & Smith, P. K. (1998). The long-term effectiveness of anti-bullying work in primary schools. *Educational Research*, 40, 203–218.

Eslea, M., Menesini, E., Morita, Y., O'Moore, M., Mora-Merchán, J. A., Pereira, B., & Smith, P. K. (2004). Friendship and loneliness among bullies and victims. Data from seven countries. *Aggressive Behavior*, 30, 71–83.

Espelage, D. L. & Swearer, S. M. (Eds.) (2004). *Bullying in American Schools: A Social-Ecological Perspective on Prevention and Intervention*. Mahwah, NJ: Lawrence Erlbaum Associates.

Fauth, R. C., Leventhal, T., & Brooks-Gunn, J. (2005). Early impacts of moving from poor to middle-class neighborhoods on low-income youth. *Applied Developmental Psychology*, 26, 415–439.

Fekkes, M., Pijpers, F. I. M., & Verloove-Vanhorick, S. P. (2005). Bullying: Who does what, when and where? Involvement of children, teachers and parents in bullying behavior. *Health Education Research: Theory & Practice*, 20, 81–91.

Finnegan, R. A., Hodges, E. V. E., & Perry, D. G. (1996). Preoccupied and avoidant coping during middle childhood. *Child Development*, 67, 1318–1328.

Finnegan, R. A., Hodges, E. V. E., & Perry, D. G. (1998). Victimization by peers: Associations with children's reports of mother-child interaction. *Journal of Personality and Social Psychology*, 75, 1076–1086.

Finkelhor, D. & Dziuba-Leatherman, J. (1994). Victimization of children. *American Psychologist*, 49, 173–183.

Finkelhor, D., Ormrod, R., Turner, H., Hamby, S. L. (2005). The victimization of children and youth: A comprehensive, national survey. *Child Maltreatment*, 10, 5–25.

Flannery, D. J., Vazsonyi, A. T., Liau, A. K., Guo, S., Powell, K. E., Atha, H., Vesterdal, W., & Embry, D. (2003). Initial behavior outcomes for the PeaceBuilders universal school-based violence prevention program. *Developmental Psychology*, 39, 292–308.

Flouri, E. & Buchanan, A. (2002). Life satisfaction in teenage boys: The moderating role of father involvement and bullying. *Aggressive Behavior*, 28, 126–133.

Forgatch, M. S. (2003). Implementation as a second stage in prevention research. *Prevention & Treatment*, 6, No Pagination Specified (DOI: 10.1037/1522–3736.6.1.624c).

Fraser, M. W., Galinsky, M. J., Smokowski, P. R., Day, S. H., Terzian, M. A., Rose, R. A., & Guo, S. (2005). Social information-processing skills training to promote social competence and prevent aggressive behavior in the third grades. *Journal of Consulting and Clinical Psychology*, 73, 1045–1055.

Frey, K. S., Hirschstein, M. K., Snell, J. L., Edstrom, L. V. S., MacKenzie, E. P., & Broderick, C. J. (2005) Reducing playground bullying and supporting beliefs: An experimental trial of the Steps to Respect Program. *Developmental Psychology*, 41, 479–491.

Graham, S. & Juvonen, J. (1998). Self-blame and peer victimization in middle school: An attributional analysis. *Developmental Psychology*, 34, 587–599.

Hanish, L. D. & Guerra, N. G. (2000). Predictors of peer victimization among urban youth. *Social Development*, 9, 521–543.

Haselager, G. J. T., Hartup, W. W., van Lieshout, C. F. M., & Riksen-Walraven, J. M. (1998). Similarities between friends and nonfriends in middle school. *Child Development*, 69, 1198–1204.

Haynie, D. L., Nansel, T., Eitel, P., Crump, A. D., Saylor, K., Yu, K., & Simons-Morton, B. (2001). Bullies, victims, and bully/victims: Distinct groups of at-risk youth. *Journal of Early Adolescence*, 21, 29–49.

Hazler, R. J. (1996). *Breaking the Cycle of Violence: Interventions for Bullying and Victimization*. Washington, DC: Accelerated Development.

Hazler, R. J., Hoover, J. H., & Oliver, R. (1991). Student perceptions of victimization by bullies in school. *Journal of Humanistic Education and Development*, 29, 143–150.

Hewitt, J. (1995). Sources of variance affecting receipt of aggression. *Perceptual and Motor Skills*, 81, 751–754.

Hodges, E. V. E. & Perry, D. G. (1999). Personal and interpersonal consequences of victimization by peers. *Journal of Personality and Social Psychology*, 76, 677–685.

Hodges, E. V. E., Malone, M. J., & Perry, D. G. (1997). Individual risk and social risk as interacting determinants of victimization in the peer group. *Developmental Psychology*, 33, 1032–1039.

Hodges, E. V. E., Boivin, M., Vitaro, F., & Bukowski, W. M. (1999a). The power of friendship: Protection against an escalating cycle of peer victimization. *Developmental Psychology*, 35, 94–101.

Hodges, E. V. E., Finnegan, R. A., & Perry, D. G. (1999b). Skewed autonomy-relatedness in preadolescents' conceptions of their relationships with mother, father, and best friend. *Developmental Psychology*, 35, 737–748.

Hodges, E. V. E., Card, N. A., & Isaacs, J. (2003). Learning of aggression in the family and in the peer group. In W. Heitmeyer & J. Hagan (Eds.) *International Handbook of Violence Research* (pp. 495–510). Netherlands: Kluwer Academic Publishers.

Hubbard, J. A., Dodge, K. A., Cillessen, A. H. N., Coie, J. D., & Schwartz, D. (2001). The dyadic nature of social information processing in boys' reactive and proactive aggression. *Journal of Personality and Social Psychology*, 80, 268–280.

Hughes, J. N., Cavell, T. A., Meehan, B. T., Zhang, D., & Collie, C. (2005). Adverse school context moderates the outcomes of selective interventions for aggressive children. *Journal of Consulting and Clinical Psychology*, 73, 731–736.

Jacobson, J. L. & Wille, D. E. (1996). The influence of attachment pattern on developmental changes in peer interaction from the toddler to the preschool period. *Child Development*, 57, 338–347.

Juvonen, J., Nishina, A., & Graham, S. (2000). Peer harassment, psychological adjustment, and social functioning in early adolescence. *Journal of Educational Psychology*, 92, 349–359.

Kallestad, J. H. & Olweus, D. (2003). Predicting teachers' and schools' implementation of the Olweus Bullying Prevention Program: A multilevel study. *Prevention & Treatment*, 6, No Pagination Specified. (DOI: 10.1037/1522–3736.6.1.621a).

Kellam, S. G., Ling, X., Merisca, R., Brown, C. H., & Ialongo, N. (1998). The effect of the level of aggression in the first grade classroom on the course and malleability of aggressive behavior into middle school. *Development and Psychopathology*, 10, 165–185.

Kochenderfer, B. J. & Ladd, G. W. (1996). Peer victimization: Cause or consequence of school maladjustment? *Child Development*, 67, 1305–1317.

Ladd, G. W. & Kochenderfer-Ladd, B. (1998). Parenting behaviors and parent-child relationships: Correlates of peer victimization in kindergarten? *Developmental Psychology*, 34, 1450–1458.

Ladd, G. W. (2005). *Children's Peer Relations and Social Competence: A Century of Progress*. New Haven, CT: Yale University Press.

Ladd, G. W. & Troop-Gordon, W. (2003). The role of chronic peer difficulties in the development of children's psychological adjustment problems. *Child Development*, 74, 1344–1367.

Lagerspetz, K. M. J., Björkqvist, K., Berts, M., & King, E. (1982). Group aggression among school children in three schools. *Scandinavian Journal of Psychology*, 23, 45–52.

La Greca, A. M. & Harrison, H. M. (2005). Adolescent peer relations, friendship, and romantic relationships: Do they predict social anxiety and depression? *Journal of Clinical Child and Adolescent Psychology*, 34, 49–61.

Little, T. D., Bovaird, J. A., & Card, N. A. (Eds.) (2007). *Modeling Ecological and Contextual Effects in Longitudinal Studies*. Mahwah, NJ: Lawrence Erlbaum Associates.

Ma, X. (2002). Bullying in middle school: Individual and school characteristics of victims and offenders. *School effectiveness and school improvement*, 13, 63–89.

McCabe, K. A. & Martin, G. M. (2005). *School Violence, the Media, and Criminal Justice Responses*. New York: Peter Lang.

Mellor, A. (1990). *Bullying in Scottish Secondary Schools*. Edinburgh: Scottish Council for Research in Education.

Menesini, E., Eslea, M., Smith, P. K., Genta, M. L., Giannetti, E., Fonzi, A., & Costabile, A. (1997). Cross-national comparison of children's attitudes towards bully/victim problems in school. *Aggressive Behavior*, 23, 245–257.

Metropolitan Area Child Study Research Group. (2002). A cognitive-ecological approach to preventing aggression in urban settings: Initial outcomes for high-risk children. *Journal of Consulting and Clinical Psychology*, 70, 179–194.

Mrazek, P. J. & Haggerty, R. J. (Eds.). (1994). *Reducing Risks for Mental Disorders: Frontiers for Preventive Intervention Research*. Washington, DC: National Academy Press.

Nansel, T. R., Overpeck, M., Pilla, R. S., Ruan, W. J., Simons-Morton, B., & Scheidt, P. (2001). Bullying behaviors among US youth: Prevalence and association with psychosocial adjustment. *Journal of the American Medical Association*, 285, 2084.

Nation, M., Crusto, C., Wandersman, A., Kumpfer, K. L., Seybolt, D., Morrissey-Kane, E., & Davino, K. (2003). What works in prevention: Principles of effective prevention programs. *American Psychologist*, 58, 449–456.

Neary, A. & Joseph, S. (1994). Peer victimization and its relationship to self-concept and depression among schoolgirls. *Personality and Individual Differences*, 16, 183–186.

Newman, R. S. & Murray, B. J. (2005). How students and teachers view the seriousness of peer harassment: When is it appropriate to seek help? *Journal of Educational Psychology*, 97, 347–365.

Olweus, D. (1978). *Aggression in the Schools: Bullies and Whipping Boys*. Washington, DC: Hemisphere.

Olweus, D. (1991). Bully/victim problems among schoolchildren: Basic facts and effects of a school based intervention program. In D. Pepler & K. Rubin (Eds.), *The Development and Treatment of Childhood Aggression* (pp. 411–448). Hillsdale, NJ: Erlbaum Associates.

Olweus, D. (1993). *Bullying at School: What we Know and what we can Do*. Malden, MA: Blackwell Publishing.

Olweus, D. (2001). Peer harassment: A critical analysis and some important issues. In J. Juvonen & S. Graham (Eds.), *Peer Harassment in School: The Plight of the Vulnerable and Victimized* (pp. 3–20). New York: Guilford Press.

O'Moore, A. M. & Minton, S. J. (2005). Evaluation of the effectiveness of an anti-bullying pro-gramme in primary schools. *Aggressive Behavior*, 31, 609–622.

O'Moore, A. M., Kirkham, C., & Smith, M. (1997). Bullying behavior in Irish schools: A nation-wide survey. *The Irish Journal of Psychology*, 18, 141–169.

Orpinas, P., Home, A. M., & Staniszewski, D. (2003). School bullying: Changing the problem by changing the school. *School Psychology Review*, 32, 431–444.

Österman, K., Björkqvist, K., Lagerspetz, K. M. J., Kaukiainen, A., Huesmann, L. R., & Fraczek, A. (1994). Peer and self-estimated aggression and victimization in 8-year-old children from five ethnic groups. *Aggressive Behavior*, 20, 411–428.

Parker, J. G. & Gamm, B. K. (2003). Describing the dark side of preadolescents' peer experiences: Four questions (and data) on preadolescents' enemies. In E. V. E. Hodges & N. A. Card (Eds.), *Enemies and the Darker Side of Peer Relations, New Directions for Child and Adolescent Development*, 102, 55–72. San Francisco: Jossey-Bass.

Parke, R. D. & Slaby, R. G. (1983). The development of aggression. In P. H. Mussen (Series Ed.) & E. M. Hetherington (Volume Ed.), *Handbook of Child Psychology* (4th edition, Vol. 4, pp. 547–641). New York: Wiley.

Peebles-Wilkins, W. (2005). Zero tolerance in educational settings. *Children and Schools*, 27, 3.

Pellegrini, A. D. (1995). A longitudinal study of boys' rough-and-tumble play and dominance during early adolescence. *Journal of Applied Developmental Psychology*, 16, 77–93.

Pellegrini, A. D., Bartini, M., & Brooks, F. (1999). School bullies, victims, and aggressive victims: Factors relating to group affiliation and victimization in early adolescence. *Journal of Educational Psychology*, 91, 216–224.

Percy-Smith, B. & Matthews, H. (2001). Tyrannical spaces: Young people, bullying and urban neighborhoods. *Local Environment*, 6, 49–63.

Perren, S. & Hornung, R. (2005). Bullying and delinquency in adolescence: Victims' and perpe-trators' family and peer relations. *Swiss Journal of Psychology*, 64, 51–64.

Perry, D. G., Kusel, S. J., & Perry, L. C. (1988). Victims of peer aggression. *Developmental Psychology*, 24, 807–814.

Perry, D. G., Hodges, E. V. E., & Egan, S. K. (2001). Determinants of chronic victimization by peers: A review and new model of family influence. In J. Juvonen & S. Graham (Eds.), *Peer Harassment in School: The Plight of the Vulnerable and Victimized* (pp. 73–104). New York: Guilford.

Pierce, K. A. & Cohen, R. (1995). Aggressors and their victims: Toward a contextual framework for understanding children's aggressor-victim relationships. *Developmental Review*, 15, 292–310.

Pope, A. W. & Bierman, K. L. (1999). Predicting adolescent peer problems and antisocial activities: The relative roles of aggression and dysregulation. *Developmental Psychology*, 35, 335–346.

Prinstein, M. J., Boergers, J., & Vernberg, E. M. (2001). Overt and relational aggression in ado-lescents: Social-psychological adjustment of aggressors and victims. *Journal of Clinical Child Psychology*, 30, 479–491.

Rigby, K. (1993). School children's perceptions of their families and parents as a function of peer relations. *Journal of Genetic Psychology*, 154, 501–513.

Rigby, K. (2001). Health consequences of bullying and its prevention in school. In J. Juvonen, S. Graham (Eds.), *Peer harassment in school. The plight of the vulnerable and the victimized* (pp. 310–331). New York: Guilford.

Rodkin, P. C. & Hodges, E. V. E. (2003). Bullies and victims in the peer ecology: Four questions for psychologists and school professionals. *School Psychology Review*, 32, 384–400.

Roland, E. (2000). Bullying in school: Three national innovations in Norwegian schools in 15 years. *Aggressive Behavior*, 26, 35–143.

Salmivalli, C. & Issacs, J. (2005). Prospective relations among victimization, rejection, friendless-ness, and children's self- and peer-perceptions. *Child Development*, 76, 1161–1171.

Salmivalli, C. (2001). Group view on victimization: Empirical findings and their implications. In J. Juvonen & S. Graham (Eds.), *Peer Harassment in School: The Plight of the Vulnerable and the Victimized* (pp. 398–419). New York: Guildford Press.

Salmivalli, C., Lagerspetz, K. M. J., Bjorkqvist, K., Osterman, K., & Kaukiainen, A. (1996). Bullying as a group process: Participant roles and their relations to social status within the group. *Aggressive Behavior*, 22, 1–15.

Salmivalli, C., Huttunen, A., & Lagerspetz, K. M. J. (1997). Peer networks and bullying in schools. *Scandinavian Journal of Psychology*, 38, 305–312.

Salmivalli, C., Kaukiainen, A., & Voeten, M. (2005). Anti-bullying intervention: Implementation and outcome. *British Journal of Educational Psychology*, 75, 465–487.

Schwartz, D. & Proctor, L. (2000). Community violence exposure and children's social adjustment in the school peer group: The mediating roles of emotion regulation and social cognition. *Journal of Consulting and Clinical Psychology*, 68, 670–683.

Schwartz, D., Dodge, K. A., & Coie, J. D. (1993). The emergence of chronic peer victimization in boys' play groups. *Child Development*, 64, 1755–1772.

Schwartz, D., Dodge, K. A., Pettit, G. S., & Bates, J. E. (1997). The early socialization of aggressive victims of bullying. *Child Development*, 68, 665–675.

Schwartz, D., Hopmeyer Gorman, A. H., Toblin, R. L., & Abou-ezzedine, T. (2003). Mutual antipathies in the peer group as a moderating factor in the association between community violence exposure and psychosocial maladjustment. In E. V. E. Hodges & N. A. Card (Eds.), *Enemies and the Darker Side of Peer Relations, New Directions for Child and Adolescent Development* (Vol. 102, pp. 39–54). San Francisco: Jossey-Bass.

Sheridan, S. M., Warnes, E. D., & Dowd, S. (2004). Home-school collaboration and bullying: An ecological approach to increase social competence in children and youth. In D. L. Espelage & S. M. Swearer (Eds.), *Bullying in American Schools: A Social-Ecological Perspective on Prevention and Intervention* (pp. 245–268). Mahwah, NJ: Erlbaum.

Shields, A. & Cicchetti, D. (2001). Parental maltreatment and emotion dysregulation as risk factors for bullying and victimization in middle childhood. *Journal of Clinical Child Psychology*, 30, 349–363.

Siann, G., Callaghan, M., Lockhart, R., & Rawson, L. (1993). Bullying: Teachers' views and school effects. *Educational Studies*, 19, 307–321.

Siann, G., Callaghan, M., Glissov, P., Lockhart, R., & Rawson, L. (1994). Who gets bullied? The effect of school, gender and ethnic group. *Educational Research*, 36, 123–134.

Slee, P. T. (1995). Bullying in the playground: The impact of inter-personal violence on Australian children's perceptions of their play environment. *Children's Environments*, 12, 320–327.

Smith, P. K. & Shu, S. (2000). What good schools can do about bullying: Findings from a survey in English schools after a decade of research and action. *Childhood*, 7, 193–212.

Smith, P. K., Morita, Y., Junger-Tas, D., Olweus, D., Catalano, R. F., & Slee, P. T. (Eds.) (1999). *The Nature of School Bullying: A Cross-National Perspective*. New York: Routledge.

Smith, P. K., Cowie, H., Olafsson, R. F., & Liefooghe, A. P. D. (2002). Definitions of bullying: A comparison of terms used, and age and gender differences, in a fourteen-country international comparison. *Child Development*, 73, 1119–1133.

Smith, P. K., Ananiadou, K., & Cowie, H. (2003). Interventions to reduce school bullying. *Canadian Journal of Psychiatry*, 48, 591–599.

Smith, J. D., Schneider, B. H., Smith, P. K., & Ananiadou, K. (2004). The effectiveness of whole-school antibullying programs: A synthesis of evaluation research. *School Psychology Review*, 33, 547–560.

Spilsbury, J. C. (2005). Children's perceptions of the social support of neighborhood institutions and establishments. *Human Organization*, 64, 126–134.

Stephenson, P. & Smith, D. (2002). Why some schools don't have bullies. In M. Elliot (Ed.), *Bullying: A Practical Guide to Coping for Schools* (pp. 12–25). London: Pearson Education.

Stevens, V., De Bourdeaudhuij, I., & Van Oost, P. (2000). Bullying in Flemish schools: An evaluation of anti-bullying intervention in primary and secondary schools. *British Journal of Educational Psychology*, 70, 195–210.

Tolan, P., Gorman-Smith, D., & Henry, D. (2004). Supporting families in a high-risk setting: Proximal effects of the SAFEChildren preventive intervention. *Journal of Consulting and Clinical Psychology*, 72, 855–869.

Tolan, P. H., Guerra, N. G., & Kendall, P. C. (1995). Introduction to Special Section: Prediction and prevention of antisocial behavior in children and adolescents. *Journal of Consulting and Clinical Psychology*, 63, 515–517.

Troy, M. & Sroufe, L. A. (1987). Victimization among preschoolers: Role of attachment relationship history. *Journal of the American Academy of Child and Adolescent Psychiatry*, 26, 166–172.

Verkuyten, M. & Thijs, J. (2002). Racist victimization among children in The Netherlands: The effect of ethnic group and school. *Ethnic and Racial Studies*, 25, 310–331.

Wandersman, A. & Florin, P. (2003). Community interventions and effective prevention. *American Psychologist*, 58, 441–448.

Whitney, I. & Smith, P. K. (1993). A survey of the nature and extent of bullying in junior/middle and secondary schools. *Educational Research*, 35, 3–25.

Wolke, D., Woods, S., Stanford, K., Schulz, H. (2001). Bullying and victimization of primary school children in England and Germany: Prevalence and school factors. *British Journal of Psychology*, 92, 673–696.

Chapter 8
Assessment of Childhood Sexual Abuse: Clinical Measures, Evaluation, and Treatment

Mark V. Sapp

Childhood sexual abuse (CSA) is a global problem of epidemic proportion affecting children of all ages, races, and economic and cultural backgrounds. Research over the past several decades has focused on documenting prevalence rates, improving tools for medical and psychological evaluations, and understanding the short- and long-term consequences of CSA. A better understanding of the populations at greatest risk and a greater awareness of the short- and long-term effects of CSA will ultimately lead to improved outcomes for all victimized children.

Many problems and challenges however remain. Greater focus on the relationship between teenage violence and sexual assault and the impact child and adolescent victimization has on the patients, their families, and communities is needed. Medical curricula on a national level are now addressing sexual abuse and are stressing the need for multidisciplinary teams, including law-enforcement, social service workers, and medical and mental health personnel, as mandatory first responders in the management of child and adolescent sexual assault. A well-coordinated multidisciplinary approach fosters open communication between all disciplines serving the child victims and maximizes opportunities for assessment and intervention. Although the field of child and adolescent sexual abuse has expanded tremendously over the past several decades, this growth only recently has begun to focus on the greater awareness and services which are needed for improved management and treatment of all sexual abuse survivors. Sexual abuse, assault, and sexual victimization, particularly of children and adolescents, remains but one area of child abuse work still in great need of enhanced research and services (Heger et al., 2000).

Defining the Problem

Understanding the definition of childhood sexual abuse, sexual assault, rape, acquaintance rape, date rape, and statutory rape are important not only for the identification of victims but also to ensure appropriate treatment and management of the adolescent victim (American Academy of Pediatrics, 2001). Prevalence rates for child sexual abuse are difficult to obtain and estimates of prevalence vary widely. Although clinical and nonclinical population-based studies have been documented, no accepted methodology for estimating prevalence exists (Gorey & Leslie, 1997). Many young victims may be particularly reluctant to report sexual assault because of embarrassment, fear of retribution, feelings of guilt, or a lack of knowledge regarding victim's rights. The adolescent victim may also feel he or she contributed to the abuse or may not identify what happened as rape because the experience did not fit a popular concept of sexual assault (The Commonwealth Fund, 1997). Many developing countries may lack the economic resources to maintain reporting systems and manage cases of sexual abuse (Johnson, 2004).

Sexual Abuse

Sexual abuse is generally defined as any sexual activity (including vaginal/anal intercourse, oral–genital contact, genital–genital contact, fondling, and exposure to pornography or to adults engaging in sexual activity) involving a child who is unable to give consent (Johnson, 2002). In the United States (USA), all states receiving federal government funding are required to report data regarding the maltreatment of children, including reporting all cases of alleged sexual abuse. In the year 2000, 879,000 children from 34 states (representing 78.1% of the child population in the USA) were estimated to have been maltreated. Of that total, 10.1% or 88,000 children were victims of sexual abuse (US Department of Health and Human Services, 2002). Three decades of research estimate the overall prevalence of CSA world-wide to range from 11% to 32% for females and 4% to 14% for males (Gustafson & Sarwer, 2004). Meta-analysis of studies conducted in North America between 1969 and 1991 found that 22.3% of women and 8.5% of men reported experiencing CSA (Gorey & Leslie, 1997).

Prevalence rates of CSA internationally suggest that the problem is global in scope (Lalor, 2004). The incidence of sexual abuse in Europe has been estimated as 6–36% in females and 1–15% in males younger than 16 years of age (Johnson, 2002). Other regions of the world are plagued by political unrest and economic instability with little resources for government-funded social service programs. A South African population-based study reported nearly one-third of all adolescent females as victims of rape or sexual coercion (Jewkes & Abrahams, 2002). The number of children exploited through child prostitution is also unknown though some estimates are as high as 1–10 million children worldwide (Willis & Levy, 2002). Researchers are challenged to use these data to support the development of sexual abuse intervention and prevention programs which can be implemented worldwide (Lalor, 2004).

Sexual Assault

The National Institute of Justice estimates ~1 million new cases of sexual assault and rape each year in the USA alone. A significant percentage of these cases are adolescent and child victims. A survey of American high school students found

20% of all students questioned reporting at least one episode of forced sexual contact (Greydanus et al., 1987). A study conducted in Canada on female adolescents found similar results, with 23% of the young women reporting at least one episode of unwanted sexual contact (Bagley et al, 1997). Researchers estimate that ~74% of women who had sexual intercourse before age 14 and 60% of women who had sex before age 15 likely had sex involuntarily at some earlier time point in their lives (Alan Guttmacher Institute, 1994).

The American Academy of Pediatrics defines sexual assault as any situation in which there is sexual contact with or without penetration that occurs because of physical force or psychological coercion (American Academy of Pediatrics, Committee on Adolescence, 1994). Sexual assault is also defined as forced or coerced (1) vaginal or anal penetration by an object, finger, or penis, (2) oral sex, (3) breast or genitalia fondling, or (4) forced or coerced touching of another person's genitalia (Kilpatrick et al., 2003). The National Survey of Adolescents found 8% of 4,023 adolescents interviewed reported being victims of at least one sexual assault, representing 13% of the females and 3.4% of the males completing the survey (Kilpatrick et al., 2000). The National Victims Center (1992) and the Department of Justice (Langan, 1994) report that adolescents have the highest reported rates of sexual assault, more than 50–60% of all cases. Emmert and colleagues found girls at the highest risk were between the age of 11and 15 years having a stepfather in the home, although most girls older than 15 years were assaulted by a stranger. More than 25% of the adolescent assault victims showed signs of physical trauma, with face and neck as the most common sites of contact. A total of 17.5% reported threats of violence or use of a weapon, and 9.7% of assault encounters had alcohol as an influencing factor (Emmert & Kohler, 1998).

Studies reveal that as many as 95% of the sexual assault victims do not report their unwanted sexual encounter to the authorities, although three-quarter of the victims do tell another person (Fisher et al., 2000). In a broader analysis on sex crimes against women and an analysis of intimate partner violence, about four-fifth (80%) of rapes were unreported to the police (Tjaden & Thoennes, 2000, 1998). In comparison to adult rape victims, adolescent rape victims are more likely to have used alcohol or drugs and are less likely to be physically injured, as perpetrators of adolescent sexual assault are less likely to use weapons. Adolescent female victims are also more likely to delay seeking medical care and are less likely to press charges than adult victims (Peipert & Domagalski, 1994; Muram et al., 1995).

Rape

From both a legal and clinical perspective, rape is defined as "forced sexual intercourse" that occurs because of physical force or psychological coercion. Rape involves vaginal, anal, or oral penetration by the offender and may include penetration with a foreign object, such as a bottle, or situations in which the victim is unable to give consent because of intoxication or developmental disability (American Academy of Pediatrics, Committee on Adolescence, 1994; Perkins & Klaus, 1996).

Like sexual assault, a large percentage of rapes are never reported to the police and more than 50% of rape victims tell no one of their abuse. Only 5% of rape victims visit a rape crisis center (Bureau of Justice statistics, 1996; Koss & Harvey, 1991). Rape is also a crime against many children and adolescents as studies have shown that estimates are as high as 50% of all rape victims being under the age of 18 and 16% under the age of 12 years (Langan, 1994). More than 75% of adolescent rapes are committed by an acquaintance of the victim, with less than 25% committed by a stranger (National Victim Center, 1992; Heise, 1993). Historically, the definition of rape has been gender specific, referring to the forced penetration of a female by a male assailant. Many states have now abandoned this concept in favor of the gender-neutral term of sexual assault. Thus, the legal definition of criminal sexual assault is any genital, oral, or anal penetration by a part of the accused's body or by an object, using force or without the victim's consent (American Medical Association, 1995).

Acquaintance Rape

Intimate partner violence occurs at a staggering rate of 4.4 million women assaulted by male partners at some point during adulthood (National Institute of Justice, 1998). Research indicates that adolescents are not immune to intimate partner violence and ~45.5% of females and 43.2% of male high school students report that they have been victims of physical aggression by dating partners at least once (O'Keefe et al., 1986; O'Keefe & Treister, 1998). Other studies conducted in US high schools have revealed that a substantial number of adolescents have experienced some from of sexual assault in a dating relationship. The Sexual Experience Survey, administered to 6,159 women and men enrolled in 32 higher education institutions across the USA, revealed that since the age of 14 years, 27.5% of college women had experienced an act that met the legal definition of rape and 7.7% of college men had committed such an act (Koss et al., 1987). The vast majority of sexual assaults committed on college campuses are perpetrated by boyfriends, friends, or acquaintances of the victim, with more than 59% occurring on a date (Abbey, 1991). Acquaintance rape among younger adolescents is frequently incestuous, with United States Bureau of Justice Statistics reporting 20% of rape victims aged 12–17 years were attacked by a family member (Langan & Harlow, 1994).

Frequency and severity of violence among intimate partners have been shown to increase if the pattern has been established in adolescence (Feld & Straus, 1989). Psychological abuse defined as monopolization, degradation, and isolation that occurred at least once in a relationship was reported by 82% of girls and 76% of boys in a recent study looking at adolescent violence and sexual coercion (Jackson et al., 2000). By definition, acquaintance rape refers to sexual abuse committed by someone known to the victim, such as a date, teacher, employer, or family member. Assault by a perpetrator related to the victim is generally defined as incest. Although incest refers to sexual intercourse among family members, or those legally barred from marriage, this definition has been broadened to also include step-relatives and parental figures living in the home (Hibbard & Orr, 1985). The highest incidence of acquaintance rape seems to be among girls in the 12th grade and young women in the first year of college.

Date Rape

Date rape is considered a subset of acquaintance rape and generally refers to forced or unwanted sexual activity that occurs within a dating relationship (Hibbard & Orr, 1985). Researchers at the Harvard School of Public Health have reported an increased incidence of intimate partner violence among sexually experienced adolescent girls. Adolescent girls intentionally hurt by a date or intimate partner in the previous year were found to be more likely to experience sexual heath risks, including increased vulnerability to human immunodeficiency virus (HIV) infections and other sexually transmitted infections (STIs) (Silverman et al., 2001). Other studies found similar results regarding the associations of both severe dating violence and sexual abuse history with pregnancy and sexual risks among adolescents (Coker et al., 2000; Raj et al., 2000; Shrier et al., 1998). Adolescent victims of dating violence were less likely to use condoms consistently or negotiating condom use, suggesting a possible coercive role on the part of the male dating partner, resulting in an increased incidence of unsafe sex practices (Wingood et al., 2001).

Drug-Facilitated Sexual Assault

In the past decade, the phenomenon of drug-facilitated sexual assault has surfaced and receiving significant media coverage. Alcohol and drug use immediately before a sexual assault has been reported by more than 40% of adolescent victims and adolescent assailants (Seifert, 1999). Victims, often young women, are given a drug surreptitiously, or in some cases may have taken the drug recreationally causing stupor and even an unconsciousness state. Victims may also experience significant amnesia, making it difficult for a victim to recall any of the details of what happened. The young woman is then raped while under the influence of certain drugs often with little to no recollection of the assault. Illicit drugs commonly identified in this context are flunitrazepam (Rohypnol, "roofies"), gamma-hydroxybutyrate (GHB), ketamine (special K), and other benzodiazepines such as clonazepam (Gaensslen & Lee, 2001; Nicholson et al., 2001). The effects of flunitrazepam begin 30 min after ingestion, peaks within 2 h, and can persist for up to 9–12 h. Drug effects include somnolence, decreased anxiety, muscle relaxation, and profound sedation (Seifert, 1999; Schwartz & Weaver, 1998; Anglin et al., 1997; Druid, 2001). The Drug-Induced Rape Prevention and Punishment Act of 1996 increases penalties for those who use controlled substances to commit rape (Drug Induced Rape Prevention and Punishment Act of 1996).

Statutory Rape

Statutory rape is defined as consensual sexual intercourse between a person 18 years or older and a person under the age of legal consent (American Academy of Pediatrics, Committee on Adolescence, 1994). Statutory rape laws are based on the premise that until a person reaches a certain age, he or she is legally incapable of consenting to sexual intercourse. The age at which an adolescent may consent to sexual intercourse varies from state to state and ranges from 14 to 18 years. The consent of an individual younger than this age range is legally irrelevant because he or she is defined as being incapable of consenting. Data from the National Maternal and Infant Health Survey indicate that 24% of births to 17-year-old women, 27% of births to 16-year-old girls, and 40% of births to 14-year-olds were fathered by men at least 5 years older (Small & Kerns, 1993; Donovan, 1997).

Earlier concerns over a possible link between statutory rape and teen pregnancy led many states to enact legislature requiring mandatory reporting of statutory rape as child abuse. In 1996, Congress enacted amendments to the federal Child Abuse Prevention and Treatment Act (CAPTO) which changed the definition of rape to include some forms of statutory rape. Clinicians and health care providers have voiced concern about the impact increased statutory rape reporting and enforcement may have on the adolescents' access to health care. Researchers have looked at the effects of increased criminalization of statutory rape and have not found any associated improvement in the child welfare system or health care access involving adolescents (Teare & English, 2002). Furthermore, researchers have found no proven link or relationship between expanded statutory rape laws, increased mandatory reporting, and the incidence of teenage pregnancy (Teare & English, 2002). Concern remains that the new laws and mandatory reporting statutes may have a significant impact on the interaction between the health care providers and the adolescent patient. Some adolescents may refuse to seek medical care or disclose personal risk information because of possible reporting of the sexual partner (Ford & Millstein, 1997; Donovan, 1997).

Populations at Risk

Sexual Exploitation/Prostitution

Teenage prostitution is one of the nation's least recognized public health epidemics (Wurbacher et al., 1991). It is estimated that at any given period ~325,000 children nationwide are sexually exploited through prostitution and/or pornography (Nadon, 1998; English, 2006 (Yates et al., 1991a). By some accounts, this number is as high as 900,000 (Monte, 2004). Criminal justice data estimates that 25% of all individuals involved in sex work are under the age of 18, with an estimated age of entry into sexual exploitation as young as 13 (Nadon et al., 1998). Research suggests that nearly one-third of this nation's runaway youth (yearly estimate of 1.5 million) have had some involvement or exposure to prostitution or pornography (English, 2006). This sector of America's youth is not only a divers group representing all races, economic and cultural backgrounds, but these young individuals are seriously underserved with limited available medical resources (English, 2006; Willis & Levy, 2002; Barrett, 1999; Roy et al., 2004; Unger et al., 1998). Sexually exploited youth sustain life and daily living through high-risk behaviors with little or no direct medical care. Data on the global health problems associated with child prostitution identify infectious disease, pregnancy, mental illness, substance abuse, violence, and malnutrition as the major adverse health effects of childhood prostitution (Willis & Levy, 2002).

Work in the sex industry place youth at a high risk for sexually transmitted diseases (STDs) and HIV (Yates et al., 1991b; Tyler et al., 2004). Annual estimates worldwide are as high as 2 million cases of STIs in prostituted children. Three hundred thousand cases of HIV infection, 500,000 cases of hepatitis B virus (HBV), and 4.5 million new cases of human papilloma virus (HPV) are estimated annually worldwide (Willis & Levy, 2002). Morbidity and mortality associated with these infections is staggering and only likely to increase in large part secondary to the paucity of adequate and accessible medical services available to this high-risk population of children. Prostituted children who are infected with an STI that causes genital ulcers, such as syphilis or chancroid, have a fourfold increased risk of HIV infection, and a single act of unprotected sex with an HIV-infected person can result in transmission to that youth (The Alan Guttmacher Institute, 1999; World Health Organization, 2000). Lack of medical services for children with STDs only increases their risk of acquiring both HIV and additional STDs since the majority of these children will remain untreated. The US accounts for ~15% of the world's exploited children and thus we are facing a health care crisis located in our own backyard and not limited simply to third world underserved countries. Currently most sex work has a strong economic basis, primarily as a source of income not only for sex workers but also for dependent kin and associates, including pimps, managers, and ancillary workers (Aral et al., 2003).

IV Drug Use/ Incarceration

Prevalence rates for sexual abuse are higher in other vulnerable populations such as intravenous (IV) drug users, incarcerated youth, and homeless and runaway teens. Studies evaluating both prevalence of sexual assault and factors associated with sexual violence found that 36% of IV drug-using men and women had a lifetime history of sexual violence (68% for women and 19% for men), with the prevalence of sexual assault being 21% (33% for women and 13% for men) (Braitstein et al., 2003). Among incarcerated youth, another vulnerable sample, victimization and perpetration rates of sexual abuse were also found to be higher than in the general population (Morris et al., 2002). For those with a history of sexual assault at any age, victimization was strongly associated with a variety of HIV risk factors such as prostitution and knowingly using HIV-infected equipment. A significantly high prevalence rate of HIV in those with a history of sexual assault (25.3%) compared to those individuals without assault histories (19.1%) is well documented (Morris et al., 2002).

Street Youth

Many young people in the USA run to the street with dreams of finding jobs and new lives away from dysfunctional and abusive families. Running away today is often associated with a child or youth's desire to escape a place and a life where he or she feels abused, rejected, or unwanted. Life in the street, however, is often a life characterized by hunger, prostitution, chronic illness, violence, and the threat of HIV/AIDS (Shane, 1989). Research among street youth 12–19 years of age who were recruited from the streets in Denver, New York City, and San Francisco as part of an HIV/AIDS prevention program found prevalence rates for sexual abuse for female respondents at 35% and males at 24%. The mean age of first sexual abuse encounter was 9.0 years for females and 9.9 for males. This study also found that respondents were more likely to report sexual abuse while living at home than while living on the street. Of the youth studied who reported positive histories of sexual abuse, 85% reported sexual abuse while living at home, 48% reported sexual abuse while living on the street, and 33% of this study cohort reported abuse both at home and on the street. Significantly higher rates of suicide attempts among homeless and runaway youth who were sexually abused or physically abused before leaving home were also noted (Molnar et al., 1998). Whatever the motivation or reason for leaving home, compelling research begs for enhanced medical and social interventions to ultimately decrease the overall morbidity and long-term medical and mental health sequelae which frequently accompany life on the streets (Kral et al., 1997).

Adolescent Perceptions and Attitudes

Adolescence is a time of rapid physical growth and social development and many teens have not yet acquired the skills needed to recognize and avoid potentially danger-ous dating or social situations. Because some teens are viewed as a voluntary sexual participant until an assault occurs, aggressive behaviors may be viewed by some as normative in this context (Kershner, 1996; Small & Kerns, 1993). Adolescent males and females may bring different expectations to dating situations and attribute different meanings to the same behaviors based on past experiences (Hibbard & Orr, 1985). Cassidy et al. found that adolescents who were presented a vignette of unwanted sexual activity accompanied by a photograph of the victim dressed in provocative clothing were more likely to conclude that the victim was in part responsible for the assault, was more likely to view the assailant's behavior as justified, and was less likely to interpret the unwanted sexual experience as rape (Cassidy & Hurrell, 1995). In a separate study addressing adolescent attitudes toward violence and sex, 32% of the women surveyed believed forced sex was acceptable if the couple had been dating a long time, 31% believed the unwanted sexual activity was acceptable if the woman agreed to have sex with her partner but later changed her mind, and 27% of the females believed forced sex was acceptable if the women "led him on." In the same study, 54% of the young men questioned believed that forced sex was acceptable if his date or young woman said "yes" even though she later changed her mind. Forty percent of these men also believed that forced sex was acceptable if the man had spent a lot of money on the date (Parrot, 1989). The acquaintance rape/date rape phenomenon has presented new challenges and opportunities to providers and individuals who work with teens and young adults, sounding the wake-up call for increased education and guidance around physical, sexual, and social development and behavior.

Indicators of Possible Sexual Abuse and Assault

The diagnosis of sexual abuse is generally based on the child or adolescent's history and not confirmatory findings on physical examination (Hornor, 2004). As many as 96% of sexual abuse evaluations will have normal genitalia with no evidence of abuse on the physical exam (Johnson, 2004). Thus it is essential for primary care providers (PCP), emergency room staff as well as school and community personnel to have a clear understanding of both the behavioral and medical indicators that can signal possible histories of sexual abuse. Since the majority of sexual abuse survivors either never disclose their abuse histories or wait months or even years to report their experiences, early recognition of sexual abuse indicators can prevent delays in diagnosis and management of these children.

Behavioral Indicators

Changes in behavior noted by parents, friends, and teachers can often signal or raise concerns for possible sexual abuse. Behaviors of concern however can be markedly different depending on the age, development, and cognitive level of the child. Older adolescents are more likely to change friends in school and often change the way they dress and talk. There is also significant literature suggesting an increase in high-risk sexual practices as a key indicator for possible unwanted sexual activity or abuse. In younger children, the behaviors themselves are often sexual in nature and prove very anxiety-provoking to parents (Sanford & Cohens-Kettens, 2000). However, sexual behavior is a normal part of childhood development, expected in all children and includes a wide range of behaviors (Sanford & Cohens-Kettens, 2000).

Cause for concern is raised when certain aspects of the child's behavior are outside the expected bounds of normal sexual development. Children with problematic sexual behavior will often continue the behavior even after being told to cease (Heiman et al., 1998). Preschool children rarely depict sexual acts through insertion of objects and rarely attempt physical engagement in explicit sexual contact with other children. In contrast, sexually abused prepubertal children tend to exhibit sexual behaviors considered advanced and age inappropriate (Hornor, 2004). Age-inappropriate behaviors may indicate likely prior exposure to explicit sexual behavior or materials in or out of the home. For this reason it is recommended that parents monitor their children for exposure to sexual materials and establish open lines of communication allowing discussions of childhood development and sexuality. PCPs are encouraged to discuss openly with both parents and patients issues surrounding human sexuality as a part of routine anticipatory guidance (Heiman et al., 1998). When confronted with behaviors that raise concern, the PCP should obtain a complete behavioral and sexual history as well as refer the individual to child protective services and appropriate mental health providers for further evaluation (Heiman et al., 1998).

Childhood sexual behaviors of concern

- Repeated object insertion into vagina and/or anus
- Age-inappropriate knowledge of sex
- Child asking to be touched/kissed/etc. in the genital area
- Sex play involving one or more of the following

    - Oral–genital contact
    - Anal–genital contact
    - Genital–genital contact
    - Digital penetration of vagina/anus
    - Object penetration of vagina/anus
    - Four years or greater age difference between children
    - Use of force, threats, or bribes

- Common sexual behavior with features that cause concern

    - Increasing frequency of the behavior
    - Preoccupation with the behavior
    - Talk and language during the behavior (Hornor, 2004)

While many behaviors may very well just be part of expected adolescent development, parents and teachers should be aware of the possibility of an abusive and/or violent dating relationship when particular behavioral patterns are noted. Many such behaviors may serve as red flag for sexual coercion or partner abuse. Be aware of sudden changes in clothes or makeup, falling grades or dropping out of school, avoiding or changing friends, sudden changes in mood, and sudden changes in sleep and eating habits. Adolescents may appear depressed or anxious and may even entertain suicidal ideations and attempts (American Academy of Pediatrics,

1999; Nicoletti, 2000) There is also a high incidence of illicit drug use which often impairs the individual's ability to make sound and safe decisions when faced with a sexual encounter (Nicoletti, 2000).

Adolescent behaviors of concern

- Sudden change in mood and personality
- Anxiety
- Depression
- Falling grades and problems in school
- Change in eating or sleeping habits
- Sudden change in appearance, clothes, makeup, and hair
- Sexual behaviors and high-risk sexual practices
- Substance use and abuse (American Academy of pediatrics, 1999)

PCPs are encouraged to discuss openly with both parents and patients issues surrounding human sexuality as a part of routine anticipatory guidance (Hornor, 2004). When confronted with behaviors that raise concern, the provider should obtain a complete behavioral and sexual history as well as refer the individual to child protective services and appropriate mental health providers for further evaluation based on his or her assessment and evaluation (Hornor, 2004b).

Medical Indicators

Just as certain behaviors may lead one to suspect sexual abuse in a child or adolescent, physical findings on medical exams may also lead the health care professional to entertain a diagnosis of sexual abuse (Adams, 2001). Noncontact CSA (e.g., viewing pornography) as well as contact sexual abuse, touching, and light rubbing may not result in physical findings visible on examination (Johnson, 2004). Even minor abrasions and erythema may heal in a matter of hours to days (Johnson, 2004). If suspicion of CSA is not raised as a result of the child's history or behavior, CSA may go undetected for weeks, months, or even years. Normal or nonspecific examinations should not lessen suspicions of abuse or detract from the patient's history when a child alleges that sexual abuse has occurred. The presence of STIs can support and often confirm a diagnosis of CSA. Sexually transmitted diseases that are considered definitive evidence of sexual abuse or sexual contact are postnatally acquired gonorrhea or syphilis (Adams, 2001). A positive genital culture for Chlamydia or herpes, or a positive wet mount for trichomonas, is evidence of probable sexual abuse (Adams, 2001). Anogenital warts are one of the most common STIs in adults and have serious medical, social, and legal implications when discovered in children. However, because of the multiple modes by which warts may be transmitted and the long latency period from time of exposure to manifestation of clinical symptoms, great care and caution must be given to any case of suspected sexual abuse based on the presence of genital warts alone (Hornor, 2004a).

Possible medical complaints or findings that may suggest a history of past or acute sexual abuse in an adolescent include chronic abdominal pain, chronic pelvic pain, breast pain, STIs, chronic headache, and pregnancy (American College of Obstetricians and Gynecologists 1997. Medical findings that may overlap all ages from childhood to adolescence include anal–genital trauma, bleeding, discharge, pain, and itching; burning on urination; STIs; enuresis and encopresis; recent urinary tract infections; and abdominal pain and chronic constipation (American Academy of Pediatrics, 1999)

Assessment of Sexual Abuse and Assault

Crisis Response Team

The initial evaluation for any allegation of child and adolescent sexual abuse should be a coordinated effort between medical and psychological services, provided in a safe, protected environment. The primary goal of this evaluation involves assessment and treatment of medical injuries, detection and prophylaxis of STDs and pregnancy, forensic evidence collection, emotional support, referral for further psychological services, and guidance through legal services should a patient decide to pursuer prosecution of the assailant (Bechtel & Podrazik, 1999). In attempt to minimize additional trauma which may be relived during the investigation and assessment, case management should be conducted by sexual abuse experts in a coordinated effort between all medical and hospital staff, mental health providers, police, legal investigators, victim advocacy agencies, and forensic scientists. The guiding principle behind this coordinated effort is to ensure that rape victims receive comprehensive, consistent medical treatment and evidentiary examinations, emotional support, and appropriate referral for further medical and psychological therapy. Rape protocols are now available and considered standard of care in most medical centers, thus providing a consistent process for evaluation, treatment, and collection of forensic evidence (Bechtel & Podrazik, 1999). Guidelines are now available through the American College of Emergency Physicians suggesting not only physician supervision but also the training and utilization of non-MD trained medical personnel to address the care and evidence collection of rape victims. In smaller communities where sexual assault response teams are not available, the pediatrician can serve to help orchestrate the medical evaluation and integration of mental health, social service agencies, and legal providers who are essential components of any rape or abuse evaluation team (Volker, 1996).

Defining roles of all providers involved in the assault evaluation should be clearly stated in attempt to minimize repetition questioning, assessment, and evaluation. A careful history should be obtained in a sensitive, nonjudgmental fashion and documented using the victim's own words as often as possible. Most programs reserve forensic interviewing to trained specialists and medical providers are cautioned from becoming a "Private Investigator" when working with cases of alleged abuse and assault (Bechtel & Podrazik, 1999).

Clinical History

Pertinent historical information should include general demographic information such as the name of the alleged perpetrator and relationship to the victim, the circumstances of assault such as the location of the alleged abuse, physical violence used, physical and behavioral symptoms after the assault, any relevant medical history such as menarche, last menstrual period, previous consensual sexual activity, possibility of preexisting pregnancy, previous history of STDs, physical injuries or sexual assault, and the use of alcohol or drugs by the patient or the assailant before the assault (Bechtel & Podrazik, 1999). It is generally necessary to obtain informed consent of the patient prior to any examination or treatment. It is also necessary to obtain consent to release physical evidence collected for forensic examination to the police or legal authorities for use in the forensic science laboratory. Other consents may also be needed for further testing as in the case of STD screening and HIV testing. All injuries should be clearly documented through written descriptions, anatomical drawings, labels, and photographic pictures (Gaensslen & Lee, 2001).

Patterns of Injury

Over the past several decades, significant work in the field of child abuse and neglect has focused on defining patterns of physical injuries which result from child and adolescent sexual abuse (McCann et al., 1992). Results from these studies now serve as the foundation for much of the medical and legal procedures currently used daily across this country in sexual abuse treatment programs. The Hegar study (Heger et al., 2002) conducted between 1985 and 1990 involved 2,384 children and adolescents in a tertiary referral center who were evaluated for possible sexual abuse. Children were referred after a disclosed sexual abuse, because of behavioral changes suggestive of possible abuse or because of exposure to an abusive environment. A small fraction of patients, 182 or 7.6%, were referred for medical or physical findings indicating possible sexual abuse. A total of 96.3% of all children referred for evaluation had normal medical physical examinations. Of the 182 children referred for evaluation because of a concerning medical condition, only 92% were found to be normal at the time of the examination (Heger et al., 2002). While initial studies reported normal exams in ~96% of the patients, when looking specifically at the adolescent population it is believed that slightly higher rates of genital injury may be found if the examination is performed within 24h of the assault (Sugar et al., 2004). Younger children are more often victims of prolonged abuse and thus the chronicity of this abuse and the delay in reporting may account for the smaller percentage of physical findings documented when looking at a broader age range of sexual abuse victims inclusive of all children and adolescents.

Caution should be exercised to prevent the focus of any medical assessment from shifting away from the child to a preoccupation for the presence or absence of medical findings diagnostic of penetrating trauma. The history from the child remains the most important part of any assessment. The absence of compelling laboratory data or medical findings suggestive of penetrating trauma should not preclude the medical professional's ability or the ability of the system charged with the protection of the child to provide healing and safety for each child (Heger et al., 2002). However, individuals without medical knowledge and physicians without expertise more often expect physical evidence to support a history of abuse and believe that a doctor can determine from a vaginal examination whether a woman or child is a virgin (Underhill & Dewhurst, 1978). "It's normal to be normal," (Adams et al., 1994) and the expert must relay the additional caveat that while the exam may be normal, "Normal" does not mean that "nothing happened" (Kellogg et al., 2004).

Forensic Examination

A forensic evaluation is conducted when the patient is medically stable and consent obtained. The forensic examination is crucial not only to the criminal justice system but also to fulfill an important obligation to the victim and society by documenting that a sexual assault has occurred. Standard protocol for any sexual abuse assessment dictates that the forensic examination, together with a complete physical examination, be conducted in a deliberate, considerate manner, with the utmost respect for the patient. If, for example, the examiner is male and the patient is female, a female chaperone should be present during the examination. The adolescent patient may request a family member or a friend to remain in the room during the examination and the examiner should provide a clear and succinct explanation of each part of the assessment to prepare the patient for the examination (Jenny, 1992). While forensic protocols may vary from state to state, collection of clothing and DNA material, screening for STD along with the comprehensive physical examination should be standard for any abuse evaluation. Counseling regarding potential adverse consequences of abuse should be provided and appropriate referrals for follow-up should be given.

Medical and Psychological Consequences of Sexual Abuse

Childhood sexual abuse is often accompanied by wide-ranging physical and mental adverse outcomes (Beautrais, 2000). A strong relationship exists between sexual abuse and the development of pain disorders, infectious diseases, and multiple psychiatric conditions such as depression, anxiety, sleep disturbances, low self-esteem, suicidality, and substance abuse (Beautrais, 2000). In the USA the incidence of psychiatric diagnoses occurring over a lifetime is 56% for women and 47% for men who have reported histories of CSA. The rates of psychiatric diagnoses when no history of CSA is reported are significantly lower at 32% for women and 34% for men (Martin et al., 2004). The prevalence of women with lifetime alcohol dependence was 15.6% among those reporting CSA, compared with 7.6% among those not reporting CSA. The equivalent percentages among men were 38.7% and 19.2% (Kessler et al., 1994). Unwanted sexual experiences in adolescence has also led to gender-reversal patterns such as internalizing behaviors in males (e.g., bulimia) and externalizing behaviors such as fighting in females (Shrier et al., 1998). Other associations between adolescent rape and behavioral changes include younger age of first voluntary sexual intercourse, increased seeking and receipt of psychological services, and greater amounts of illegal drug use (Miller et al., 1995; Nagy et al., 1995).

Medical Consequences

Sexually Transmitted Diseases and HIV

One-half of high school students in the USA have engaged in sexual intercourse, and ~900,000 US adolescents become pregnant each year (Grunbaum et al., 2002). Behaviors conferring vulnerability to STIs and pregnancy are disproportionately higher among US adolescents compared with adolescents from other industrialized nations. Approximately 1 in 16 (6.2%) girls becomes pregnant and ~8 million cases of non-HIV-related STDs are diagnosed each year among persons 13–24 years of age in the USA (Centers for Disease Control and Prevention, 2002b). More than 31,000 persons were reported to have AIDS in the USA within this same age bracket (Centers for Disease Control and Prevention, 2002a). Among adolescents, new HIV infections are more common among girls than among boys (61% versus 39%) and adolescent girls are far more likely to be infected through heterosexual intercourse than are boys (45% versus 9%).

The diagnosis and management of STDs is an important treatment question for the assault victim. Accurate risk assessment for contracture of STDs after sexual assault has been complicated by regional variations in the prevalence of STDs. One study of 204 adolescent victims found that 43% had at least one preexisting STD (Jenny et al., 1990). The most common infections acquired after rape include bacterial vaginosis, trichomonas, and chlamydia. The Centers for Disease Control and Prevention (CDC) estimates the risk of acquiring an STD post sexual assault in adults as 6–12% for *Neisseria gonorrhea* (GC), 4–17% for Chlamydia, 0.5–3% for syphilis, and <1% for HIV (Schwartz & Whittington, 1990). CDC data also state that HIV seroconversion has occurred in persons whose only known risk factor was sexual assault or sexual abuse, but the frequency of this occurrence is probably low. In consensual sexual activity, the risk for HIV transmission from vaginal intercourse is 0.1–0.2% and for receptive anal intercourse is 0.5–3%. The risk for HIV transmission from oral sex is substantially lower. Specific circumstances and characteristics of an assault might increase the risk for HIV transmission and it is postulated that children might be at a higher risk for transmission because child sexual abuse is frequently associated with multiple episodes of assault which might result in multiple episodes of mucosal trauma (www.CDC.gov).

Alarming rates for both sexual abuse and HIV/AIDS in sub-Saharan Africa have been reported in recent CSA studies (Lalor, 2004). The incidence of HIV/AIDS in the general population of South Africans between the ages of 15 and 49 years is 19.94%, 25.06% of 15–49-year-olds in Zimbabwe and 35.8% of 15–49-year-olds in Botswana (Lalor, 2004). Coupling the HIV/AIDS data with the prevalence rate for penetrative sexual abuse of 5% will result in an estimated HIV exposure and transmission risk for 1% of all children living in this region of the world. In Botswanna where HIV/AIDS is even more prevalent, nearly 2 out of every 100 children will experience penetrative sexual abuse by an HIV positive perpetrator (Lalor, 2004). The potential for life-threatening infections and systemic illness as a result of CSA has tremendous health and economic implications for these developing countries and their people. This study mandates the development of CSA treatment and prevention programs for developing countries as well as developed countries.

STD Screening Protocols

The STD work-up of any sexual assault victim should be guided by the details provided in the history and findings on physical exam. Routine screening of all prepubertal girls who present with a history of sexual abuse is not routinely recommended unless findings on physical exam are suggestive of such an infection. Guidelines for adolescent screening, however, are stronger in recommending all victims of sexual assault undergo complete STD screening including screening for HIV (Linden, 1999; Petter & Whitehill, 1998; Hampton, 1995). Testing should include culture sampling of appropriate sites for GC and *Chlamydia trachomatis*. Vaginal secretions should be microscopically examined for *Trichomonas* species. Specimen should be tested for herpes virus if there is clinical indication. Blood should be collected for testing of syphilis, hepatitis B and C virus (HBV and HCV), and HIV. When tested in the acute setting, these results may serve as the baseline indicating the presence or absence of any STD in the victim at the time the assault occurred. This testing however is controversial for some who prefer performing the initial STD screening 2 weeks after the assault as not to taint the history or character of the alleged victim. Medical follow-up is mandatory and standard of care dictates repeating syphilis and HBV tests in 2 weeks and a repeat of HIV screening in 3–6 months.(Linden, 1999; Petter & Whitehill, 1998; Hampton, 1995).

STD Prophylaxis

Current recommendations for STD prophylaxis postsexual abuse vary depending on the circumstances and the age of the child. Prepubertal females appear to be at lower risk for ascending infections than are adolescents or adult women, and often regular follow-up can be ensured (Center for Disease Control and Prevention, 2006). HIV prophylaxis is not universally recommended but should be considered on the basis of history and physical exam and if there was mucosal exposure (oral, vaginal, and anal). When deciding whether or not to prophylax for HIV, providers should consider the risk and benefits of the medical regimen, whether there was repeated abuse or multiple perpetrators, if the perpetrator is known to be HIV positive or if there is a high prevalence of HIV in the geographic area where the sexual assault occurred (Linden, 1999; Petter & Whitehill, 1998; Hampton, 1995). Medical providers are recommended to search the CDC website for the most up to date recommendations regarding STD prophylaxis and treatment of STDs in cases of sexual assault against women, men, children, and adults (www.CDC.gov).

Pregnancy

Overall risk of pregnancy following sexual assault is estimated to be as high as 5% and thus postassault pregnancy prophylaxis is recommended (American Academy of Pediatrics, Committee on Adolescence, 1994) (Holmes et al., 1996). Pregnancy prevention and postcoital contraception should be addressed with every adolescent female rape and sexual assault victim. The discussion should include risks of failure and options for pregnancy management. Always obtain a baseline urine pregnancy test during the initial abuse evaluation because the adolescent could be pregnant from sexual activity that occurred prior to the assaults (Linden, 1999; Petter & Whitehill, 1998; Hampton, 1995). Several forms of emergency contraception are available for women who are victims of sexual assault. The side effect profile and complication risk associated with intrauterine devices (IUDs) however relegates the adolescent assault victim to hormonal therapy as the safest option for emergency contraception. It is incumbent upon all providers to explain the risks and possible benefits of emergency contraception and frequent side effects which may be experienced. Multiple drug combination regimen are available but more recently, high-dose progesterone has been employed with reported decrease in adverse side effects and an 89% efficacy rate in prevention of unwanted pregnancy. Plan B, for example, is an FDA-approved high-dose progesterone only emergency contraceptive that can prevent a pregnancy after contraceptive failure, unprotected sex, and in cases of sexual assault if taken within 72 h of the unwanted sexual contact. Plan B is not RU-498 (the abortion pill) and does not work if you are already pregnant. Plan B, like other hormone preparations, does not protect against HIV and other STDs, but when used as instructed, serves as an effective method for prevention of unwanted pregnancies resulting from sexual assault and abuse (www.go2planb.com; Trussell et al., 1996).

Nonsexual Physical Injury

The most common injuries reported in cases of comorbid physical violence, dating violence, and sexual abuse are scratches, bruises, welts, black eyes, swelling or busted lips, and sore muscles, sprains, and pulls. Victims experiencing multiple forms of violence report greater numbers of injuries than do victims of a single form of violence (Amar & Gennaro, 2005). While victims often sustain major physical injuries and emotional distress, it is known that less than half of those injured in sexual violence seek health care for injuries and less than 3% will see a mental health professional (Amar & Gennaro, 2005). Work in the field of chronic pain has sought to identify possible relationships between chronic back pain, chronic pelvic pain, and sexual abuse histories in childhood and adolescence (Reiter & Gambone, 1990; Reiter et al., 1991; Rapkin et al., 1990). When questioned, patients with chronic pain, regardless of the location of pain, typically had childhoods characterized by an atmosphere of violence, physical and sexual abuse, and emotional neglect (Walker et al., 1992). In one study, 22% of patients with chronic pelvic pain were sexually abused before the age of 15 years, significantly more than patients with back pain alone or no pain at all. Women with chronic pelvic pain were exposed more frequently to physical violence (38%) and suffered more emotional neglect (25%) during childhood than did women in the pain-free control group. There appears to be a significant association between sexual victimization before the age of 15 and the later development of chronic pelvic pain and this finding only strengthens the association between a variety of physical maladies in adulthood and histories of CSA (Lampe et al., 2000).

Psychological Consequences

Over the past three decades, research in the field of CSA has identified multiple associated adverse mental health outcomes. Sexual abuse has been specifically linked to depression in all age groups, anxiety disorders, panic attacks, phobias, substance abuse, and post-traumatic stress disorder (Cheasty et al., 1998; Silverman et al., 1996; Fergusson et al., 1996; Widom, 1999). Childhood sexual abuse often co-occurs with other adverse family conditions, including marital conflict, parental substance abuse problems, and domestic violence; however, even when taking these factors into account, CSA remains a powerful independent predictor of psychopathology (Mullen et al., 1996; Briere & Runtz, 1990).

Mood Disorders/PTSD/Anxiety

Many child and adolescent victims of sexual abuse experience feelings of guilt, shame, and humiliation and often blame themselves in part for the assault, especially when drugs or alcohol were involved (Widom, 1999). Both male and female victims are at an increased risk for developing adverse social and psychological outcomes (Boney-McCoy & Finkelhor, 1996; Neumann et al., 1996).

The risk of youth suicide is strongly associated with a history of psychiatric disorders and adverse childhood experiences. A recent study looking at the relationship between sexual abuse and youth suicide surveyed 2,485 eighth- through tenth-grade students in 27 Southern Australian schools (Martin et al., 2004). Students completed a self-administered questionnaire including items on sexual abuse and suicidality as well as measures of depression, hopelessness, and family functioning. The study revealed an increased incidence of suicidal thoughts, plans, threats, and attempts in both males and females; however, this relationship existed independent of depression, hopelessness, and family functioning in males only. Boys who reported high levels of distress about sexual abuse had a tenfold increased risk for suicide plans and threats and a 15-fold increased risk of suicide attempts when compared to nonabused males (Martin et al., 2004). Girls reporting histories of CSA and concurrent high levels of distress about their abuse experiences had a threefold increase in thoughts or plans for suicide. Fifty-five percent of the males and 19% of the females reporting prior sexual abuse experiences had attempted suicide (Martin et al., 2004). All adolescents should be screened for experiences of sexual abuse and suicidal behaviors as part of routine well child care. Practitioners should be aware of the increased risk of suicidality in all sexually abused adolescents. Practitioners should also be aware of gender differences and understand that when controlling for depression, hopelessness, and family functioning, males are at a significantly greater risk for suicidal behaviors than are females (Martin et al., 2004).

Posttraumatic stress disorder (PTSD) occurs in up to 80% of rape victims (Pynoos & Nader, 1992). Results from The National Survey of Adolescents indicated that sexual assault was a significant risk factor for a range of comorbid disorders, including comorbid PTSD and major depression, comorbid PTSD and substance abuse, and comorbid major depressive episodes of substance abuse (Kilpatrick et al., 2003; Brady et al., 1994). Many rape and sexual assault survivors will experience the Rape Trauma Syndrome. This syndrome is characterized by an initial phase lasting days to weeks during which the victim experiences disbelief, anxiety, fear, emotional liability, and guilt. The reorganization phase may last months to years where the victim progresses through a period of adjustment, integration, and recovery (Petter & Whitehill, 1998). In general, the adolescent may feel that his or her trust has been violated, experience increased self-blame, less positive self-esteem, anxiety, alcohol abuse, and adverse effects on sexual activity, including increased sexual risk behaviors (Miller et al., 1995; Smith et al., 1996; Moore et al., 1989). Appropriate mental health services are crucial at this time to help the adolescent survivor deal with the acute and more long-lasting mental health and physical adverse outcomes that often accompany sexual assault.

Substance Abuse and Dependence

Research has consistently demonstrated the over-representation of both adult women and adolescent girls who are survivors of childhood abuse among females with alcohol and drug use problems. Women and girls with sexual abuse histories were found to have elevated rates of substance use problems whether they were sampled from populations of mental health treatment facilities, medical clinics, elementary or high school students or the general community at large (Simpson &

Miller, 2002). PTSD is thought to mediate the relationship between early abuse and the use of alcohol and drugs later in life (Epstein et al., 1998). Alcohol and drug use may serve as a coping mechanism and a means of self-medication for painful reexperiencing and arousal symptoms associated with PTSD (Simpson & Miller, 2002). Thus when childhood abuse is associated with PTSD, the likelihood that a woman will have difficulties with alcohol or drugs is greater than in cases where PTSD is absent (Simpson & Miller, 2002).

Eating Disorders

Eating disorder behaviors have been reported at higher rates among adolescent girls who have experienced dating violence and rape. Studies have also found increased rates of internalizing disorders such as bulimia in boys and have found that both types of victimization, physical and sexual abuse, were associated with diet pill and laxative use, vomiting, and binge eating.(Ackard & Neumark-Sztainer, 2002). Other studies evaluating 2,600 girls between the ages of 14 and 18 regarding sexual assault experiences and current dietary practices found girls who experienced sexual assault were almost five times more likely to practice purging and two-and-a -half times more likely to take diet pill than those with no sexual abuse history (Thompson et al., 2001). Enhanced screening of young women and men attending eating disorder clinics is thus mandated such that treatment programs can be tailored toward both the eating disorder behavior and the comorbid mental health sequelae which may exist as a result of past childhood abuse.

Revictimization

In addition to the physical, psychological, and social consequences of child and adolescent sexual abuse, there is growing evidence that these individuals are at an increased risk for revictimization. By definition, revictimization is the occurrence of at least one incident of CSA followed by a subsequent incident of sexual victimization. Studies have shown that 15–79% of women with CSA histories were raped as adults (Roodman & Clum, 2001). Girls who experience violence and physical assaults are significantly more likely to be sexually assaulted in the same year (Follette et al., 1996). Victims of sexual revictimization are more likely to meet criteria for lifetime PTSD and dissociative disorders, experience higher levels of distress and anxiety, and demonstrate higher levels of risk-taking sexual behaviors and consequences (Wyatt et al., 1992). Victims of sexual revictimization are also more likely to have negative personal perceptions, lower self-esteem, and limited range of interpersonal expectations, and tended to expect others to be hostile and dominant (Cloitre et al., 2002). The adverse psychological consequences of sexual abuse are long lasting and there is growing evidence that these psychological effects of interpersonal violence including sexual assault are cumulative in nature (Follette et al., 1996).

Prevention, Intervention, and Education

The key to sexual abuse prevention relies on education and training in early detection, diagnosis, and management of sexual abuse cases. Parents can help prevent CSA through open discussions of normal sexual development with their children. The pediatrician and health care provider is in an ideal position to both aid parents in these discussions and to incorporate sexual development and abuse prevention into routine anticipatory guidance (Thomas et al., 2004). The American College of Obstetrics and Gynecology recommends that all physicians who evaluate victims of sexual assault provide resources and referrals for mental health and psychological services as well as perform case-oriented medical and forensic examinations. Providers should be comfortable and knowledgeable talking to victims about his or her rights, be able to direct victims to obtain legal assistance, and be able to discuss preventive strategies for future problems and victimization (American College of Obstetricians and Gynecologists, 1997).

Child Advocacy Center

Sexual abuse prevention initiatives should be coordinated efforts through community-based programs and facilities. Child Advocacy Centers (CACs) and Child Abuse Assessment Centers (CAACs) provide a safe environment for the diagnosis, treatment, and prosecution of sexual abuse cases (Joa & Goldberg Edelson, 2004). Evaluation teams consist of medical professionals, mental health workers, and representatives of law enforcement. Approximately 400 centers in existence today help to coordinate the variety of services that are needed for the appropriate management of CSA cases (Jackson, 2004). The primary goal of all CACs is to ensure that children are not further victimized by the systems that are designed to protect them. Program objectives include the following:

- Developing a comprehensive multidisciplinary, developmentally and culturally appropriate response to child abuse which is designed to meet the needs of children and their families in a specific community;
- Establishing a neutral, child-friendly facility where interviews and/or services for abused children can be provided;
- Preventing trauma to the child caused by multiple, duplicative contacts with different professionals;
- Providing needed mental health treatment and other services to children and families;
- Maintaining open communication, information sharing, and case coordination among community professionals and agencies involved in child protection efforts so that case decision-making and policy development are enhanced;
- Coordinating and tracking investigative, prosecutorial, child protection, and treatment efforts so that cases do not "fall through the cracks";

- Holding more offenders accountable through improved prosecution of child abuse cases;
- Enhancing professional skills necessary to effectively respond to cases of child abuse through cross-disciplinary and cross-cultural training and support;
- Enhancing community awareness and understanding of child abuse (www. nationalCAC.org).

Recent studies looked at the legal outcomes of sexual abuse cases handled through CAACs and compared case results with outcomes of non-CAAC investigations (Joa & Goldberg Edelson, 2004). The study revealed a higher likelihood of charges filed against perpetrators when cases were investigated and managed through the CAAC. Guilty verdicts were also more frequent in CAAC cases (Joa & Goldberg Edelson, 2004). The multidisciplinary team of specially trained professionals is optimal for evaluation of children in both emergency room at time of presentation and in outpatient settings such as CACs and CAACs. Providers who work with children and adolescents are encouraged to locate and notify local abuse centers when suspected CSA cases arise.

Sexual Assault Nurse Examiners

National trends toward centralized multiagency assessment and treatment facilities has in part led to the development of the Sexual Assault Nurse Examiner (SANE) program. These specialized nurses trained in the care and management of adult and adolescent victims of sexual abuse and sexual violence are becoming integral members of the first-response team and are often the first individual to have contact with an adolescent after a sexual assault has occurred. These agencies and specialized staff can provide a strong safety net for the traumatized teens (Pharris & Nafstad, 2002). Qualified nurses can not only provide expert medical assessment and forensic evidence collection but they are also able to mediate the often emotional responses of fear and feelings of blame and guilt that many adolescents emote following a sexual assault. Training programs are available for nurses specializing in adolescent sexual-assault responses and many states and communities have embarked upon development of pedi-SANE programs to provided similar care and management targeting cases of child sexual abuse (Ledray, 2001).

Programs for At Risk Teens

Whereas the exact numbers of sexually exploited youth in the Unites States is unknown, we do know that few cities and states have the resources to provide dedicated medical service aimed at intervention and prevention of sexual exploitation of teens and youth. It is essential that all sexually exploited children receive appropriate HIV and STD screening, education, and subsequent referral to appropriate medial providers to prevent additional mobility and potential mortality as a result of their abuse and life circumstances. The SAGE Project (Standing Against Global Exploitation Project), Inc., was founded by Norma Hotaling in 1992 in the San Francisco/Bay Area as an organization aimed at providing survivor-center care and services for men, woman, and youth involved in commercial sex exploitation (CSE) and prostitution (www.sagesf.org). Over the past 15 years, the SAGE project has served as one of the country's leading programs advocating for client services, community outreach, and legislative reform. The program also serves as a model by which other communities and municipalities may build and develop programs to address CSE in their own neighborhoods. The SAGE mission is to improve the lives of individuals and victims of CSE or individuals at risk for CSE. Program projects include but are not limited to trauma recovery, substance abuse treatment, vocational training, housing assistance, and legal advocacy. To accomplish project goals, SAGE works closely with law enforcement, public health, and social service agencies as well as local merchants and volunteers. SAGE is also aware of the great need to reach out to community youth at risk since a large percentage of adult victims of CSE and prostitution were victims of child sexual abuse and trafficked into sex trade as children. One example of SAGE's work is the STAR Center—SAGE Trauma and Recovery Center. Center services are twofold with a harm reduction unit and a day treatment program. SAGE conducted interviews with prostitutes and sex workers and found that an overwhelming number of sex workers wanted a safe place to learn about reducing risk such as hepatitis, HIV, and physical and emotional violence. The Day Treatment program is a 26-week day program which incorporates peer counseling, life skills for girls, medial screening and referrals, psychological and mental health counseling, rape and sexual abuse counseling, and substance abuse counseling (www.sagesf.org). As SAGE has grown and expanded to meet community needs of sex work survivors in the San Francisco/ Bay area, it has served as the gold standard encouraging the development of new programs in other cities and communities around the country. Other such programs providing support services for exploited children and teens have been developed in cities, such as Boston's Teen Prostitution Prevention Program (TPPP) and the S. T.A.R. (Saving Teens At Risk) program in Brooklyn, NY.

Conclusion

Few patients can prove as challenging and evoke the emotion which surrounds cases of CSA. Prevalence rates are difficult to define and the reality that many cases are never reported is an alarming and disturbing fact. As child advocates, practitioners must be aware of the early indicators and signs signaling abuse and not delay the diagnosis and management of these children. Additional research is needed to better define populations at risk and target programs in attempts to minimize the late effects of CSA. While prevention remains the ultimate goal, improved awareness and education for communities and professionals alike is required to ensure appropriate and quality care for all children who are sexually abused.

References

Abbey, A. (1991). Acquaintance rape and alcohol consumption on college campuses: How are they linked. *Journal of American College Health*, 39, 165–169.

Ackard, D. M. & Neumark-Sztainer, D. (2002). Date violence and date rape among adolescents: Associations with disordered eating behaviors and psychological health. *Child Abuse Neglect*, 26, 455–473.

Adams, J. A. (2001). Evolution of a classification scale: Medical evaluation of suspected child sexual abuse. *Child Maltreatment*, 6, 31–35.

Adams, J. A., Harper, K., Knudson, S., & Revilla, J. (1994). Examination findings in legally confirmed child sexual abuse; it's normal to be normal. *Pediatrics*, 94, 310–317.

Alan Guttmacher Institute (1994). *Sex and America's Teenagers*. New York: AGI.

Alan Guttmacher Institute (1999). *Facts in Brief: Teen Sex and Pregnancy*. New York: The AGI.

Amar, A. F. & Gennaro, S. (2005). Dating violence in college women: Associated physical injury, healthcare usage and mental health symptoms. *Nursing Research*, 54(40), 235–242.

American Academy of Pediatrics, Committee on Adolescence (1994). Sexual assault and the adolescent. *Pediatric*, 94, 761–765.

American Academy of Pediatrics, Committee on Adolescence (2001). Care of the Adolescent Sexual Assault Victim. *Pediatrics*, 107, 1476–1479.

American Academy of Pediatrics (1994). Sexual assault and the adolescent. *Pediatrics*, 151–155,

American Academy of Pediatrics (1997). Sexually transmitted diseases: Sexual abuse. Report of the Committee on Infectious Diseases, pp. 112–116.

American Academy of Pediatrics (1999). Guidelines for the evaluation of sexual abuse of children: Subject review. *Pediatrics*, 103, 186–191.

American College of Obstetricians and Gynecologists (1997). *Sexual assault*. ACOG Technical Bulletin 242. Washington, DC: ACOG.

American Medical Association (1995). *Strategies for the Treatment and Prevention of Sexual Assault*. Chicago: AMA.

Anglin, D., Spears, K. L., & Hutson, H. R. (1997). Flunitrazepam and its involvement in date or acquaintance rape. *Academic Emergency Medicine*, 8, 47–61.

Aral, S. O., St Lawrence, J. S., Tikhonova, L., et al. (2003). The social organization of commercial sex work in Moscow, Russia. *Sexually Transmitted Diseases*, 30, 39–45.

Bagley, C., Bolitho, F., & Bertrand, L. (1997). Sexual assault in school, mental health and suicidal behavior in adolescent women in Canada. *Adolescence*, 32, 361–366.

Barrett, D. (1999). Reaching out to Child Prostitutes. *Nursing Standard*, 13, 22–23.

Beautrais, A. L. (2000). Risk factors for suicide and attempted suicide among young people. *Australian and New Zealand Journal of Psychiatry*, 43, 420–436.

Bechtel, K. & Podrazik, M. (1999). Evaluation of the adolescent rape victim. *Pediatric Clinics of North America*, 46, 809–823.

Boney-McCoy, S. & Finkelhor, D. (1996). Psychosocial sequelae of violent victimization in a national youth sample. *Journal of Consulting and Clinical Psychology*, 63, 726–736.

Brady, K. T., Killeen, T., Saladin, M. E., Dansky, B., & Becker, S. (1994). Comorbid substance abuse and posttraumatic stress disorder. *American Journal on Addictions*, 3, 160–164.

Braitstein, P., Li, K., Tyndall, M., et al. (2003). Sexual violence among a cohort of injection drug users. *Social Science & Medicine*, 57, 561–569.

Briere, J. & Runtz, M. (1990). Differential adult symptomatology associated with three types of child abuse histories. *Child Abuse & Neglect*, 14, 357–364.

Bureau of Justice Statistics (1996). *Criminal Victimization 1994*. Washington, DC: U.S. Department of Justice. publication no. NCJ-158022.

Cassidy, L. & Hurrell, R. M. (1995). The influence of victim's attire on adolescent's judgments of date rape. *Adolescence*, 30, 319–323.

Centers for Disease Control and Prevention (2002a). *HIV/AIDS Among U.S. Women: Minority and Young Women at Continuing risk*. Atlanta, GA: Centers for Disease Control and Prevention.

Centers for Disease Control and Prevention (2002b). *Young People at Risk: HIV/AIDS Among America's Youth.* Atlanta, GA: Centers for Disease Control and Prevention.

Center for Disease control and Prevention (2006). *2006 Guidelines for Treatment of Sexually Transmitted Diseases.* Atlanta, GA: U.S. Department of Health and Human Services.

Cheasty, M., Clare, A. W., & Collins, C. (1998). Relation between sexual abuse in childhood and adult depression: Case-control study. *BMJ,* 16, 198–201.

Cloitre, M., Cohen, L. R., & Scarvalone, P. (2002). Understanding revictimization among childhood sexual abuse survivors: An interpersonal schema approach. *Journal of Cognitive Psychotherapy,* 16, 91–112.

Coker, A. L., McKeown, R. E., Sanderson, M., Davis, K. E., Valois, R. F., & Huebner, E. S. (2000). Severe dating violence and quality of life among South Carolina high school students. *American Journal of Preventive Medicine,* 19, 220–227.

Commonwealth Fund (1997). *In Their own Words: Adolescent Girls Discuss Health and Health Care Issues.* New York: Louis Harris and Associates.

Donovan, P. (1997). Can statutory rape law be effective in preventing adolescent teen pregnancy? *Family Planning Perspectives,* 29, 30–34.

Drug Induced Rape Prevention and Punishment Act of 1996 (1996). Pub L. No. 104–305, 110 Stat. 3807 Oct 13, 1996.

Druid, H., Holmgren, P., & Ahlner, J. (2001). Flunitrazepam: An evaluation of use, abuse, and toxicity. *Forensic Science International,* 122, 136–141.

Emmert, C. & Kohler, U. (1998). Data about 154 children and adolescents reporting sexual assault. *Archives of Gynecology and Obstetrics,* 261, 61–70.

English B (2006). Leaving "the life" Boston Globe, June 21, 2006. Boston.

Epstein, J. N., Saunders, B. E., Kilpatrick, D. G., & Resnick, H. S. (1998). PTSD as a mediator between childhood rape and alcohol use in adult women. *Child Abuse & Neglect,* 22, 223–234.

Feld, S. L. & Straus, M. A. (1989). Escalation and desistance of wife assault in marriage. *Criminology,* 27, 141–161.

Fergusson, D. M., Horwood, L. J., & Lynskey, M. T. (1996). Childhood sexual abuse and psychiatric disorder in young adulthood, II: Psychiatric outcomes of childhood sexual abuse. *Journal of the American Academy of Child and Adolescent Psychiatry,* 35, 1365–1374.

Fisher, B. S., Cullen, F. T., & Turner, M. G. (2000). *Sexual Victimization of College Women, NCJ 182369.* Washington DC: Bureau of Justice Statistics.

Follette, V. M., Polusney, M. A., Bechtle, A. E., & Naugle, A. E. (1996). Cumulative trauma: The impact of child sexual abuse, adult sexual assault, and spouse abuse. *Journal of Traumatic Stress,* 9, 25–35.

Ford, C. A. & Millstein, S. G. (1997). Delivery of confidentiality assurance to adolescents by primary care physicians. *Archives of Pediatrics & Adolescent Medicine,* 151, 505–509.

Gaensslen, R. E. & Lee, H. C. (2001). *Sexual Assault Evidence: National Assessment and Guidebook.* National Institute of Justice, October 2001.

Gorey, K. M. & Leslie, D. R. (1997). The prevalence of child sexual abuse: Integrative review adjustment for potential response and measurement biases. *Child Abuse & Neglect,* 21, 391–398.

Greydanus, D. E., Shaw, R. D., & Kennedy, E. L. (1987). Examination of sexually abused adolescents. *Seminars Adolescent Medicine,* 3, 59–66.

Grunbaum, J. A., Kann, L., Kinchen, S. A., et al. (2002). Youth risk behaviors surveillance: Untied States, 2001. *MMWR Surveillance Summaries,* 51(4), 1–62.

Gustafson, T. B. & Sarwer, D. B. (2004). Childhood sexual abuse and obesity. *Obestiy Review,* 5, 129–135.

Hampton, H. L. (1995). Care of the woman who has been raped. *The New England Journal of Medicine,* 332, 234–237.

Heger, A., Emans, S. J., & Muram, D. (Eds.) (2000). *Evaluation of the Sexually Abused Child,* 2nd edition. Oxford University Press, New York.

Heger, A., Ticson, L., Velasquez, O., & Bernier, R. (2002). Children referred for possible sexual abuse: Medical findings in 2384 children. *Child Abuse & Neglect,* 26, 645–659.

Heiman, M. L., Leiblum, S., Esquilin, S. C., & Pallitto, L. M. (1998). A comparative survey of beliefs about "normal childhood sexual behavior. *Child abuse and Neglect*, 22, 289–304.

Heise, L. L. (1993). Reproductive freedom and violence against women: Where are the intersections. *The Journal of Law, Medicine & Ethics*, 21, 206–216.

Hibbard, R. & Orr, D. P. (1985). Incest and sexual abuse. *Seminars in Adolescent Medicine*, 1, 153–164.

Holmes, M. H., Resnick, H. S., Kilpatrick, D. G., et al. (1996). Rape related pregnancy: Estimates and descriptive characteristics from a national sample of women. *American Journal of Obstetrics and Gynecology*, 175, 320–325.

Hornor, G. (2004a). Ano-genital warts in children: Sexual abuse or not? *Journal of Pediatric Health Care*, 18, 165–170.

Hornor, G. (2004b). Sexual behavior in children: Normal or not? *Journal of Pediatric Health Care*, 18, 57–64.

Jackson, S. (2004). A USA national survey of program services provided by child advocacy center. *Child Abuse & Neglect*, 28, 422–421.

Jackson, S. M., Cram, F., & Seymour, F. W. (2000). Violence and sexual coercion in high school students dating relationships. *Journal of Family Violence*, 15, 23–36.

Jenny, C. (1992). The role of the physician as medical detective. In A. Heger & S. J. Emans (Eds.), *Evaluation of the Sexually Abused Child.* (pp. 51–61). Oxford University Press, New York.

Jenny, C., Hooton, T. M., Bowers, A., et al. (1990). Sexually transmitted diseases in victims of rape. *The New England Journal of Medicine*, 322, 713–716.

Jewkes, R. & Abrahams, N. (2002). The epidemiology or rape and sexual coercion in South African. *Social Science & Medicine*, 55, 1231–1244.

Joa, D. & Goldberg Edelson, M. (2004). Legal outcomes for children who have been sexually abused: The impact of child abuse assessment center evaluations. *Child Maltreatment*, 9, 263–276.

Johnson, C. F. (2002). Child maltreatment: Recognition, reporting and risk. *Pediatrics International*, 44, 554–560.

Johnson, C. F. (2004). Child sexual abuse. *Lancet*, 364, 462–470.

Kellogg, N. D., Menard, S. W., & Santos, A. (2004). Genital anatomy in pregnant adolescents: "Normal" does not mean "nothing happened". *Pediatrics*, 113, e67–e69.

Kershner, R. (1996). Adolescent attitudes about rape. *Adolescence*, 31, 29–33.

Kessler, R. C., McGonagle, K. A., Shao, S., et al. (1994). Lifetime and 12-month prevalence of DESM-III-R psychiatric disorders in the United States. Results from the National co morbidity Survey. *Archives of General Psychiatry*, 51, 8–19.

Kilpatrick, D. G., Aciemo, R. E., Saunders, B., et al. (2000). Risk factors of adolescent substance abuse and dependence: Data from a national sample. *Journal of Consulting and Clinical Psychology*, 68, 19–30.

Kilpatrick, D. G., Ruggiero, K. J., Aciemo, R. E., et al. (2003). Violence and risk of PTSD, major depression, substance abuse/dependence, and comorbidity: Results from the National Survey of Adolescents. *Journal of Consulting and Clinical Psychology*, 71, 697–702.

Koss, M. P. & Harvey, M. R. (1991). *The Rape Victim: Clinical and Community Interventions.* Newbury Park, California: Sage Publications.

Koss, M. P., Gidycz, C. A., & Wisnieqski, N. (1987). The scope of rape: Incidence and prevalence of sexual aggression and victimization in a national standard of higher education students. *Journal of Consulting and Clinical Psychology*, 55, 162–170.

Kral, A. H., Monar, B. E., Booth, R. E., & Watters, J. K. (1997). Prevalence of sexual risk behavior and substance use among runaway and homeless adolescents in San Francisco, Denver and New York City. *International Journal of STD and AIDS*, 8, 109–117.

Lalor, K. (2004). Child sexual abuse in sub-Saharan Africa: A literature review. *Child abuse & Neglect*, 28, 439–460.

Lampe, A., Solder, E., Ennemoser, A., Schubert, C., Rumpold, G., & Sollner, W. (2000). Chronic pelvic pain and previous sexual abuse. *Obstetrics and Gynelcology*, 96, 929–933.

Langan, P. A. & Harlow, C. W. (1994). *Bureau of Justice Statistics: Child Rape Victims, 1992 Crime Data Brief.* Washington, DC: U.S. Department of Justice; publication no. NCJ-147001.

Ledray, L. E. (2001). Highlights of the first national sexual assault response team training conference. *Journal of Emergency Nursing,* 27, 607–609.

Linden, J. S. (1999). Sexual assault. *Emergency Medicine clinics of North America,* 17, 685–697.

Martin, G., Bergen, H. A., Richardson, A. S., Roeger, L., & Allison, S. (2004). Sexual abuse and suicidality: Gender differences in a large community sample of adolescents. *Child Abuse & Neglect,* 28, 491–503.

McCann, J., Vois, J., & Simon, M. (1992). Genital injuries resulting from sexual abuse: A longitudinal study. *Pediatrics,* 89, 307–317.

Miller, B. C., Monson, B. H., & Norton, M. C. (1995). The effects of forced sexual intercourse on while female adolescents. *Child Abuse & Neglect,* 19, 1289–1301.

Molnar, B. E., Shade, S. B., Kral, A., Booth, R. E., & Watters, J. K. (1998). Suicide behavior and sexual/physical abuse among street youth. *Child Abuse & Neglect,* 22, 213–222.

Monte, M. A. (2004). Female prostitution, customers and violence. *Violence Against Women,* 10, 247–280.

Moore, K. A., Nord, C. S., & Petterson, J. L. (1989). Nonvoluntary sexual activity among adolescents. *Family Planning Perspectives,* 21, 110–114.

Morris, R. E., Anderson, M. M., & Knox, B. W. (2002). Incarcerated adolescents' experiences as perpetrators of sexual assault. *Archives of Pediatrics & Adolescent Medicine,* 156, 831–835.

Mullen, P. E., Marin, J. L., Anderson, J. C., Romans, S. E., & Herbison, G. P. (1996). The long-term physical emotional and sexual abuse of children: A community study. *Child Abuse & Neglect,* 20, 7–21.

Muram, D., Hostetler, B. R., Jones, C. E., & Speck, P. M. (1995). Adolescent victims of sexual assault. *The Journal of Adolescent Health,* 17, 372–375.

Nadon, S. M., Koverola, C., & Schludermann, E. H. (1998). Antecedents to prostitution. *Journal of Interpersonal Violence,* 13, 206–211.

Nagy, S., DiClemente, R., & Adcock, A. G. (1995). Adverse factors associated with forced sex among southern adolescent girls. *Pediatrics,* 96, 944–946.

National Institute of Justice (1998). *Violence by Intimates: Analyses of Data on Crimes by Current or Former Spouses, Boyfriends and Girlfriends BJS.* Publication No NCJ 167237 Annapolis, MD: Bureau of Justice statistics Clearinghouse.

National Victim Center (1992). *Rape in America: A Report to the Nation.* Arlington, Virginia: NVC.

Neumann, D. A., Houskamp, B. M., Pollock, V. E., & Briere, J. (1996). The long term sequelae of childhood sexual abuse in women: A meta-analysis review. *Child Maltreatment,* 1, 6–16.

Nicholson, K. L., & Baister, R. L. (2001). GHB: A new and novel drug of abuse. *Drug and Alcohol Dependence,* 63, 1–22.

Nicoletti, A. (2000). Perspectives of pediatric and adolescent gynecology from the allied health care professional: Recognizing teen dating violence. *Journal of Pediatric and Adolescent Gynecology,* 13, 79–80.

O'Keefe, M. & Treister, L. (1998). Victims of dating violence among high school students: Are the predictors different for males and females? *Violence Against Women,* 4, 195–223.

O'Keefe, N. K., Brockopp, K., & Chew, E. (1986). Teen dating violence. *Social Work,* 31, 465–468.

Parrot, A. (1989). Acquaintance rape among adolescents: Identifying risk groups and intervention strategies. *Journal of Social Work & Human Sexuality,* 8, 47–61.

Peipert, J. F. & Domagalski, L. R. (1994). Epidemiology of adolescent sexual assault. *Obstetrics and Gynecology,* 84, 867–871.

Perkins, C. & Klaus, P. (1996). *Criminal Victimization 1994; National Crime Victimization Survey.* Washington, DC: Bureau of Justice Statistics.

Petter, L. M. & Whitehill, D. L. (1998). Management of female sexual assault. *American Family Physician,* 58, 920–926.

Pharris, M. D. & Nafstad, S. S. (2002). Nursing care of adolescents who have been sexually assaulted. Nursing care of adolescents who have been sexually assaulted. *The Nursing Clinics of North America*, 37, 475–497.

Pynoos, R. S. & Nader, K. (1992). Post traumatic stress disorder. In E. R. McAnarney, R. E. Kreips, D. P. Orr, & G. D. Comerci (Eds.), *Testbook of Adolescent Medicine*. (pp. 1003–1009). Philadephia, PA: WB Saunders Co.

Raj, A., Silverman, J. G., & Amaro, H. (2000). The relationship between sexual abuse and sexual risk among high school students: Findings from the 1997 Massachusetts Youth Risk Behavior Survey. *Maternal and Child Health Journal*, 4, 125–134.

Rapkin, A. J., Kames, L., Darke, L., Stampler, F., & Naliboff, B. (1990). History of physical and sexual abuse in women with chronic pelvic pain. *Obstetrics & Gynecology*, 76, 92–96.

Reiter, R. C. & Gambone, J. C. (1990). Demographic and historic variables in women with idiopathic chronic pelvic pain. *Obstetrics & Gynecology*, 75, 428–432.

Reiter, R. C., Shakerin, L. R., Cambone, J. C., & Milburn, A. K. (1991). Correlation between sexual abuse and somatization in women with somatic and nonsomatic chronic pelvic pain. *American Journal of Obstetrics and Gynecology*, 165, 104–109.

Roodman, A. A. & Clum, G. A. (2001). Revictimization rates and method variance: A meta-analysis. *Clinical Psychology Review*, 21, 183–204.

Roy, E., Haley, N., Leclerc, P., Wochanski, B., Boudreau, J. F., & Boivin, J. F. (2004). Mortality in a cohort of street youth in Montreal. *Journal of American Medical Association*, 292, 569–574.

Sanford, T. & Cohens-Kettens, P. T. (2000). Sexual behavior in Dutch and Belgian children as observed by their mothers. *Journal of Psychology and Human Sexuality*, 12, 105–116.

Schwartz, R. H. & Weaver, A. B. (1998). Rohypnol: The date rape drug. *Clinical Pediatrics (Phila)*, 37, 321.

Schwartz, S. K., & Whittington, W. L. (1990). Sexual assault and sexually transmitted diseases: Detection and management in adults and children. *Review Infectious Diseases*, 12 (suppl. 6), 682–690.

Seifert, S. A. (1999). Substance use and sexual assault. *Substance Use & Misuse*, 34, 935–945.

Shane, P. G. (1989). Changing patterns among homeless and runaway youth. *American Journal of Orthopsychiatry*, 59, 208–214

Shrier, L. A., Pierce, J. D., Emans, S. J., & DuRant, R. H. (1998). Gender differences in risk behaviors associated with forced or pressured sex. *Archives of Pediatrics & Adolescent Medicine*, 152, 57–63.

Silverman, A. B., Reinherz, H. Z., & Giaconia, R. M. (1996). The long-term sequelae of child and adolescent abuse: A longitudinal community study. *Child Abuse & Neglect*, 20, 709–723.

Silverman, J. G., Raj, A., Mucci, L., & Hathaway, J. (2001). Dating violence against adolescent girls and associated substance use, unhealthy weight control, sexual risk behavior, pregnancy and suicidality. *Journal of the American Medical Association*, 286, 572–579.

Simpson, T. L. & Miller, W. R. (2002). Concomitance between childhood sexual and physical abuse and substance use problems. *Clinical Psychology Review*, 22, 27–77.

Small, S. A. & Kerns, D. (1993). Unwanted sexual activity among peers dating early and middle adolescence: Incidence and risk factors. *Journal of Marriage and the Family*, 55, 941–952.

Smith, M. D., Besharov, D. T., Gardiner, K. N., & Hoff, T. (1996). *Early Sexual experiences: How voluntary? How violent?* MenloPark, CA: Henry J Kaiser family Foundation.

Sugar, N. F., Fine, D. N., & Eckert, L. O. (2004). Physical injury after sexual assault: Findings of a large case series. *American Journal of Obstetrics and Gynecology*, 190, 71–76.

Teare, C. & English, A. (2002). Nursing practice and statutory rape. Effects of reporting and enforcement on access to care for adolescents. *The Nursing Clinics of North America*, 37, 869–885.

Thomas, D., Flaherty, E., & Binns, H. (2004). Parent expectations and comfort with discussion of normal childhood sexuality and sexual abuse prevention during office visits. *Ambulatory Pediatrics*, 4, 232–236.

Thompson, K. M., Wonderlich, S. A., Crosby, R. D., & Mitchell, J. E. (2001). Sexual violence and weight control techniques among adolescent girls. *The International Journal of Eating Disorders*, 29, 166–176.

Tjaden, P. & Thoennes, N. (1998). *Prevalence, Incidence and Consequences of Violence Against Women: Findings from the National Violence Against Women Survey.* NCJ 172837. Washington DC: National Institute of Justice; Center for Disease Control and Prevention.

Tjaden, P. & Thoennes, N. (2000). *Extent, Nature and Consequences of Intimate Partner Violence. NCJ 181867.* Washington DC: National Institute of Justice; Center for Disease Control and Prevention.

Trussell, J., Ellertson, C., & Rodriguez, G. (1996). The Yuzpe regimen of emergency contraception: How long after the morning after? *Obstetrics and Gynecology,* 88, 150–154.

Tyler, K. A., Whitbeck, L. B., & Hoyt, D. R. (2004). Risk factors for sexual victimization among male and female homeless and runaway youth. *Journal of Interpersonal Violence,* 19, 503–520.

Underhill, R. A. & Dewhurst, J. (1978). The doctor cannot always tell. Medical examination of the hymen. *Lancet,* 1, 375–376.

Unger, J. B., Simon, T. R., Newman, T. L., Montgomery, S. B., Spike, M. D., & Albornoz, M. (1998). Early adolescent street youth with unique problems and service needs. *Journal of Early Adolescence,* 18, 325–348.

US Department of Health and Human Services (2002). *Administration on Children, Youth and Families. 11 years of Reporting: Child Maltreatment 2000.* Washington, DC: US Government Printing Office.

Volker, R. (1996). Experts hope team approach will improve the quality of rape exams. *Journal of the American Medical Association,* 275, 973–974.

www.CDC.gov/std/treatment/2006/sexual-assault.htm, February 7, 2007

www.go2planb.com/ForConsumers/AboutPlanB/WhatisPlanB.aspx, February 7, 2007

www.nationalCAC.org/professionals/model/CAC_model.html, February 7, 2007

www.sagesf.org/html/about_main.htm, February 7, 2007

Walker, E. A., Katon, W. J., Hansom, J., Harrops-Griffiths, J., Holm, L., & Jones, M. L. (1992). Medical and psychiatric symptoms in women with childhood sexual abuse. *Psychosomatic Medicine,* 54, 658–664.

Widom, C. S. (1999). Posttraumatic stress disorder in abused and neglected children grown up. *The American Journal of Psychiatry,* 156, 1223–1229.

Willis, B. M. & Levy, B. S. (2002). Child prostitution: Global health burden, research needs, and interventions. *Lancet,* 359, 1417–1422.

Wingood, G. M., DiClimente, R. J., Hubbard-McCree, D., Harrington, K., & Davies, S. L. (2001). Dating violence and the sexual health of black adolescent females. *Pediatrics,* 107, e72.

World Health Organization (2000). *Initiative on HIV/AIDS and Sexually Transmitted Infections.* March 3, 2000.

Wurbacher, K. V., Evans, E. D., & Moore, E. J. (1991). Effects of alternative street school youth involved in prostitution. *Journal of Adolescent Health,* 12, 549–554.

Wyatt, G. E., Guthrie, D., & Notgrass, C. M. (1992). Differential effects of women's child sexual abuse and subsequent sexual revictimization. *Journal of Consulting and Clinical Psychology,* 60, 167–173.

Yates, G. L., Mackenzie, R. G., Pennbridge, J., & Swofford, A. (1991a). A risk profile comparison of homeless youth involved in prostitution and homeless youth not involved. *Journal of Adolescent Health,* 12, 545–548.

Yates, G. L., Pennbridge, J., Swofford, A., & Mackenzie, R. G. (1991b). The los angeles system of care for runaway homeless youth. *Journal of Adolescent Health,* 12, 555–560.

Chapter 9
Impact of Trauma in School Violence on the Victim and the Perpetrator: A Mental Health Perspective

Lane J. Veltkamp and Amy Lawson

Introduction

Juvenile violence came into national focus during the school shootings in the 1990s. These school shootings were a wake-up call regarding the impact of violence. Shock, fear, and a desire to understand have resulted in increased awareness and numerous publications regarding this important topic. School-based risk factors and school-based protective factors have been identified which may help in the prevention of problems and in the early identification of problems and those risk factors that maintain and increase problems.

Soriano (1999) has pointed out that antisocial behavior is surging. It was estimated that 160,000 students miss school everyday in the United States because of bullying and threats. The National Association of School Psychologists (2002) has reported that bullying is the most common form of violence in our society, identifying that between 15 and 30% of students are either bullies or victims. Hoover et al. (1992) found that up to 75% of students surveyed reported being victimized and 1 out of 7 students had suffered severe trauma as a result. Nansel et al. (2001) reports that ~3.7 million youth engage in bullying and 3.2 million are victims of moderate to severe bullying. From 1994 to 1998 there were 188 violent deaths on or near school grounds (Thornton et al., 2001). Over two thirds of students believe that schools respond poorly to bullying with a high percentage of students believing that adult help is infrequent. Clearly, bullying behavior is not caused by one factor but involves personality, family, school, community, and peer group factors (Hoover et al., 1992).

Assessing Risk Factors

Of importance in the understanding of violent behavior is the relationship between trauma experienced by the child and violent behavior. Victims of trauma experience traumatic events, such as domestic violence, physical abuse, sexual abuse, and/or neglect, in different ways. Therefore, their reactions to the trauma may be expressed differently. For example, some victims will take a path where they reexperience trauma in future relationships during adolescence and adulthood. This reexperiencing may take the form of troubled, disordered, or dysfunctional relationships. It is also possible that the trauma is experienced through self-defeating/self-destructive behaviors. This could take the form of self-mutilation, destructive financial relationships, and destructive behaviors in the form of gambling, sexual addiction, or placing themselves in dangerous situations. The third option is that people who have been traumatized through victimization may do well in their life and relationships. This may be due to resilience, developing corrective positive relationships in adulthood, or achieving well-being through self-help, therapy, or by the use of a mentor early in life. In any event, these pathways offer the victim both destructive and constructive options of dealing with the traumatic events. In order to understand why and how traumatic events affect a person, we will look at risk factors within the individual, the family, the peer group, the community, and the school.

Individual Risk Factors

Many authors (Satcher, 2001) have contributed to the identification of risk factors in the community, the peer group, the school, and the family. Children who engage in overt, aggressive behaviors on school grounds are more likely to be of the male gender; they are often older than their victims, who are typically males as well (Sprague & Walker, 2005). Gray (2000) has suggested that children who engage in aggressive or bullying behaviors have a drive for power and control or the need to dominate others. In order to receive what they desire during their interactions with their peers, these children may inflict pain and demonstrate a lack of empathy for others. Perhaps an underdeveloped ego fuels the impulsive behaviors of the child who is not mature enough to fully consider reality and make rational decisions. Without a fully developed ego, the child not only seeks instant gratification through aggression but also demonstrates errors in thinking. For example, the aggressor or bully often has an unrealistically favorable view of the self, despite the fact that others often contradict these beliefs. It has also been noted that these children often believe that "everyone is out to get them" and/or that the victim provoked them or "had it coming." Along with an underdeveloped ego, research has shown that children who engage in aggressive behaviors typically have lower academic competence or intellectual achievement scores than their nonviolent peers (Gray, 2000).

Although the perpetrators of aggressive or violent acts are irritable, have a negative mood in general, and are slow to adapt to new situations, it has been found that they establish friendships easily. In fact, bullies are often viewed by others as popular and score high on measures of social acceptance (Connolly & O'Moore, 2003; Dake et al., 2003; Weir, 2001). It is not uncommon for children who engage in aggressive acts to have friends, alliances, and/or supporters who not only empower the bullies but are empowered by the aggressor as well (Gray, 2000). With others by their side, the aggressive behaviors of the perpetrators are reinforced. Both he and his peers may engage in other antisocial behaviors, including the use of drugs and alcohol, which are commonly associated with violence. In fact, 39% of middle and high school students cite alcohol as a major factor in the occurrences of school violence (Prevention Institute, 2006).

Aggressive or violent acts committed on school grounds are not only the result of children who are identified as bullies, but also can often be attributed to the actions of their victims. It has been found that two thirds of the perpetrators in recent school shootings were children who felt bullied, persecuted, or threatened by peers (NASP, 2002). As a result, it is important for educators and mental health professionals to review the risk factors that are most commonly attributed to victims of aggressive or violent interactions. Similar to children who engage in aggressive behaviors, the targets are more likely to be boys and are often identified as being physically weaker than their peers. Victims also tend to be insecure and most will take a passive stance in the face of aggression. The few who strike out against their aggressors in an attempt to defend themselves will often try to interact with the bullies following the attack. These reactions are testament to the fact that victims tend to lack the appropriate means for interacting with others. It has been noted that they are often isolated from and rejected by their peers and do not have many good friends (Piskin, 2002; Bernstein & Watson, 1997; NASP, 2002). Victims of aggression may also display academic difficulties and antisocial and/or hyperactive behaviors related to their emotional problems and underdeveloped social skills, which further targets them for victimization (Johnson et al., 2002). The underdeveloped social skills may be attributed to the fact that many victims have overprotective parents or even school personnel.

Family Risk Factors

The home environment is the place where a child first encounters and learns to interact with others and plays a key role in how a child will behave within society. It has been noted that children who display aggressive behaviors on school grounds have often seen or experienced physical aggression or violence within the home (Dwyer et al., 1998; Mohandie et al. 2000). It has been found that children involved in aggressive or bullying behaviors were 2.2 times more likely to suffer from child abuse than their peers who did not display bullying behaviors (Dake et al., 2003). Along with the family discord and/or physical aggression often present in the home, research has suggested that the parents' attitude toward the child frequently leads to aggressive or bullying behaviors. Children who bully others often live with mothers who are cold and rejecting, her attitude lacking warmth and compassion toward her child. This constant rejection and negative attitude creates an anxious–avoidant attachment between the parent and child. In such an environment, the child learns the role of both the victim and aggressor (Bernstein & Watson, 1997). Without a healthy attachment, the child does not experience emotional support or engage in positive, effective communication, two factors that are vital in developing positive coping, social, and/or personal skills (Connolly & O'Moore, 2003).

When a parent is emotionally uninvolved and/or physically absent, appropriate boundaries are not established for the child. Boundaries help the child learn socially appropriate behaviors and how to control impulses (Connolly & O'Moore, 2003; Bernstein & Watson, 1997). Research also has suggested that the frequency and severity of the aggressive or violent behaviors that may follow maltreatment are directly related to the amount of adult supervision that the child receives (2002). When an adult is not readily available or present in the home, it is likely that the child is not consistently punished for aggressive behaviors. Inconsistent discipline not only demonstrates a tolerance for aggression by the parents but also reinforces the inappropriate actions of the child (Connolly & O'Moore, 2003; Bernstein & Watson, 1997; Mohandie et al. 2000; NASP, 2002).

Although the evidence of an uninvolved parent may suggest a lack of discipline, it has been found that aggressive children often emerge from homes with authoritarian parents. The adults are likely to use harsh and aggressive physical punishment and negative messages to establish order. The punishment may reach the point of physical and emotional mistreatment (Connolly & O'Moore, 2003; Dake et al., 2003; Piskin, 2002; NASP, 2002). The children may not be the only victims of the aggressive behaviors in the home: It is likely that the adults also use aggressive behaviors when interacting with one another. In such an environment, the child is unable to build a positive self-concept and develop self-control that will carry him forward into the future. Instead, the child may feel the need to attack others before he or she is assaulted and learns to handle his or her own anger and conflict with aggression.

The home environment as well as the parent–child relationship also plays a key role in the social, emotional, and behavioral development of children who become targets of peer aggression. It has been found that the parents of victims tend to be intrusive and demanding, displaying control over most social situations instead of allowing their children to freely interact with others. This overprotective nature, found especially among the mothers, hinders the development of age-appropriate social skills and fosters the passive personality that many victims display. This overly protective parent–child relationship has been found to be particularly troublesome for boys (Dake et al., 2003; Bernstein & Watson, 1997; NASP, 2002).

Although the parents of these children are more actively involved compared with the parents of bullies, victims may have trouble bonding with their caregivers. The victims experience periods of intense interest as well as rejection, creating an unstable bond or insecure attachment between the parents and children. A child living under such conditions does not give up on the relationship; instead, he or she will continuously strive to please his or her parents, hoping that doing so will elicit attention. Growing and developing in the midst of wavering affection not only creates an unhealthy relationship between the parent and the child but also teaches the youth the role of a victim (Bernstein & Watson, 1997).

Peer Group Risk Factors

Children who display aggressive behaviors often interact with peers who advocate, support, or promote such actions (NASP, 2002). With the group standing behind him or her, personal responsibility for the inappropriate behaviors is often diffused (Mohandie et al. 2000). Some of these groups can be identified as official gangs or hate groups. Interestingly, the child does not have to be affiliated with or obtain membership in a certain group to adopt their antisocial values and behaviors. Instead, the child may admire the group from the periphery and engage in behaviors advocated by the group. (Dwyer et al., 1998).

Community Risk Factors

Research (Mohandie et al. 2000) has shown that children who grow up in impoverished families and neighborhoods have an increased likelihood of engaging in aggressive and/or violent behaviors. Within these areas, the unemployment rate is high and they lack the resources that could offer needed assistance to families. Being surrounded by substandard schools and housing facilities contributes to feelings of hopelessness and the belief that society does not care about their needs. Violence then becomes an expression of the anger, frustration, and alienation that these children struggle with on a daily basis (Prevention Institute, 2006; Mohandie et al., 2000).

School Risk Factors

It has been noted that aggressive or bullying behaviors thrive more readily in an environment in which the students receive negative feedback and/or attention from the school staff than in a more positive climate that sets high standards for interpersonal behaviors and respect (NASP, 2002). Furthermore, it has been hypothesized that school-related stress, school size, and class size are factors that contribute to the prevalence of bullying behaviors within the educational system. However, it does not appear that such issues significantly increase the risk of aggressive behaviors within the school (Natvig et al., 2001; Olweus, 2003). Instead, it was found that school alienation, or the degree to which a student finds the work at school meaningless and unchallenging, is more likely to influence the frequency of bullying behavior. When a child is not challenged or does not see the relevance of issues addressed at school, he or she is more likely to engage in aggressive behaviors (Natvig et al., 2001).

Along with the school environment and the quality of assignments, research has indicated that a teacher's attitude and/or response to aggressive situations influence the occurrence of these behaviors. It has been noted that although teachers generally display negative attitudes toward bullying behaviors, 25% do not feel that aggressive behaviors and verbal attacks are wrong (NASP, 2002). Although the majority of educators agree that aggressive and violent actions should not be tolerated, research has found that only 4% intervene when such behaviors or situations arise (Dake et al., 2003; NASP, 2002). A lack of action can be contributed to the fact that teachers often do not know how to act in an aggressive situation or fear the child who has instigated the situation. In addition, the teacher may not find fault with the aggressor's behavior, claiming that boys will be boys. Without consequences that are enforced by the adults, aggressive actions are reinforced and continue to escalate.

Television and Video Game Violence

Research has estimated that the average child watches 23–28 h of television a week and that by age 18 he or she has witnessed 200,000 acts of television violence, including 40,000 murders (Hurst, 2004). A child's contact with violence can be increased through other multimedia venues, such as video games, the Internet, music, and movies. This heavy exposure to violence can lead children to accept aggressive behaviors as an appropriate way of interacting and/or resolving differences with others (Hurst, 2004; Prevention Institute, n.d.). These images will also desensitize children to future violence that they experience in reality and on television. Interestingly, the violence that children experience through the media not only encourages such behaviors as a means of coping but also may increase their fear of being victimized. In order to protect themselves from falling victim to others' aggressive and/or violent behaviors, children may begin to carry weapons or engage in violence themselves (Hurst, 2004; Prevention Institute, 2006).

The Importance of Early Identification

Early identification is a key factor in the success of treatment, improving the possibility that treatment will be effective in rehabilitating the victim as well as the offender.

When aggressive behavior occurs on school grounds, it is often identified as bullying. Many teachers and other educational staff remain unaware of the direct (i.e., physical actions and verbal insults) and indirect (i.e., shunning from the group) bullying behaviors that occur around them. Understanding the risk factors that can contribute to aggressive behavior in children is just the beginning; school staff should also receive training so that they will be more adept at identifying the bullying or aggressive behaviors that are occurring in the classrooms, in the halls, and on the school grounds (National Association of

State Boards of Education [NASBE], 2006). A portion of the training should also address the warning signs that teachers and other school staff should recognize. Although these warning signs are present in most cases of school violence, their existence does not necessarily indicate that a child will become violent (Dwyer et al., 1998). It has been noted that most children who display aggressive or violent behaviors exhibit multiple warning signs with increased intensity over time. Therefore, as teachers and other school staff assess the children in the classrooms, they must use caution. School personnel must work to ensure that their actions on behalf of the student do not cause harm. The warning signs should not be used to isolate, stereotype, or mislabel children; instead, researchers have identified these indicators to increase the likelihood that the child will receive assistance before they engage in violence. As a result, educators should attempt to understand a child's aggressive or violent behavior in the context of these risk factors while regarding the youth's developmental level. This results in school personnel forming a more objective conclusion (Dwyer et al., 1998).

Indicators that a child is struggling and may need support include excessive feelings of isolation and rejection (Dwyer et al., 1998). Many children and adolescents experience rejection as they search for their individual identities; those who are troubled, however, are often isolated from their mentally healthy peers. In light of these deep feelings of rejection and isolation, it is not uncommon for the child to withdraw from social interactions with their peers. Often these emotions are accompanied by depression, a lack of confidence, and a feeling of always being picked on or persecuted. Children who are consistently the target of teasing, humiliation, and physically aggressive behaviors are likely to withdraw socially. In addition, they may eventually vent their frustration and anger in inappropriate ways which may include violence.

Although many children withdraw from their peers as they struggle with negative emotions, some will have difficulty controlling their anger and frustration. When a child frequently lashes out at others, using mild forms of aggression, such as hitting and intimidation, it is cause for concern (Dwyer et al., 1998). The same is true for individuals who have a history of discipline problems. These patterns of aggressive behaviors are often an expression of emotional turmoil. If the emotional as well as the behavioral issues are not addressed by caring adults, they may escalate to the point where the child engages in violence. It has been noted that this risk increases for children who display antisocial behaviors within multiple environments, such as school, community, and home.

Researchers (Dwyer et al., 1998) have noted that children who display aggressive or violent behaviors tend to associate with other individuals who display and support such actions. Although many of these social groups are not recognized as gangs or hate groups, teachers and other school staff should note that it is a possibility. An intense prejudice or willingness to victimize certain populations should raise concern and prompt school personnel to offer additional supports to the child. Even if a child is not officially affiliated with a gang, he or she may identify with its members and imitate the behaviors of its members. The delinquent behaviors that the child and his or her peer group perform may include the consumption of alcohol and other drugs. These substances lower the youth's inhibitions and self-control, making it more likely that he or she will engage in violent behaviors. The risk also increases if the child has access to firearms or other weapons. In addition, children who have access to or possession of firearms also have a higher risk of becoming the victim of violence.

A child's behavior among his or her peers is only one aspect of the risk factors that can indicate that he or she may need additional supports from school staff or mental health professionals. The youth's academic performance can also raise concern. If a child is not expressing interest in school or is continuously performing poorly, it may indicate that he or she is at risk for violent behavior (Dwyer et al., 1998). Again, caution must be used when evaluating the student because these two factors can be caused by a number of events. However, it has been noted that when a low-achieving student feels frustrated, chastised, or worthless, he or she is at a greater risk for aggressive or violent behavior. Within the realm of academics, a consistent expression of violence in drawings or written material may indicate the potential for violence. If a teacher notices these themes among a student's work, he or she should seek assistance from a mental health professional, especially if the child has targeted a specific individual as a potential victim. A verbal threat of violence, especially those that incorporate a specific plan, should be considered a reliable indicator that future violence will occur if a supportive adult does not intervene (Dwyer et al., 1998).

These warning signs can be early indicators that a child may engage in violent behavior in the future and should be cause for concern. When the frequency and intensity of some of the high-risk behaviors mentioned above increases, they are identified as imminent warning signs. Again, these signs do not necessarily indicate that violence will occur, especially if only one is present; however, they do require teachers and other school staff to take immediate action. The imminent warning signs, as identified by Dwyer et al. (1998), include the child experiencing severe rage for what appear to be minor reasons. The intensity of these emotions can lead the child to engage in the destruction of property and in serious physical altercations with peers or family members. School personnel should also immediately seek assistance on behalf of a child if he or she engages in self-injurious behaviors or verbalizes a threat of suicide and/or expresses a detailed threat of lethal violence. If the child possesses and/or has used firearms and other weapons, it not only increases the concern for the child and the school community but also requires that teachers and school staff react immediately to prevent the possibility of violence. As the teachers and other school staff move to de-escalate the situation, they must contact the child's parents as well as outside agencies that might be able to intervene and/or offer support to the child and his or her family (Dwyer et al., 1998).

Selecting Appropriate Interventions

Resilience

Before the most appropriate intervention can be selected, an assessment of the level of resilience should be made. Resilience is defined as the capacity to rebound from hardship experienced early in life. Wolin and Wolin (1993) report that hardships not only cause pain but also encourage uncommon strength. Becoming resilient allows the individual to master painful memories, to accept painful remarks, to take revenge by living well instead and breaking the cycle of blaming and finding fault, and to put the past in its place. In addition, they identify seven strengths or resiliencies that can be used by children, adolescents, and adults in developing a more resilient self. These resiliencies are particularly useful for adolescents and adults (Wolin & Wolin, 1993). Once the level of resilience has been established, the most appropriate intervention can be selected.

Behavior Management

Although children are continuously interacting with teachers and peers, providing them with opportunities to learn and practice appropriate social skills, some children need additional support and instruction. Behavior management programs that target children who engage in aggressive and/or violent behaviors provide assistance to children with both their anger control and problem-solving skills (Dwyer et al., 1998). With time and practice, these programs teach the children alternative and socially appropriate replacement responses that will allow them to positively engage their peers and form more healthy relationships. In addition, some schools incorporate interventions that enhance interpersonal and conflict resolution skills (Dwyer et al., 1998).

Parent Training

Parent training is often based on the belief that juveniles engage in criminal activities because they lack the skills for obtaining rewards by appropriate means (Dwyer et al., 1998). It has also been suggested that parents, with the proper instruction, can alter their children's behaviors. Research has demonstrated that parent training may not only reduce the aggressive behaviors of the targeted child but also increase the frequency of acceptable behavior. In addition, the frequency of inappropriate behaviors expressed by the aggressor's siblings might be reduced as a result of the parent training.

Along with changes in the parents' attitudes and responses to the aggressive child, it has been noted that these families should be encouraged to make sure that firearms are out of the child's reach (Dwyer et al., 1998). In order to reinforce such behavior, law enforcement officers could be asked to provide the families with information regarding safe firearm storage.

Therapy for the Child

In addition to parent training programs, therapy for the aggressive child and his or her family may reduce the antisocial or inappropriate behaviors. Two programs that are commonly thought of when addressing the issue of children with behavioral problems are therapeutic wilderness programs and boot camps. Wilderness programs attempt to produce positive attitudes and behaviors and teach problem-solving skills through the use of physical challenges. It is assumed that the skills established and practiced during the course of the program will be transferred to the various settings that the child encounters in his or her everyday life. Like wilderness programs, boot camps focus on delinquent behaviors. Since these two types of programs do not address the underlying causes found in the child's everyday environment, the skills taught during the camps are not easily transferred to the home or community settings. Therefore, researchers have found that both wilderness programs and boot camps do not have lasting effects on the attitudes or behaviors of children (Tarolla et al., 2002).

Peer group counseling is another common intervention strategy used in schools and juvenile correctional facilities. At this point, research has shown little support for its effectiveness. In fact, group counseling has been known to be detrimental to a delinquent when he or she is treated with other children with behavior problems. If the group involves nondelinquent peers, however, the results may be more promising (Tarolla et al., 2002).

Interventions with more of a systemic approach, on the contrary, have been shown to be more effective at maintaining the positive effects of therapy. For example, family therapy that focuses on the maladaptive patterns in the family unit that not only cause but also maintain the aggressive behaviors of the targeted youth has proven effective in reducing the conduct problems. In addition, it has been found that this type of family therapy improves concentration and problem solving. Another program that has been shown to reduce violent and criminal activity is multisystemic therapy. It uses multiple established treatment modes to address the causes of delinquent behaviors as well as how the family, school, and community influence the maintenance of such actions. The Juvenile Counseling and Assessment Program (JCAP) uses multiple approaches when treating court-referred children and their families. It often includes individual, group, and family counseling, as well as training in problem solving, social skills, anger management, lifestyle, and career decisions. Thus far, JCAP has shown positive results for reducing recidivism (Tarolla et al., 2002).

Cognitive-behavioral treatment has shown some promise in improving violent youths' social problem-solving skills and impulse control. This method is based on the premise that antisocial behaviors are mediated by cognitive deficiencies and distortions. Therefore, the youths work to identify and modify maladaptive thoughts and behaviors through behavior modification strategies, rehearsal, role taking, and cognitive reinforcement. The children also work on developing appropriate anger management and coping skills (Tarolla et al., 2002).

Safety Plan

The National Association of School Boards of Education developed a policy update regarding bullying and schools and has identified descriptions and definitions of common forms of bullying including verbal, physical, direct, indirect, and typed. They report that effective school programs

- Provide early intervention.
- Offer balanced discipline with behavioral supports.
- Support parents' efforts to teach their children good social skills.
- Train school staff with prevention and intervention skills.
- Change attitudes toward bullying.
- Empower students to support each other.
- Create a positive school environment.

They point out that parents can be aware of changes in a child's attitude and behavior and let the schools know if their child is being bullied. In addition, parents should teach their child strategies to counter bullies and their effect by teaching the child to stand up for himself verbally, to walk away from bullies, and to use humor. Parents should begin teaching good social skills early, foster positive social relationships and activities, and use alternatives to physical punishment.

Legal Complexities and Treatment and Solutions

The state of Oregon has developed laws to address bullying as well as harassment within the school system. For example, it requires each school district to develop policies prohibiting harassment, intimidation, and bullying. In Oregon House Bill 3403, emphasis is placed on identification of the problem and handling the problem specifically and clearly. In addition to strong policies and laws, the Bill offers a straightforward approach by law enforcement and clear-cut consequences by the courts, which provides a clear message in communities that there is a zero tolerance for behavior that involves bullying, intimidation, and harassment.

Child and Adolescent Psychiatry and Alerts (2002) has identified a number of treatments for offenders. Therapeutic wilderness programs were found to be ineffective and boot camps had few long-term effects. Family systems therapy focused on maladaptive family patterns that cause and maintain delinquent behavior. These patterns include poor family organization and cohesion, ineffective parent supervision and discipline, the use of aggression or coercion, and failure to support positive behaviors in children. The therapeutic techniques used involve improving communications between parents and children, behavior contracting, rule making, and positive reinforcement, as well as broader systemic approaches. The authors report that literature reviews and meta-analyses suggest that family therapy is effective in reducing conduct problems in children. Along with assistance from a mental health professional, the NASBE has found a number of helpful interventions, including supporting parents' efforts to teach their children good social skills, equipping children and school staff with prevention and intervention skills, changing attitudes toward bullying, empowering students to support each other, and creating a positive school environment.

In summary, it is important that there is zero tolerance within the community for bullying, harassment, and intimidation. It is important to first identify the problem, take the problem seriously, and provide consequences in the community for offenders. In addition, it is necessary to identify treatment programs that have been proven successful and to provide support for victims. Courts must monitor offender's behavior and monitor the effectiveness of treatment programs.

What Schools Can Do

A quick response is crucial in the form of early identification. Most schools respond to violent behaviors with reactive interventions and policies, which tend to reinforce the negative feedback and attention that the children receive. Instead, the NASP suggests that educational staff establish prevention programs that build a more positive environment not only within the school but in the community as well. Such a program requires dedication from teachers, parents, and students, as well as from other members of the community. The program should be established and implemented in elementary or middle school, although it could begin as early as preschool. The following components should be implemented:

- Problem students should be in social skills training counseling, or other interventions should be offered for both the aggressor and the victim when bullying occurs.
- When aggressive acts occur, clear and consistent consequences should be present and known to all children.
- The intervention should address not only the behavior but also the underlying causes.
- Parents must learn to model and reinforce the positive behavioral patterns that their children display, including interpersonal encounters.
- School personnel must support the parents in their efforts to teach their children good social skills by keeping the lines of communication open among the parents, child, and school staff.

Dwyer et al. (1998) emphasize that it is necessary for schools to consider both prevention and intervention, providing staff with access to a team of specialists who are trained in evaluating serious behavioral and academic concerns. It is also critical to have a coordinated service system involving families and communities, child and family service agencies, law enforcement, juvenile justice, mental health agencies, businesses, and faith and ethnic leaders. In addition to collaborating with members of the community, the school should involve parents as soon as possible in safety and response plans, informing them about school discipline policies, procedures, and rules, and routinely updating them about their child's behavior both negative and positive. Students should be encouraged to take responsibility for their actions and actively engaged in the planning, implementation, and evaluation of violence prevention initiatives. It is important to simplify requests for urgent assistance because children who are at risk of endangering themselves or others cannot be placed on a waiting list. Therefore, interventions should be available as soon as possible, referrals made as promptly as possible, and feedback provided to the referring professional quickly and efficiently. Violence prevention and response is also enhanced by providing the entire community, including teachers, students, parents, and support staff, with training and support in responding to imminent warning signs, preventing violence, and intervening safely and effectively.

Analyzing the context in which the violence occurs will help determine the appropriate course of action or intervention (Dwyer et al., 1998). It is important to consider the child's age, cultural background, and family experience and values. Interventions should be comprehensive and multidisciplinary. Special education evaluations for troubled children should be provided when necessary. Safety can be enhanced by supervising access to the building and the grounds, reducing class size, and reducing school size, adjusting the schedule to minimize time in hallways or potentially dangerous locations, conducting safety audits, and closing school campuses during lunch periods. It is necessary to have a plan to channel students away from areas where incidents are likely to occur, thereby prohibiting them from congregating where they are likely to engage in rule-breaking or aggressive behaviors. It is also necessary for adults to be visible throughout the building, to stagger dismissal times and lunch periods, to monitor surrounding school grounds, and coordinate with local police to ensure safe routes to and from school (Dwyer et al., 1998).

Schools with effective prevention programs in place focus on academic achievement (Dwyer et al., 1998). They convey to students they believe that they can meet both the academic and the behavioral standards set forth for students. Expectations should be communicated in ways that are easily understood by students and also possible for students to integrate. Family members, particularly parents, should be supported and feel free to express their concerns regarding their children. Positive relationships should be emphasized between students and staff and opportunities should be available for students to spend quality time with adults in the school. Also, positive relationships among students should be encouraged and effective strategies to deal with feelings, particularly anger, taught so that students are able to handle conflict constructively. Students not only need to learn to be responsible for their actions but also need to feel safe expressing their emotions to school staff in order to reduce feelings of isolation, rejection, and disappointment. School personnel should have a system in place for referring children who are suspected of being mistreated or neglected to both health care and mental health care facilities. Students should be supported in making the transition from their adolescence to adult life as well as the workplace (Dwyer et al., 1998).

All school personnel should be offered training and receive training to prevent and intervene in aggressive incidents. The training program should include elements that will assist staff members:

- To quickly identify and respond to potentially dangerous victimization.
- To teach them to implement positive feedback and modeling to foster good social interactions.
- To help to change the attitude that many in the community have toward bullying behaviors.
- To see the aggressive acts as potentially dangerous rather than mere immaturity.
- To teach children to work together to stand up to the bully instead of being part of an accepting crowd of observers.
- To reach out to excluded peers and celebrate acts of kindness (NASP, 2002).

The response plan should also include some provisions for responding when a crisis has occurred. Dwyer et al. (1998) suggest that professionals both within the school and in the community can be involved to assist parents in understanding their children's reaction to the violence. These professionals should also be available for the teachers and other staff as they are dealing with their own reactions. Debriefing and grief counseling is very important at this point. Mental health counseling should be available as the staff and students adjust following a crisis. Since some victims or offenders may have been removed from the school, assist the victims and family members to reenter the school environment. This may help to make it easier for both the victim and classmates to adjust when the victim returns to the classroom. The staff should coordinate with individuals from the juvenile detention facility or mental health facility to make the return as uneventful as possible (Dwyer et al., 1998).

What Parents Can Do

Parents have several options to consider. Parents should be aware of any changes that occur in their children. Frequently, children will display behavioral, physiological, or psychological symptoms of the anxiety that they experience as a result of the bullying behavior. Victims often become withdrawn or reluctant to attend classes; they might also complain about headaches, stomachaches, or problems sleeping, as well as other somatic complaints. Parents should talk with children about their concerns and then reassure them that they will work with the school staff to stop the bullying behavior. Parents should also teach their child strategies to counter the bullying behavior, such as standing up for themselves verbally, walking away, using humor, thinking of positive images or statements about themselves to bolster self-esteem, and getting help from an adult. In addition, parents should begin teaching good social skills early on in childhood, praising the child for appropriate social behaviors and model interactions that do not involve aggression. Encourage the child to support the peers or catch the child doing something good and offer positive reinforcement. Parents should monitor television watching and video games. Parents can help their children identify peers with whom they get along and offer suggestions for social interactions. They should also pay attention to the activities that their children enjoy doing and encourage them to help build self-esteem. Parents should use alternatives to physical punishment. Adults should intervene when the bullying behavior occurs (NASP, 2002). The school's discipline policy should be discussed with the child, including the reasons they are in place. Parents should involve the child in setting rules for appropriate behavior in the home and be involved with what their children are watching on television. They should talk with them about the violence they see on television, in video games, or the neighborhood and help them understand the consequences of violence. Parents can also help their child express anger in ways that do not include verbal or physical aggression. Parents should keep the lines of communication open, know their child's friends, and be involved in their child's school life by supporting and reviewing homework, talking with his or her teacher, and attending school functions (Dwyer et al., 1998).

What Students Can Do

Dwyer et al. (1998) expressed a number of creative ideas for students. Students should listen when their friends share troubling thoughts or feelings and encourage them to seek help from a trusted adult. Children should share their own concerns with their parents. Students can also create, join, or support student organizations that combat violent behaviors, like peer mediation or conflict resolution programs, and organize a school assembly to address ideas about how to deal with violence, intimidation, and bullying. Children should work with teachers and administrators to create a safe process for reporting bullying behavior, weapon possession, drug selling, gang activity, graffiti, and vandalism. The school might even consider inviting law enforcement to share safety tips with both staff and students and conduct a safety audit. School staff should encourage students to volunteer to be a mentor to younger students or tutor peers and to model responsible behavior and avoid being part of the onlooking crowd when fights break out (Dwyer et al., 1998).

Some Final Thoughts

It is important for parents, school staff, students, and other community members to have the ability to identify the problem and understand the relationship between traumatic experiences and how the anger acted out harms others. Both adults and children should also recognize that interventions can be successful. In order to both identify and understand problem behaviors, individuals must be aware of the risk factors that can contribute to aggression and/or violence. It is also important for parents, teachers, and students to be able to identify at-risk feelings, attitudes, and behaviors early so that effective or successful interventions can be selected.

References

Bernstein, J. Y. & Watson, M. W. (1997). Children who are targets of bullying. *Journal of Interpersonal Violence, 12*(4), 483–498.

Connolly, I. & O'Moore, M. (2003). Personality and family relations of children who bully. *Personality and Individual Differences, 35(3)*, 559–567.

Dake, J. A., Price, J. H., & Telljohann, S. K. (2003). The nature and extent of bullying at school. *The Journal of School Health,* 73(5), 173–180.

Dwyer, K. P., Osher, D., & Warger, C. (1998). *Early warning timely response: A guide to safe schools.* Washington, D.C.: U.S. Department of Education.

Gray, C. (2000, Winter). Gray's guide to bullying part I: The basics. *The Morning News,* 12(4), 243–247.

Hoover, J. H., Oliver, R., & Hazler, R. J. (1992). Bullying: Perceptions of adolescent victims in the Midwestern USA. *School Psychology International,* 13(1), 5–16.

Hurst, M. D. (2004, November 17). Researchers target impact of television violence. *Education Weekly,* 24(12), 8.

Johnson, H. R., Thompson, M. J. J., Wilkinson, S., Walsh, L., Balding, J., & Wright, V. (2002). Vulnerability to bullying: Teacher-reported conduct and emotional problems, hyperactivity, peer relationship difficulties, and prosocial behavior in primary school children. *Educational Psychology,* 22(5), 553–556.

Mohandie, K., et al. (2000). Suicide and Violence Risk in Law Enforcement: Practical Guidelines for Risk Assessment, Prevention, and Intervention. *Behavioral Science and the Law,* 17(3), 357–376.

Nansel, T. R., Overpeck, M., Pilla, R. S., Ruan,W. J., Simons-Morton, B., & Scheidt, P. (2001). Bullying behaviors among US youth: Prevalence and association with psychosocial adjustment. *Journal of the American Medical Association,* 285(16), 2094–2100.

National Association of School Psychologists. (2002). *Bullying prevention: What schools and parents can do.* Bethesda, MD: National Association of School Psychologists.

National Association of State Boards of Education. (2003, June). Bullying in schools. *NASBE Policy Update,* 11(10).

Natvig, G. K., Albrektsen, G., & Qvarnstrøm, U. (2001). School-related stress experience as risk factor for bullying behavior. *Journal of Youth and Adolescence,* 30(5), 561–575.

Olweus, D. (2003). A profile of bullying at school. *Educational Leadership,* 60(6), 12–17.

Piskin, M. (2002). School bullying: Definition, types, related factors and strategies to prevent bullying problems. *Educational Sciences: Theory and Practice,* 2(2), 555–562.

Satcher, D. (2001). *Youth violence: A report by the surgeon general.* Washington, D.C.: U.S. Department of Health and Human Services.

Soriano, M. (1999, Winter). The family role in violence precaution and response. *School Safety*, 12–16.

Sprague, J. R. & Walker, H. M. (2005). *Safe and healthy schools.* New York: The Guilford Press.

Tarolla, S. M., Wagner, E. F., Rabinowitz, J., & Tubman, J. G. (2002). Understanding and treating juvenile offenders: A review of current knowledge and future directions. *Aggression and Violent Behavior,* 7(2), 125–143.

Thornton, T. N., Craft, C. A., Dahlberg, L.L., Lynch, B. S., Baer, K. (2001). *Best Practices of Youth Violence Prevention: A Sourcebook for Community Action.* Atlanta: US Department of Health and Human Services, Centers for Disease Control.

Weir, E., (2001). The health impact of bullying. *CMAJ: Canadian Medical Association Journal,* 165, 1249.

Wolin, S. J. & Wolin, S. (1993). *The resilient self: How survivors of troubled families rise above adversity.* New York: Random House Inc.

Chapter 10
Boundary Violations: Harassment, Exploitation, and Abuse

Thomas W. Miller and Lane J. Veltkamp

Introduction

Violence in the school environment may take several forms. Bullying, exploitation, sexual harassment, and sexual boundary violations have become the focus of exploitation and abuse experts as a serious concern (Olarte, 1991; Veltkamp & Miller, 1994; Miller & Veltkamp, 1989; Crisci, 1999). The spectrum of sexual boundary violations range from tainted jokes, unwanted sexual advances, and inappropriate educator–child relationships to sexual harassment. During the last decade, many organizations have endorsed rules of ethical conduct that prohibit sexual contact between professionals and clients and advised members on the importance of setting sexual boundaries (American School Boards; American Psychiatric Association, 1995; American Psychoanalytic Association, 1993; American Psychological Association, 1995; National Association of Social Workers, Inc., 1990; Jordan & Walker, 1995). Major efforts have also been made to clarify and prohibit sexual contact in the workplace but those have only begun to read the educational setting. There is a dearth of research on sexual harassment or contact in either setting.

The purpose of this chapter is to elucidate the specific spectrum of sexual boundary violations that professionals must be aware of in the course of providing school-based services. It offers the reader an understanding of the triggers for potential sexual boundary violations, a perpetrator profile and victim profile, the exploitation of the victim in the school setting and the "Trauma Accommodation Syndrome," and a legal case which has signatures for school-based professionals.

Clinician Gabbard (1991) suggested that violations of sexual boundaries between educators and students can occur when the perpetrator confuses his or her own need to be loved with the needs of the victim. The perpetrator fantasizes that love in and of itself may cure his or her psychopathology. The tendency for incestuous sexual experiences—based, perhaps, on the perpetrator's past—to be reenacted in the perpetrator–victim dyad, and the close link between incest and the desire to be helpful and parental, reflects the immaturity and psychopathology of the perpetrator.

Perpetrators often act out their anger and frustration through the sexual exploitation of others. Olarte (1991) identified characteristics of perpetrators who violate sexual boundaries in the school setting. Such perpetrators are often middle aged, going through some type of personal distress or conflict, professionally isolated, likely to overvalue their professional capacity, unorthodox in their moral decision-making processes, likely to overpersonalize the teacher–student relationship, and likely to ignore or deny any ethical responsibility to the victim, society, or to their professional code of conduct.

Case Example

Among recent cases in the public domain is the case of a Florida teacher, Debra LaFave, who was charged with several counts of having illegal sexual relations with a minor in 2005. The teacher claimed she was raped by a schoolmate at age 13 and this resulted in her promiscuous behavior with school-aged children in her school. The teacher's history notes that she sang professionally, did some modeling, and had several relationships before marrying. Her history also notes that after a high school lesbian affair was discovered, she entered therapy for a brief period of time. The teacher was highly popular with the students; she sometimes dressed inappropriately, sometimes wearing a very short skirt or a low-cut blouse showing cleavage. The teacher met a 14-year-old student at an after-school tag football game. The relationship developed over a period of weeks. Shortly after school ended for the year, she drove the boy to her home and performed fellatio on him. Over several encounters the relationship became intimate and they had sex in the back of her sports utility vehicle (SUV) while it was being driven by the boy's cousin. The boy's mother soon learned of the affair and notified the police. They tape-recorded conversations between the lovers, then arrested LaFave when she drove to the boy's home to pick him up. The boy gave police an accurate description of her tattoos, tan lines, and pubic area. This teacher is currently serving probation until 2015 and her teaching certificate has been revoked. In testimony given in court, the teacher attributed her indiscretions to bipolar disorder, previously known as manic depression, which is associated with intense and irregular mood swings and with hypersexuality and poor judgment during manic episodes.

School administrators, teachers, school counselors, and others recognize sexual boundary violations as a form of school violence. Sexual boundary violations are defined as spectrum of activities that may include but not be limited to self-disclosure of information about one's life, one's family, one's experiences or feelings—including positive and negative reactions to a student. In the school environment, accompanying a student to any destination outside the school or a school-sponsored activity may exceed boundary issues. Accepting or giving a gift can all be forms of moving beyond the boundary of one's professional school-related activities. All of these instances have been identified in civil and licensing board litigation cases as evidence of the existence of an inappropriate relationship between teacher and student (Brodsky, 1989; Miller & Veltkamp, 1989; Megana, 1990). Unfortunately, there is a dearth of research on sexual contact in the school setting, even though in the health care field, some self-reporting surveys reveal that 7–12% of counselors have committed sexual boundary violations and engaged in sexual relationships (Schoener & Milgram, 2004).

Teachers, like other professionals, are often confronted with duality of role issues with their students. Sexual boundary violations have become an important focus in understanding the spectrum of abuse and a serious concern for the mental health profession (Brodsky, 1989; Olarte, 1991). Within the construct of sexual boundary violations are unwanted sexual discussion and advances, educator–child relationships, and issues related to sexual harassment.

The American Medical Association has reinforced the Hippocratic Oath with a specific rule stating "sexual contact between a physician and a patient is unethical because it violates the trust necessary in the physician-patient relationship" (American Medical Association, 1991).

Incidence and Prevalence Data

While major efforts to clarify and prohibit sexual contact in health-related and educational settings have been made, there are educators and clinicians who continue to engage in sexual or sexualized contact with their students and clients. In the health care arena, some self-reporting surveys reveal that 7–12% of therapists have engaged in sexual relationships with at least one patient (Schoener et al., 1989). One study found that 80% of therapists reporting any sexual involvement with patients became intimate with the patient. One study regarding psychiatrists found that 65% have counseled at least one patient who has been sexually abused by a previous professional (Gartrell et al., 1987; Kluft, 1990).

Clinical studies indicate that up to 90% of clients who engage in sexual contact with their therapists were psychologically harmed as a result. There is clinical research (Cantrell et al., 1989) which argues that the resulting impact and injuries may include sexual dysfunction, anxiety disorder, psychiatric hospitalization, increased risk of suicide, dissociation, depression, internalization, and feelings of guilt, anger, shame, fear, confusion, hatred, and worthlessness (Pope, 1986). In addition, the abuse by a therapist may exacerbate the patient's presenting illness and may create new psychopathology such as posttraumatic stress disorder in the client or student (Jorgenson, 1994). Among other issues, patients are vulnerable when they enter treatment. There is a significant power imbalance: the therapist over the patient. Often, patients lack self-esteem and are fearful. Sexual contact with clients constitutes misuse of the therapist's power and places the patient in a vulnerable/helpless position.

Prevalence data related to sexual boundary violations is vague and there is a dearth of studies in the school setting. Much of the data are derived from questionnaire surveys of clinicians–client relationships requesting respondents to be honest and truthful about unethical behavior. Several national surveys have been completed, suggesting prevalence in the range of 12% among male therapists and 3%

among female therapists (Kluft, 1990). The study which surveyed three major mental health professions, including psychiatry, clinical psychology, and clinical social work, found no differences among the mental health disciplines in the incidents of such sexual boundary violations. The professions have also made considerable efforts to understand the origins and process of sexual boundary crossings and violations.

Elliott (1990), addressing the issue of abuse-related counter-transference and the therapist as an abuse survivor, suggests that clinicians are even more likely than other professionals to have been sexually or physically abused and to have come from homes where substance abuse was a problem for parents. Unresolved child abuse issues can impede or interfere with therapeutic effectiveness with patients. Sexual boundary violations are, perhaps, the most dangerous form of abuse-related counter-transference. Boundary incursion by a person entrusted to be a therapeutic agent may not only revisit the abuse-related issues for the patient but also reinforce abuse-related trauma in the survivor client. Megana (1990), researching this area, has concluded that researcher sexual abuse survivors who are sexually revictimized by their therapists suffer greater symptoms than cohorts who were molested as children but not during therapy.

Gabbard (1991) addressed the psychodynamics of such violations wherein perpetrators who transgressed sexual boundaries with victims show considerable confusion of their own needs with that of victims' needs or experience a sense of love. Most notable among these psychodynamics themes are confusion of one's own need to be loved with those of the victim, particularly when one is vulnerable due to personal problems; the fantasy that love in and of itself may by curative; the proneness of the perpetrator–victim dyad to reenact incestuous sexual involvement from the victim's past; the close linkage between wanting to be helpful and sexual involvement; and the tendency of some perpetrators to act out their hostility through sexual exploitation of the victim. In addition, the perpetrator may sexually exploit a victim simply because he or she wants to or because he or she has the opportunity.

Whether unwanted discussion or advances, sexual boundary violations, or the medium of sexual harassment in the school setting, three main methodologies have been utilized to collect data on the characteristics of the perpetrator. Olarte (1991) identifies these data summaries as including the following:

1. Composites of the descriptions of such perpetrators based on their treatment.
2. Profile descriptions of perpetrators extrapolated from research surveys that guarantee anonymity to the professional.
3. A detailed classification and description of offenders based on voluntary evaluations of such offenders by national centers that specialize in the diagnosis and treatment of victims of physical and sexual abuse.

Olarte (1991) reports that characteristics frequently seen include a young to middle-aged perpetrator, usually a male but with increased frequency of female perpetration, who is undergoing some type of personal distress, who was isolated professionally, who tends to overvalue his or her healing capacity, who is unorthodox about his or her therapeutic methods, who frequently personalizes the teacher–student relationship, and who ignores or denies his or her ethical responsibility to his or her victim.

Symptom Indicators of Sexual Harassment or Boundary Violations

In some cases of sexual exploitation or sexual abuse, the victim will notice that a precursor to these behaviors may involve sexually suggestive or other inappropriate behaviors. Both behavioral and physical symptoms are summarized in Table 10.1.

Often these behaviors are confusing and subtle and can be identified by the student because they often feel uncomfortable. Examples of warning signs in educational settings may include the following:

1. Faculty, staff who tell sexually tainted jokes or stories
2. Giving the potential victim seductive looks and flirting

Table 10.1 Behavioral and physical indicators often seen in victims of exploitation and abuse*

Behavioral indicators
Apprehension, fearfulness
Withdrawn, inhibited behavior
Compulsive behaviors
Anger
Anxiety
Phobias
Mistrust
Hyperactivity
Withdrawal
Poor peer relationships
Hostility/aggression
Physical Indicators
Sleep disturbances—insomnia, nightmares
Difficulty concentrating
Exaggerated startle response
Apprehension, anticipatory anxiety
Phobias, obsessions
Drug/alcohol abuse
Precocious sexual behavior
Sophisticated sexual knowledge beyond the child's age
Irritability
Depression
Guilt
Suicidal thoughts and/or attempts
Mood swings

*Developed through the Department of Psychiatry, College of Medicine, University of Kentucky, by Dr. Thomas W. Miller and Lane J. Veltkamp, Director, Family Violence Clinic, 1997.

3. Discussing the staff member's personal sex life and details regarding intimate relationships to students
4. Sitting too close to students, showing affection, and inappropriate touching

In addition, other warning signals include (1) a teacher giving a student special status by scheduling after-school appointments, (2) making out of school appointments, (3) using the victim as a confidant or for personal support, (4) giving or accepting gifts, and (5) getting involved in giving money or offering substances of abuse to the student.

A Classic Legal Case Brief

The case, *Davis V. Monroe County Board of Education (1999)*, involves a fifth grader who alleges that a male student harassed her eight times during a 6-month period. The harassment included attempts to touch the student's private areas, sex-related vulgarities, and sexually suggestive behavior. All the alleged incidents occurred in the school setting.

The student reported the incidents to three teachers. She also reported the last incident to the principal, who allegedly had learned of one previous incident from a teacher. The teacher took only one remedial action—assigning the harasser to a different seat in the classroom—and the principal threatened disciplinary action. After the last incident, the perpetrator was charged with sexual battery, to which he pleaded guilty. The female student alleged that she suffered mental anguish, that her grades dropped, and that she wrote a suicide note.

The student's mother sued, claiming that the failure of school officials to prevent her daughter's sexual harassment violated Title IX. The Federal District Court dismissed the lawsuit, and the Circuit Court of Appeals affirmed that decision. Both courts concluded that a school district is not liable under Title IX for failing to prevent student-on-student, or peer, sexual harassment. After the two lower courts dismissed the case, the family appealed to the US Supreme Court, which found that Title IX damages may be found against a school board in cases of student-on-student harassment where the school was deliberately indifferent to sexual harassment so severe, pervasive, and objectively, offensive that the victim has deprived access to the school's educational opportunities and benefits. In that the Plaintiff won, they will now have the right to return to District Court for a trial for their suit on its merits.

This case involving sexual harassment, which is another form of sexual boundary violation, is critically important to school districts across the country. For the first time, the high court ruled on the contentious issue of a school board's liability for student-on-student harassment. The ruling has now set a national standard. The case has become a litmus test for sexual boundary violations and for many women's and children's rights advocates, who argue that children deserve protection from physical and verbal abuse at school—the same protections employees are afforded in the workplace setting.

The National School Board Association (NSBA), joined by several other education organizations, supports the Georgia school board's position. It contends in a friend-of-the-court brief that schools should not be held financially liable for peer sexual harassment unless the school purposefully discriminated against the student. While most school boards and administrators acknowledge that sexual harassment is a growing concern—recent studies suggest that at least 50% of all public school students are sexually harassed—they realize that striking the right balance in the classroom can present a challenge.

Prevention/Intervention in the School Environment

Prevention requires the recognition of and appropriate response to sexual boundary violations by persons in educational settings, as well as clearly defined approaches to the needs of both potential victims and perpetrators (Miller, 1998). The following policy guidelines will help educators address the issues of sexual boundary violations in the school setting:

Provide awareness training designed to help educators recognize sexual boundary violations, with special attention given to the psychological, legal, and medical needs of the student victim.

Establish policies and procedures that are designed to help administrators and staff manage and monitor sexual boundary issues; making sure that they include clearly defined reporting procedures.

Identify areas of potential risk within the school setting that encompass student–educator relationships.

Utilize multidisciplinary professionals in the form of an advisory board within the school system and community to address the effect of sexual boundary violations and evaluate monitoring policies and procedures.

Prepare incident reports and submit them to the Department of Education and Health and Human Services, as well as other appropriate licensing agencies, as required by state law.

For therapists and counselors seeking resources, fortunately there have been countless guides published in articles and books, helping clinicians carefully weigh the factors, values, and possibilities in trying to arrive at the best possible decision about whether entering into various kinds of relationships with a client makes clinical and ethical sense. In addition to the more general decision-making aids, there are resources for virtually every kind of specialty practice and context (e.g., a 3-level model for family therapists involved with religious communities to negotiate dual relationships; a decision-making model for social dual-role relationships during internships). One of the most frequently cited general models is Mike Gottlieb's "Avoiding Exploitive Dual Relationships: A Decision-Making Model" (Gottlieb, 2001). Another is Jeff Younggren who has published an 8-step model: "Ethical Decision-making and Dual Relationships" (Younggren, 2002).

There may, of course, be times—even with such helpful models—when therapists hit an impasse and are unsure whether to enter a complex dual (or multiple) relationship or try an intervention that involves similar boundary issues. Pope outlines 10 steps that therapists may find useful in addressing such impasses and thinking through whether to begin the potential dual relationship or intervention (Pope, 1986). Pope (1986) confronts a diverse set of situations, each with its own shifting questions, demands, and responsibilities. Every clinician is unique in important ways. Every client is unique in important ways. Ethics that are out of touch with the practical realities of clinical work and with the diversity and constantly changing nature of the therapeutic venture are useless (Pope, 1986). The value in using these scenarios and questions to consider nonsexual dual or multiple relationships and other forms of boundary crossings may be in direct proportion to the ability… to disclose responses that may be politically incorrect, 'emotionally incorrect,' or otherwise at odds with group norms or with what some might consider the 'right' response (Pope, 1986).

The Processing of the Boundary Violation

The impact of victimization can be both short and/or long term based on a number of factors including (1) the duration of the abuse or exploitation, (2) whether there was a use of threat or intimidation within the context of the abusive behavior, and (3) the degree to which the abusive behavior occurred. However, even the most minimal forms of sexual exploitation can cause substantial psychological damage to students. For example, many children will (1) feel a sense of shame; (2) feel guilty even though it's the educator's responsibility to prevent such exploitation; (3) have mixed feelings toward the educator, for example, betrayal, love, anger, or feeling protective; (4) feel isolated and empty; (5) feel unable to trust one's own feelings or to judge trustworthiness in other people; (6) fear that no one will believe them or understand what's happened or fear that others will find out; (7) have posttraumatic stress-related symptoms, including unexpressed rage, numbness, nightmares, obsessive thoughts, depression, suicidal thoughts, or flashbacks; (8) have confusion about dependency, control, and power.

Perpetrator/Victim Profiles

Composites of perpetrators which emerge include individuals who show impaired reality testing and poor social judgment, sociopathy and narcissism, ignorance and naiveté, anxiety, depressive symptoms, and impulsiveness. Schoener et al. (1989) have identified psychiatric data received in the voluntary evaluation of offenders. They classified sexually exploitative persons into clusters, based on their years of clinical experience rather than through systematic research. Their categories include the following:

1. Uninformed naive—These individuals lack knowledge of the expected ethical standards or lack understanding of professional boundaries and confuse personal and professional relationships.
2. Healthy or mildly neurotic—These perpetrators know the professional standards, actual contact with students tends to be limited or isolated, situational stressors foster a slow erosion of professional boundaries, and the perpetrators often show remorse.
3. Severely neurotic and socially isolated—These individuals have long-standing emotional problems such as low self-esteem, depression, feelings of inadequacy, and social isolation.
4. Impulsive character disorder—These persons have long-standing problems with impulse control in many areas of their life, their judgment is poor, and they tend to abuse more than one victim.
5. Sociopath or narcissistic character disorder—These perpetrators have long-standing serious personal pathology that expresses itself in most aspects of their lives and these perpetrators manipulate victims and colleagues to protect themselves from their unethical behavior.
6. Psychotic or borderline personality—Impaired reality testing and poor social judgment of these perpetrators hinder their ability to apply their knowledge of ethical standards or a clinical understanding of professional boundaries.

Schoener et al. (1989) believe that the uninformed naive and the mildly neurotic have a good prognosis, while the last four have a poorer prognosis. The search for a perpetrator profile must take into consideration the realization that the perpetrator bears the burden of responsibility for his or her behavior, including ethical and legal considerations, a moral code, and constraints. Wohlberg (1990) has suggested that after an extensive literature review, there is little support for a single profile for patients involved in sexual boundary violations. Gender and age combinations provide a range of diagnostic categories for both parties. What does emerge is what is referred to as commonalities representing recurring themes encountered in working with both perpetrators and victims. The central commonality is the vulnerability factor noted in both the victim and the perpetrator.

Stone (1982), examining the issue of vulnerability to sexual exploitation and sexual boundary violations, examined a sample of 46 females who had terminated with male therapists and who were divided by criteria into four groups. The groups included those who were sexually intimate, those who were sexually propositioned, those who were prematurely terminated, and those who successfully completed therapy. The study found that women who had been sexually involved with therapists had the strongest anxious attachment to significant others while there were no significant differences realized between groups and the amount of ego strength.

In another study, Averill et al. (1989) developed a profile of the victim who might be commonly vulnerable to sexual relations with a perpetrator. These researchers suggest that the typical victim may include those individuals with borderline personality disorder who have complained of loneliness or emptiness in their lives. They are often seen in treatment as resistant or actively self-defeating.

These individuals tend to show a pattern of instability in interpersonal relations, in their self concept, and are often impulsive.

In assessing the issue of outcome with respect to perpetrators, the prognosis is more favorable if the perpetrator

1. Recognizes the problem
2. Takes responsibility for the problem
3. Enters into treatment
4. Remains in treatment until behavior change occurs and avoids denial and/or projection

The Diagnostic and Statistical Manual of Mental Disorders, 4th Edition, (DSM IV) and Diagnostic Implications

As noted in the Diagnostic and Statistical Manual of Mental Disorders, 4th Edition DSM IV criteria (American Psychiatric Association, 1995), individuals sexually abused or exploited by professionals including educators may have transient stress-related paranoid ideation, inappropriate and intense anger, affective instability due to marked reactivity of mood, impulsivity in the areas of sex, spending, substance abuse, identity disturbance and unstable self-image, associations with feelings of imagined abandonment, and a general pattern of unstable interpersonal relationship with alternating extremes of idealization and devaluation.

Borderline personality disorder features may also be present in the perpetrator. These features generally demonstrate a pattern of instability in interpersonal relationships, poor self-concept, and impulsivity, and may include some of the following features:

- Identity disturbance often marked by unstable self-concept or sense of self.
- A pattern of unstable and intense interpersonal relationships that are often marked by alternating extremes of devaluation and idealization.
- Impulsive behavior that tends to be potentially self-damaging and may include self-mutilating behavior and recurrent gestures of suicidal ideation and intent.
- Unstable affective mood and chronic feelings of emptiness.
- Inappropriate and intense anger and poor management of anger and resulting behavior.
- Stress-related paranoid ideation with frantic efforts to avoid real or imagined loss or abandonment.

Numerous authors have indicated a history of abuse in the life of these individuals, which may include previous sexual abuse. Herman et al. (1989) have suggested that abuse victims may learn seductive behavior as a medium by which they tend to relate and reinforce the relationship with the perpetrator. Similarly, other clinician-researchers (Veltkamp & Miller, 1994; Veltkamp, Miller, & Silman, 1994) have noted that individuals who experience abuse in childhood may be more likely to enter abusive situations in adulthood, resulting in poor adaptation to adult life and poor survivor skills.

There may also be clinical features which suggest the presence of a personality disorder and a history of abuse as comorbid factors. Herman et al. (1989) found that 68% of the victims of abuse were diagnosed as borderline and were also sexually abused as children. The authors note that this event may indeed play a critical causative role in the formation of symptoms and the vulnerability factor noted in sexual boundary violations. The dynamic of repetition compulsion is seen as critically important as understanding the dynamics of the sexual boundary violations from the victim's perspective. While most school systems and administrators acknowledge that sexual harassment is a growing concern—estimates suggest that at least 50% of all public school students are sexually harassed–they realize that striking the right balance in the classroom can present a challenge.

Lessons Learned

Examined in this chapter are critical factors in addressing sexual boundary violations in the school environment. Identified initially are the several triggers that serve to put at-risk teachers and students in the traps of sexual boundary violations ranging from sexually tainted jokes to discussing personal sexual lives with students. Specific victim and perpetrator features are reviewed with an emphasis on recognition and empowerment to address such symptoms when they are observed in the school environment. The role of sexual boundary violations as an exploitative process involves an understanding of such activity within the context of the trauma accommodation syndrome. Vulnerable and immature human beings may fall prey to those who choose to sexually exploit them and this results in the traumatization of the victim or victims. A case example involving a current Supreme Court case provides insight into the issues involved in sexual boundary violations in the school setting and the subsequent implications for school administrators, teachers, and school-based professionals. Finally, a series of suggestions and recommendations are offered to provide a prevention model for sexual boundary violations in the school setting.

Prevention requires the *recognition* of and *appropriate response* to sexual boundary violations by persons in educational settings, as well as clearly defined approaches to the needs of both potential victims and perpetrators (Clark & Walker, 1995; Miller, 1998).

Issues and Implications in the Educational Setting

Recognition and response to the issues related to sexual boundary violations by persons in educational settings require well-defined approaches to addressing the needs of both the victim and the perpetrator. Suggested as essential guidelines in addressing sexual boundary violations in the schools include the following:

1. Recognizing and interrupting the sexual boundary violations and addressing the legal and medical needs of the student
2. Establishing policies and procedures that manage and monitor sexual boundary issues in the schools
3. Identifying areas of potential risk within the school setting and all student–educator relationships
4. Utilizing multidisciplinary professionals within the school system and in the community to address the impact and monitoring of sexual boundary violations and the evaluation of policy and procedures
5. Preparing reports of incidents as required by state law and submitting appropriate reports to the Department of Education, Health and Human Services and other appropriate licensing agencies, as mandated by law

Acknowledgments The authors acknowledge the assistance of Jill Livingston MLS, Tagalie Heister MLS, and Betty L. Downing, Department of Psychiatry, University of Kentucky, Linda Brown, Dale Dubina, and Brenda Frommer for their assistance in the preparation of this manuscript. Portions of this chapter appear in Miller, T. W. and Veltkamp, L. J. (1997). *Clinical Handbook of Adult Abuse and Exploitation*, published by International Universities Press, Inc.

References

American Medical Association (1991). The Council on Ethical and Judicial Affairs, American Medical Association, "Sexual misconduct in the practice of medicine." *Journal of the American Medical Association*, 266, 25–38.

American Psychiatric Association (1995). *Principles of Medical Ethics and Annotations Especially Applicable to Psychiatry*. Washington D.C.: American Psychiatric Association.

American Psychoanalytic Association (1993). *Principles of Ethics for Psychoanalysis and Provisions for Implementation of the Principles of Ethics for Psychoanalysis*. New York: American Psychoanalytic Association.

American Psychological Association (1995). *Ethical Principles of Psychologists*. Washington D. C.: American Psychological Association.

Averill, S. C., Beale, D., & Benfer, B. (1989). Preventing staff-patient sexual relationships. *Bulletin of the Menninger Clinic*, 53(2), 384–393.

Brodsky, A. M. (1989). Sex between patient and therapist: Psychology's data and response. In: Gabbard (Ed.), *Sexual Exploitation in Professional Relationships* (pp. 15–25). Washington D.C.: American Psychiatric Press Inc.

Cantrell, K., Harmon, J., Olarte, S., Philstein, J., & Lacilio, T. (1989). Psychiatrists-patient sexual contact: Results of a National Survey, #1, Prevalence. *American Journal of Psychiatry*, 143(2), 1126, 1131.

Clark, J. & Walker, R. (1995). Approaches to clinical supervision: Warning signs of boundary problems: What to do about them! Unpublished document, University of Kentucky: Society of Clinical Social Work.

Crisci, G. S. (1999). When no means no! *The American School Board Journal*, 186(6), 25–30.

Davis V. Monroe County Board of Education (1999). 120 F 3rd 1390. Argued January 12, 1999—Decided May 24, 1999 (97–843).

Elliott, D. M. (1990). The Effects of childhood sexual abuse on adult functioning in a national sample of professional women. Unpublished doctoral dissertation, Biola University, Rose Mead School of Professional Psychology, Los Angeles, CA.

Gabbard G. O. (1991). Psychodynamics of sexual boundary violations. *Psychiatric Annals*, 21(4), 651–655.

Gartrell, N., Herman, J., Olarte, S., Feldstein, M., & Localio, R. (1987). Reported practices of psychiatrists who knew of sexual misconduct by colleagues. *American Journal of Orthopsychiatry*, 57(3), 287–289.

Herman, J. L., Perry, J. C., & Van der Kolk, B. A. (1989). Childhood trauma in borderline personality disorder. *The American Journal of Psychiatry*, 146(2), 490–495.

Jordan, C. & Walker, R. (1995). Responding to complaints of sexual misconduct by licensed and certified professionals. Guidelines for Licensure Boards. Frankfort Kentucky: Bureau of Occupations and Professions, Commonwealth of Kentucky.

Jorgenson, L. M. (1994). Sexual boundary violations. *Treatment Today*, 6(2), 18–24.

Kluft R. P. (Ed.) (1990). *Incest-Related Syndromes of Adult Psychopathology*. (pp.263–288). Washington, D.C.: American Psychiatric Press Inc.

Megana, D. (1990). The impact of client therapist sexual intimacy and child sexual abuse on psychosocial and psychological functioning. Unpublished doctoral dissertation, University of California, Los Angeles, CA.

Miller, T. W. & Veltkamp, L. J. (1989). The adult non-survivor of child abuse. *Journal of the Kentucky Medical Association*, 87(3), 120–124.

National Association of Social workers Inc. (1990). Code of Ethics and the National Association of Social Workers.

Olarte, S. W. (1991). Characteristics of therapists who become involved in sexual boundary violations. *Psychiatric Annals*, 21, 657–660.

Pope, K. S. (1986). Research and laws regarding therapist-patient sexual involvement: Implications for therapists. *American Journal of Psychotherapy*, 40, 564.

Schoener, G., Milgram, J., Gonsiorek, E., Luepker, J., & Conroe, D. (1989). Psychotherapists' sexual involvement with clients: Intervention and prevention. 142(3), 1181–89.

Schoener G. R. & Milgram J. H. (2004). Sexual contact between psychologists and patients. *Journal of Aggression, Maltreatment and Trauma*, 11(1–2), 205–239.

Stone, L.B. (1982). A study of the relationship amongst anxious attachment, ego functioning and female patients' vulnerabilities to sexual involvement with their male psychotherapists. Los Angeles, Calif: California School of Professional Psychology, 1980. Doctoral dissertation. *Dissertation Abstracts International*. 42, 789B.

Veltkamp, L. J. & Miller, T.W. (1994). *Clinical Handbook of Child Abuse and Neglect*. Madison Connecticut: International Universities Press Inc.

Veltkamp, L. J., Miller, T. W., & Silman, M. (1994). Adult non-survivors: A failure to cope with victims of child abuse. *Child Psychiatry and Human Development*, 24(4), 231–243.

Wohlberg, J. (1990). The psychology of therapist sexual misconduct. Panel discussion: Psychological aspects of therapist sexual abuse. Presented at the Boston Psychoanalytic Society and Institute, February 10, 1990.

Younggren, J. (2002). Dual relationships; Personal and professional boundaries among rural social workers. *British Journal of Social Work*, 185, 38–46.

Chapter 11
Cliques and Cults as a Contributor to Violence in the School Environment

Thomas W. Miller, Thomas F. Holcomb, and Robert F. Kraus

Introduction

School-aged children and adolescents seek various forms of social bonding experiences and the school setting provides the opportunity for such an experience. In the popular movie *Mean Girls*, the "Plastics" are the social pinnacle of the high school hierarchy, immortalized through the barrage of teen-themed movies focused on this issue. Clearly embedded in our social consciousness, there is a perceived hierarchy that is characterized by altered behavior and appearances that include designer purses, chemically altered appearances, and copious amounts of pink color. The theme projected in several of the movies on the subject is that Hollywood asserts that normal people hate cliques only because they just want to be included in them but are not. In the school environment, certainly some students convey a sense of superiority, but most do not seem to care depending on their age, current social ties, and sense of self. On the other hand, for some students cliques exist for security (Allen 1965). They are something to hold on to as both males and females venture beyond the comfort zone of childhood and family. They serve as a safety zone for students to feel like they belong to a group and have found in that group some level of acceptance. Cliques are often composed of similar types of students—they tend to think and behave alike. They find in others, similar likes and dislikes.

A crucial dimension of school, beyond striving for the higher grades and overloading on extracurricular activities, is establishing one's self-identity. It involves developing one's self independently, without preconceived expectations from peers or stifling parental supervision. Students usually do not want to be boxed into strictly established, exclusive groups of friends. Rather, they want a school environment that offers an opportunity and a challenge to meet new friends and gain attention, acceptance, and support from peers. Part of that challenge is finding oneself as an individual and then finding others who reflect some of those individual characteristics. Cliques are based not only on superficial characteristics but also on characteristics that the search for self-identity has realized in each of us (Espejo, 2002).

The purpose and value of cliques are not always negative or elitist. It provides a meaningful experience for students to develop and understand themselves and their relationships with other in a microcosm shared by adults who may provide role models for them. Without cliques, the first fragile friendships formed as a freshman would be a lot tougher and the first weeks at school would be a lot more daunting. In the school setting, cliques may be inevitable. The context of one's clique shifts from the strictest school structure to a more casual model as one progresses through school. Most cliques at school are more like social groups. The size of the school and the evolved purpose of cliques lead to an amorphous structure of the social scene, eroding the image of labeled groups, ranked according to merit or strata. While cliques still exist, the manipulative authority they wielded in the school setting is diminished as one progresses through school grades and gains a greater self-confidence in the self.

It is usually the clique that introduces students to both the positive and the negative aspects of society, such as friendships, common interests, shared conflict, and prejudice. It is clear that members of cliques often share the same values and exhibit the same behavior. Although it has been known that cliques form in elementary school, they are commonly associated with middle and high school students. In a nationwide survey of teenage girls' views of cliques, 96.3% of the respondents claimed that cliques existed in their schools (Espejo, 2002). In addition, 84.2% of the respondents reported that most of their classmates belonged to cliques. There are common characteristics of cliques which often include appearance, athletic ability, academic achievement, social or economic status, talent, and ability to attract the opposite sex. The prominent characteristic of a clique usually becomes the clique's label. The label is significant as it is an external identity that binds the group. A group of self-assured, varsity-jacketed male students might be known as "jocks" while another group's unkempt appearance and spacey demeanor could earn them the "stoner" or "druggie" label. There are strong incentives for children and adolescents to join cliques. Students use cliques to ease their way through large peer groups. Cliques and peer groups help adolescents establish an identity (Espejo, 2002).

American schools have treated cliques as a normal and relatively harmless youth phenomenon. However, the perception that domineering high school cliques can worsen many students' feelings of depression, alienation, and rage emerged strongly after the Columbine High School shooting in Littleton, Colorado. On April 20, 1999, seniors Eric Harris and Dylan Klebold shot and killed 12 students, a teacher, and wounded 23 others before they turned the guns on themselves. The two students were part of the Trench Coat Mafia, a clique of Columbine students that did not mesh well with the rest of Columbine's student body. The Trench Coat Mafia's penchant for black clothing, fingernail polish and makeup, industrial rock music, and alleged involvement with Nazism, Satanism, and homosexuality elicited criticism from their peer groups (Espejo, 2002).

The tragedy of Columbine and the other reported school shootings summarized elsewhere in this volume have generated much criticism of high school cliques. Cliques can be socially counterproductive because they create hierarchies that alienate some students. Adolescents who are persecuted or rejected by popular or mainstream cliques may react and form cliques that defy the entire school, such as the Trench Coat Mafia. Others claim that most cliques are not exclusive and create a sense of belonging for their members. Zinn (1999) believes that cliques may prepare adolescents for the complex social structures of the real world and contends that cliques teach teenagers how to socialize in a society that is "dominated by hierarchies." The role of cliques in school violence was one of many issues raised in the aftermath of the Columbine tragedy. The elements of popular culture, video games, movies, entertainment, gun control, and bullying have also been examined in light of school shootings and remain sources of debate.

The importance of cliques is generally contingent on the innate values and security of the individual, not on an externally enforced social structure (Espejo, 2002). The student who finds it difficult to bond at the clique level may move to a more serious and vulnerable form of bonding in school through cults.

Among the various forms of bonding are cults. The word "cult" in its original sense is a broad and generic term used to describe a system of distinctive religious belief and worship. Generally, the word "cult" has taken on a negative meaning and is often used to describe groups that have asocial practices and beliefs. Cults are generally defined by their orientation and behavior. Cults are groups of individuals that freely use unethical and deceptive techniques to recruit and control members' thinking and behavior. So by definition, a cult is a system or community of ritual-obsessive devotion to or veneration for a person, principle, or thing (American Heritage Dictionary, 2004).

Cults in our society take several forms. A small group of bullies aligning to harass a peer with a chronic disability or a more organized group of peers who continually badger a fellow student because of his academic skills provide some of the basis for understanding cult behavior with the school setting. A group of girl cheerleaders who align themselves against other girls in school and provide verbal harassment either through direct contact or through cyberspace using the Internet to spread harmful gossip and bully behavior about targeted victims. Posting pictures and/or damaging information on MySpace.com looked like another install-ment of *Girls Gone Wild*. In them, cheerleaders from a Texas high school exhibited a variety of bawdy behavior. One shot showed a bikini-clad girl sharing a bottle of booze with a friend. Another featured a cheerleader and several other girls in risqué poses offering glimpses of their panties. But the most infamous photo of all was taken in a "Condoms-To-Go" store. Five smiling cheerleaders dressed in uniform posed with large candles shaped like penises. At least one of them appeared to be simulating fellatio. Streamlining video of students bulling, assaulting, or beating other students has also appeared in cyberspace. Posting of condescending state-ments about teachers, school administrators, or fellow students provided the basis for and other example of violence-provoking behavior, teacher and peer victimiza-tion, in the school environment.

There were incidents of bullying behavior toward teachers by the cheerleaders as well as toward fellow students who were not members of the cheerleaders' squad. The cheerleaders had reportedly been a menace long before the condom-store episode. When one teacher told a squad member to quit chatting on her cell phone in class, the girl with the support of fellow group members harassed the teacher with vulgarities and bully-type behavior. On other occasions, members of the cheerleading group offered disrespectful comments and slang in response to teacher and administrator control. Some teachers equated their behavior to gang members, while others observed more cult-like activities believing that some of their activities were initiation into the group. The girls' behavior was not limited to the classroom as they also were disruptive, vulgar, and disrespectful to their coaches in their cheerleading activities. This led to as many as five cheerleader coaches to quit in a 3-year period because of the behavior and control these cheerleaders had both in and out of the classroom.

Accounts of the "Mean Girl Cheerleaders" in McKinney, Texas, provide such an example of cult-related behavior as does the infamous vampire cult which emerged in Western Kentucky in the late 1990s. This cult, which preyed on students in a local rural high school, was made up of several school dropouts and others who were affecting the school environment. The focus of this group of young adults reflected on an interest in being disruptive to the school and community environment. The group focused on several destructive, violent, and bully-type behaviors that reflected their interest in several games and myths as well as new age computer technology and computer games that are outgrowths of *Dungeons & Dragons* of the previous two decades. Their focus was on blood and this led to an identity with vampirism. Such conceptual framework leads to the need to understand the psychological dimensions behind such thinking.

In reviewing the literature, psychodynamic explorations of blood and vampirism in cults or group-related behavior have drawn attention to Abraham's (1946) biting oral stage during which the infant uses his teeth with a vengeance, to Klein's (1948) description of children's aggressive fantasies, and to Fairbairn's (1993) notion of intense oral sadistic libidinal needs formed in response to actual maternal deprivation. While there is a speculative nature to these theoretical approaches, and regardless of whether early psychological and/or physical abuse actually took place, it is interesting to note that patients with psychotic features often manifest persecutory delusions of incorporation, introjections, devouring, and destruction. The psychodynamics of vampirism are quite different for the cases featuring psychopathic and perverse personality traits. As noted by Cleckley (1976) and later by Hare (1986), sociopathy is a personality disorder, perhaps schizotypal, characterized by grandiosity, egocentricity, manipulative behavior, dominance, shallow affect, poor interpersonal bonding, and lack of empathy, anxiety, and guilt. Among the most contrasting persons with elements with schizotypal features displaying overt vampirism are the psychopathic and perverse personalities carry out more integrated and organized behavior and reality testing appears somewhat intact.

The writings of Bourguignon (1977), emphasizing the strong libidinal component in vampirism and its related behaviors, labels it a perversion. The perverse aspects can be observed in few cases of vampirism, specifically when the subject apparently draws sexual satisfaction from drinking a live victim's blood. Within the sociopath and related clinical cases, depending on the actual circumstances of the vampirism, the strong desire to control the victim may be the most prominent feature. This aspect may account for the popularity of sadomasochistic scenarios involving aspects of vampirism.

What Is the Attraction to Cults?

Considerable interest as to why individuals are drawn to cults has become the focus of several studies. Deutsch and Miller (1983) examined four female cult members and found all of them to have certain attitudes including difficulties with heterosexual relations, idealism, and the wish to serve or unify with others, a spiritual world view, and a tendency to deny negative or threatening stimuli, which the investigators suggested had attracted them to the lifestyle and doctrines of a cult. Levine (1981) concluded from a series of studies that (1) alienation, (2) demoralization, and (3) low self-esteem made some individuals particularly vulnerable to cults.

Galanter (1989), having studied such "charismatic groups" as the Unification Church, the Divine Light Mission, and Alcoholics Anonymous, argued that people join these groups primarily to relieve "neurotic distress" and because of a desire for contentment, or as a result of the intolerable consequences of perceived social oppression.

The psychological aspects of the cult behavior and indoctrination are discussed by West (1980) who suggests that the following features may occur in cults:

- Sudden, drastic alteration of the members value system;
- Reduction of cognitive flexibility and adaptability;
- Narrowing, blunting, or distortion of affect;
- Psychological regression in both thinking and behavior
- Physical changes, including weight loss, deterioration in physical appearance, mask-like facial expression, often with a blank stare or darting, evasive eyes, or a puppet-like cheeriness;
- In some cases, clear-cut psychopathology exists with noted changes that may include symptoms of dissociation, obsessive thoughts and ruminations, delusional thinking, hallucinations, and various other psychiatric signs and symptoms.

MacHovec (1989) indicates that frequently reported efforts to frighten victims into silence are achieved by threats of harm or death to pets, parents, friends, or that the home will be burned down. Some report that perpetrators have dressed in costume as trusted figures (doctors, nurses, police) or fantasy figures (movie or cartoon characters) to elude detection and discredit victim reports of indoctrination. Some abused children have associated cult ritual with religious practice and fear going to religious services or funerals. If drugs are used, children may have a phobic reaction to medicine, alcohol, or "poisoned candy." If they have been bound, locked alone, or placed in cramped places, there may be excessively fearful of being left alone, physically restrained, or being in elevators, closets, stairwells, or other enclosed places. Schein (1961) suggests that indoctrination of a cult member often includes many elements similar to political indoctrination. The following rituals and stressors are likely to increase the cult recruit's vulnerability:

- Isolation of the subject and manipulation of the subject's environment;
- Control over channels of communication and information;
- Debilitation through sleep loss, fatigue, or inadequate diet;
- Degradation or diminution of the self;
- Induction of uncertainty, fear, and confusion, with joy and certainty through surrender to the group as the goal;
- Alternation of harshness and leniency in the context of discipline;
- Peer pressure, often applied through ritualized struggle sessions, generating guilt and requiring confessions;
- Insistence by leaders that the recruit's survival, physical, mental, or spiritual, depends on identifying with group;
- Assignment of monotonous tasks or repetitive activities, such as chanting, staring while immobilized, long chains of simple responses to simple commands, and endless copying of written materials;
- Acts of symbolic betrayal or renunciation of self, family, and previously held values, designed to increase the psychological distance between the recruit and his/her previous way of life.

Walsh et al. (1995) studied a sample of 75 ex-members of cults who completed two psychological measures: the short form of the Eysenck Personality Questionnaire and the Beck Sociotropy–Autonomy Scale. Compared to the norms, the sample exhibited elevated scores on neuroticism, sociotropy, and autonomy. Results also noted that the elevated neuroticism scores increasingly approached the norm as a function of time out of the cult. Ex-members in contact with support groups showed reduced levels of neuroticism and sociotropy in comparison with those who were not. While it is not possible to draw firm conclusions from a study of this design, the results are consistent with the view that people with high autonomy scores are likely to leave or be ejected from cults or new religious movements and that doing so may cause psychological difficulties which are ameliorated by time and attendance at a support group activity.

Cult Case Study

In a small rural town in Western Kentucky, four teenagers described as members of a "vampire cult" were charged with first-degree murder in the brutal death of a Florida couple. The couple had been beaten to death in their home by the cult members. The group called themselves the "Vampire Clan," and was thought to include about 30 members. The clan surfaced during an investigation into a break-in at a local animal shelter where puppies were mutilated and their body parts taken from the shelter.

The clan had elaborate scavenger hunts and intricate games of hide and seek based on a popular game called Vampire, the Masquerade. The origins of this vampire cult were influenced by a stranger who appeared in the community about a year prior to the murders and persuaded the group of teens to plan organized cult activities and games. The group of teens subsequently named themselves the "Victorian Age Masquerade Performance Society," or VAMPS.

With this cult, the use of video games had a significant role in modeling behavior for the cult. The games referred to are a part of leisure activities based on a series of games which have emerged over the past four decades. Debate over games such as *Dungeons & Dragons* is part of the lengthy history of controversial leisure activities. Olmstead (1988) has studied several of these controversial games that include fantasy and role-playing and concluded games such as these may be harmful to vulnerable persons and they are often associated with satanic possession. Observations made by some opponents of games such as these including *Dungeons and Dragons* are that this fantasy game play is an occult activity and creates a fantasy about dragons, sorcerers, elves, slayers, and soothsayers as a part of a mystical, enchanted, dangerous voyage that players embark on during the game. Because such play may represent consorting with Satan, one should expect insidious and diabolic consequences, corrupting naive players who become involved in the game without knowing its dangerous effects. Game proponents and cultists argue that these are only "games" having little effect on players, but critics see them as powerful tools of education, indoctrination, and socialization and may result in psychological impairment in the vulnerable person in search for identity and socializing experiences.

Clinical Features

In examining the clinical profiles of cultists, there is a schizotypal personality features noted in the leader of the cult in this case. Schizotypal features according to the *Diagnostic and Statistical Manual* of the American Psychiatric Association (1994) is a pervasive pattern of social and interpersonal deficits marked by acute discomfort with and reduced capacity for close relationships. Cognitive or perceptual distortions and eccentricities of behavior are also noted which begin during early adulthood and may present themselves in a variety of contexts, as indicated by five (or more) of the following:

1. Ideas of reference (excluding delusions of reference)
2. Odd beliefs or magical thinking that influences behavior and is inconsistent with subcultural norms (e.g., superstitious belief in clairvoyance, telepathy, or "sixth sense"; in children and adolescents, bizarre fantasies or preoccupations)
3. Unusual perceptual experiences, including bodily illusions
4. Peculiar thinking and speech (e.g., vague, circumstantial, metaphorical, overelaborate, or stereotyped)
5. Suspicious or paranoid ideation
6. Inappropriate or constricted affect
7. Behavior or appearance that is odd, eccentric, or peculiar

8. Lack of close friends or confidants other than first-degree relatives
9. Excessive social anxiety that does not diminish with familiarity and tends to be associated with paranoid fears rather than negative judgments about self

Take Home Message for Clinical Management

Lessons learned from examining the attraction and indoctrination phase have been summarized by Zimbardo (1997). Among the most salient aspects are the following:

- No one ever joins a "cult." Children and adolescents are more vulnerable but generally people join interesting groups that promise to fulfill their pressing needs.
- Groups become "cults" only when they are seen as deceptive, defective, dangerous, or as opposing basic values of society.
- Cults represent each society's "default values," filling in its missing functions. The cult epidemic is diagnostic of where and how society is failing its citizens.
- If you don't stand for something, you'll fall for anything. As basic human values are being strained, distorted, and lost in our rapidly evolving culture, illusions and promissory notes are too readily believed and bought without reality validation or credit checks.
- Whatever any member of a cult has done, potentially vulnerable persons could be recruited or seduced into doing—under the right or wrong conditions. The majority of "normal, average, intelligent" individuals can be led to engage in immoral, illegal, irrational, aggressive, and self-destructive actions that are contrary to their values or personality—when manipulated situational conditions exert their power over individual dispositions.
- Cult methods of recruiting, indoctrinating, and influencing their members are not exotic forms of mind control, but only more intensely applied mundane tactics of social influence practiced daily by all compliance professionals and societal agents of influence.

Clearly, three key aspects in the clinical management of these cases include prevention, early detection, and treatment. Prevention should include preventing children access to cults, prevention of neglect occurring over a long period of time, and prevention of sustained abuse over time. Early detection is critical because neglect and abuse is associated with attachment disorder, the precursor to conduct disorder, anti-social personality disorder, and other personality disorders.

Specific treatment strategies should be aimed at treatment of the "core problem," specifically the traumas in early life, including neglect, abandonment, and abuse which is often associated with attraction to cult-related experiences (Summit & Lanning, 1990).

Additional strategies useful in clinical management include the following:

1. Medical intervention and specifically hospitalization when self-destructive behavior is operative and possible medication when there is an underlying depression, or other problems which can be treated through medical intervention.
2. Assess and rule out all child and adolescent patients for a current and/or past history of abuse or neglect.
3. Document clearly all abuse or neglect for reporting purposes as well as for courtroom testimony.
4. Report all suspicion of child or adult abuse to Protective Services.
5. The treatment should include the evaluation and treatment of the core problems, specifically childhood traumas and identify issues in early adulthood.
6. The parents or family members of the cult members need education and therapy in terms of how to handle the patient, their own feelings, and the stress on the family unit.
7. Encourage a strong community response to issues surrounding prevention, early detection, treatment, and willing to testify in court proceedings which involve this level of psychopathology and abuse.

Zimbardo (1997) suggests that society is in a curious transitional phase; as science and technology make remarkable advances, antiscientific values and beliefs in the paranormal abound, family values are stridently promoted in Congress and pulpits, yet divorce is rising along with spouse and child abuse, fear of nuclear annihilation in superpower wars is replaced by fears of crime in our streets and drugs in our schools, and the economic gap grows exponentially between the rich and powerful and our legions of poor and powerless.

What makes any of us especially vulnerable to cult appeals? Someone is in a transitional phase in life: moved to a new city or country, lost a job, dropped out of school, parents divorced, romantic relationship broken, gave up traditional religion as personally irrelevant. Add to the recipe, all those who find their work tedious and trivial, education abstractly meaningless, social life absent or inconsistent, family remote or dysfunctional, friends that are too busy to find time for you, and trust in governmental structures or systems that are not creditable.

Cults promise to fulfill most of those personal individual's needs and also to compensate for a litany of societal failures: to make their slice of the world safe, healthy, caring, predictable, and controllable. They will eliminate the increasing feelings of isolation and alienation being created by mobility, technology, competition, meritocracy, incivility, and dehumanized living and working conditions in our society.

Take Home Message

Social bonding in the school setting is an important ingredient in the social and personality development of all students. The school environment offers an opportunity to some students who may have a variety of home and family issues to seek the support and identity found in groups with or beyond the walls of the school. The spectrum of options for groups can range for organized school activities, cliques, to those more sinister groups that form on the fringes of respectable and acceptable societal mores. Examined have been theoretical issues related to cult formation, attraction, and indoctrination. The range of current cults can be seen in a girl cheerleading group or perhaps in a more structured vampire cult. In either case, the group meets certain needs of some students and causes detriment for both the victims and members of the groups. Current groups or cult members and their activities in the classroom profoundly impact the school environment and the effectiveness with which the process of education requires.

Acknowledgments The authors acknowledge the assistance of Linda Brown, Celena Keel, Heather Hosford, Janeen Klaproth, Shannon Nelson, Tag Heister, Deborah Kessler, and Katrina Scott, Library Services; and Virginia Morehouse and Cathy Smith, Department of Psychiatry, and Brenda Frommer for their contributions to the completion of this manuscript.

References

Abraham, K. (1946). Psychosexual differences between hysteria and dementia praecox. *Psychoanalytic Review*, 4, 351–364.

Allen, V. L. (1965). Situational factors in conformity. In L. Berkowitz (Ed.), *Advances in Experimental Social Psychiatry*, Vol. 2. New York: Academic Press.

American Heritage Dictionary (2004). New York: Houghton Mifflin Publishers. Retrieved from website: http://www.answers.com/topic/cult

American Psychiatric Association. (1994). *Diagnostic and Statistical Manual of Mental Disorders*, 4th edition., rev. Washington, DC: American Psychiatric Press.

Bourguignon, A. (1977). Situation de vampirisme et de l'autovampirisme. *Annual Medical Psychology*, 1(2), 181–196.

Cleckley, H. (1976). *The Mask of Sanity*, 5th edition. St. Louis, MO: Mosby Publishers Incorporated.

Deutsch, A., & Miller, M. J. (1983). A clinical study of four Unification Church members. *American Journal of Psychiatry*, 140, 767–770.

Espejo, R. (2002). *Teen Issues: America's Youth*. R. Espejo (Ed.), San Diego: Lucent Books, 2002. August 2004. Retrieved: 13 April 2007. http://www.enotes.com/americas-youth-article/41233.

Fairbairn, L. R. (1993). Working with cult-affected families. *Psychiatric Annals*, 20(4), 194–198.

Galanter, M. (1989). Cults: Faith, healing, and coercion. New York: Oxford University Press.

Hare, R. (1986). Twenty years experience with the Cleckley psychopath, In W.Reid, D.Dorr, & J.Bonner (Eds.), *Unmasking the Psychopath*. New York: Norton.

Klein, M. (1948). *The Psychoanalysis of Children*. London: Hogarth Publishers.

Levine, S. (1981). Cults and mental health: Clinical conclusions. *Canadian Journal of Psychiatry*, 26, 534–539.

MacHovec, F. J. (1989). *Cults and Personality*. Springfield, IL: Charles C. Thomas Publishers.

Olmstead, A. D. (1988). Morally controversial leisure. *Symbolic Interaction*, 11, 277–287.

Schein, E. H. (1961). *Coercive Persuasion*. New York: W.W. Norton.

Summit, R. & Lanning, B. (1990). Cults and rituals: Relationships to child abuse. In *The Center for Child Protection (Welcomes You to the) Health Science Response to Child Maltreatment* 1990 (Program Guide). San Diego, CA: Children's Hospital and Health Center.

Walsh, Y., Russell, R. J. H., & Wells, P. A. (1995). The personality of ex-cult members. *Personality and Individual Differences*, 19 (3), 339–344.

West, L. J. (1980). Persuasive techniques in contemporary cults. In M. Galanter (Ed.), *Cults and New Religious Movements* (pp. 165–192). Washington, DC: American Psychiatric Press.

Zimbardo, P. (1997). What messages are behind today's cults? *American Psychological Association Monitor*, 28(5), 14–65. Washington, DC: American Psychological Association.

Zinn, D. (1999). Special Report/The Littleton Massacre: What can the schools do? *Time* May 3, 153(17), 38–42.

Part II
Treatment and Prevention of Violence in the Schools

Chapter 12
Violence in Our Schools

Matt Thompson, Bobbie Burcham, and Kathy McLaughlin

A Principal's Perspective

"Gunfire Inside a School Kills 3 and Wounds 5," and "Terror in Littleton: The Overview; 2 Students in Colorado School Said To Gun Down As Many As 23 and Kill Themselves in a Siege" are both newspaper headlines of events that have occurred since 1995. These events, tragic and devastating as any act of global terrorism, form a terrifying juxtaposition because of where they took place. Schools are often referred to as hallowed halls of learning where future generations of great minds are educated and molded. They are places that are designed to keep students safe from the harsher truths of the real world until they are deemed ready to handle them. And yet they are not. The actual harsh truth is that as much as we want to believe schools are immune to shootings, bombings, and violence in general, events in Colorado, Kentucky, and Virginia, just to name a few, have proven us wrong. To enter education in this day and age is to agree that we understand school violence as a very real possibility and that part of what we do as educators is work to prevent any further occurrences of these types of violence.

It is doubtful that anyone would disagree that school violence is not a cause but an effect. Investigations into school violence have uncovered a myriad of factors which all seem to have influenced the culminating brutal events (Educational Resources Information Center, 2000). Factors such as bullying, history of violence, feelings of ostracization, problematic home lives, and few strong relationships, just to name a few, have all been common threads running through the many examples of violence resulting in deaths in our schools (Center for Effective Collaboration and Practice of the American Institutes for Research, 1998). These factors are also common links in many other kinds of violence not resulting in deaths. Yet, further investigation indicates that these factors are not truly causes either, but are additional effects of one main underlying problem: school connectedness (Blum, 2005). In most, if not all, cases of school violence that have resulted in death, the perpetrators are seen as "outside" the school community. This does not mean that they never went to the school or were never seen by anyone there, but rather, it indicates that they were not involved with anything within the school community. They rarely, if ever, participated in clubs or activities requiring a commitment

T. W. Miller (ed.), *School Violence and Primary Prevention.*
© Springer 2008

of camaraderie. They rarely, if ever, were members of an organization within the school that worked toward a common goal. In fact, there often is not much remembered about them other than they went to school and were not involved in much. We could all blame the problems on the home lives of the violent students, yet we would be ignoring the fact that most cases of school violence do not occur with students who feel connected to the school they attend (Blum, 2005). What a powerful concept. The conclusion then is that if schools focus the majority of their structures, time, and efforts on proactively working to connect all students to the school community, the chances of school violence will drastically decrease. In fact, Blum has indicated that highly connected students (those who perceive that adults care about them as individuals and about their learning) engage in less bullying, school violence, and at-risk health behaviors (drug and alcohol use, premarital sex, substance abuse) than those students who are less connected (Blum, 2005).

Imagine a school where every student feels connected to the school, the staff members, the other students, and the vision and goals of the school. That is, imagine a school where every student feels that the adults there care about them as individuals and care about their learning. That is a school in which there will be few cases, if any, of any type of violence, let alone a shooting on the magnitude that we have seen in the last 10 years. As educators, this is the type of school that we need to work to create each and every day. Such work needs to be very intentionally focused to ensure that each and every student feels valued and connected to the school community. The work toward this goal can occur in two different ways, personal modeling and creating structures within the school. Specific examples of personal modeling can be recreated on a larger scale through entire school structures and serve as a unifying force for all staff members to help students feel connected. Once these structures are in place, a net is created that helps prevent any student, regardless of race, gender, socioeconomic status, home-life situation, or even ability, from falling through the cracks and feeling unconnected. Several examples of such structures follow.

Learning Students' Names and Mentoring

The easiest way to make students feel connected in the school is by making sure that someone in the school knows them personally. As a principal, one of the things to start from day one of the school year is to learn each and every student's name. There is no better way to make sure that students know they are known in the school then by greeting them by name as they get off the bus, enter the office, pass you in the hallway, or catch your eye in the cafeteria. Purposefully positioning yourself where you can greet students as they enter the school each morning and at intersections in the hallway during transition times is an effective strategy for learning the names of hundreds of students quickly. Once students learn that you know their names, they will become more active in talking with you. They will actually seek you out and engage you in a conversation, often just to hear you say their name.

It is amazing how a simple thing like saying a student's name can cause an effect like an ear-to-ear smile, a laugh, or even just a glint in an eye. The fact that it is the principal learning the names of each student adds to the significance. It is a powerful way to begin the connection process. Now, admittedly attempting to learn the names of 500 students is a daunting challenge, but your expectations need to be realistic. Even with getting a head start by looking through a yearbook over the summer, learning everyone's name will take a few months. But with determination and a good sense of humor, it can be accomplished.

Even with one person learning every student's name there still needs to be a systematic structure for incorporating that same level of personal knowledge of the students into the everyday school culture. One way to do this is by setting up mentors for every student. Each staff member takes on 10–15 students who are not in their classes and makes sure to learn their names and check in with them on a weekly basis. The students begin to build strong relationships with the staff members and often go out of their way to try and see them throughout the day, sharing success stories, accomplishments, and great things that are happening. The focus of the interactions is on student learning and those things that assist or hinder that from happening (remember the connectedness definition: someone cares about me and my learning). The hardest part about this school-wide structure is getting it off the ground and subtly monitoring it to ensure that all students have actually been mentored on a regular basis. One way to do this is by having staff members mail home positive postcards that brag on the students. An example of such a system is shown in Fig. 12.1.

Each teacher receives a predetermined number of postcards to make sure each student receives one throughout the year. Extras are available as needed. As they mail them, staff members put their name in a weekly or monthly drawing (one entry for each postcard). The principal or other support staff member covers the winner's class for an hour providing an extra planning period. A by-product of this is that it allows the principal to be in the classrooms more, which helps to develop stronger relationships with the students and further communicate to all that learning is important.

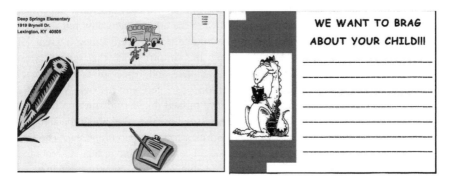

Fig. 12.1 Sample postcard sent to students by staff

Open-Door Policy and Student Surveys

Students must feel that someone is available to listen to them, no matter the context or situation. The students need to be told that an open-door policy to the principal exists for them and their families. They can talk to the principal about any problem and always know that help is available. They need to know that someone important (the principal) will listen to their issue or concern even if there is no agreement as to the final outcome. During these conversations, the students are ensured that the principal's first task is to keep everyone safe. This means keeping them safe from both getting hurt and feeling hurt. Students need to be able to talk to someone when they feel scared or threatened. This is a case of where perception is reality. If a student feels threatened, (s)he is being threatened. If a student feels bullied, they are being bullied. At least initially it does not matter if the threatening or bullying is actually happening or not. The principal needs to assume it is happening if someone feels it is. If during the conversation, it is discovered that there is not any threatening or bullying occurring and it is just either a misunderstanding of the situation (i.e., Student B told me that Student A was going to beat me up but Student A never said that) or a misconception regarding threats and bullying (i.e., I thought Student A was bothering me when (s)he happened to just be staring at me) then the principal will explain and work that out with the student. The important thing to remember, though, is that initially, the open-door policy and a listening ear is all that matters. The students have to believe and trust that you will allow them to discuss their concerns with you.

As you listen to students, much information is learned. It is vital to listen to their perspective as they have such a different view on things. In some schools there are teams of teachers who facilitate the creation of expectations and lesson plans for common areas of the school (hallway, cafeteria, playground, etc.). In the process of developing these plans and expectations, a point is made to request feedback from multiple groups including staff members, parents, and students via carefully developed safety surveys (Sprick et al., 2002). Often, the information received from students is much different than from the other two groups. For example, in one school the restrooms were not as high of a priority to parents and staff as they were to the students. The students indicated that this was the area they were most concerned about. Their survey revealed that restrooms were the areas where they felt the most unsafe. The teachers were surprised as they thought they were doing a great job supervising during restroom breaks. Using this information, the school chose restrooms as a top priority and developed lesson plans and expectations to help reach the goal of having safe restrooms where everyone is treated with respect. Without the viewpoint from the students the staff may have missed this very disturbing information. Each year the staff uses student surveys to see how they feel about the safety of the school and then use that data to plan priorities for the upcoming year. The data also give an objective way to measure success. The bottom line is that students feel connected when they can freely share their thoughts, opinions, and concerns in a safe environment. School-wide structures need to be in place to allow this to happen.

Engaging, Rigorous Work and After-School Activities

Another way to help students feel connected to their school is to ensure that they are actively engaged with rigorous work during classroom instruction (Pogrow, 2005). Active, problem-solving lessons engage students even if they initially are not interested in the topic. Raising the level of instruction and expectations increases the level of communication and interest within the classroom. Rigorous work, while occasionally a source of resistance at the outset, prevents boredom and promotes active engagement. Some students, who are experts at misbehavior in the majority of school settings, have no problems whatsoever in a classroom where the teacher has built strong relationships and created engaging and interesting lessons. These students, who have the reputation of problem kids across multiple settings, spending most of their time in other classrooms out of their seats, disrupting the class, and who comprise the majority of all discipline referrals, instead become key contributors in classrooms where true instructional engagement occurs. Engaging lessons do not eliminate misbehavior and episodes of violence completely, but they do drastically decrease the likelihood of something dangerous happening by increasing school connectedness. Rigorous work also sets a precedent of high expectations for the students that encourage them to reach new heights both academically and behaviorally. While students are often fearful of ultimate success, consistently high expectations provide a structure in which success can be reached in a supportive, comforting, and safe way. The danger of failure and the frustration of potential failure are eliminated because the students know that the environment they are in supports them upward and onward toward success, albeit with much effort on their part. The end product of rigorous, engaging classroom instruction is that students feel connected and supported.

The question then becomes how to duplicate this on a school-wide level. In other words, what does the structure look like that promotes rigorous engagement for all students in other settings besides their classroom. One answer is to implement as many different extracurricular activities and clubs as possible. Although successful at the middle and high school level for decades, after-school clubs and activities do not always find support at the elementary level. In fact it almost seems that the number of extracurricular opportunities offered by schools is inversely proportional to the other strategies that are used to connect them to school. At the high school level, where there are large class sizes and students often get lost in the crowd, there are more extracurricular activities available than at any other level. However, the positive impact of early intervention is significant. Extracurricular activities if offered at the elementary level can connect students at earlier ages to school and help them find areas of expertise and interest that they never knew existed. While funding is often a problem for these activities at the elementary grades, small stipends and supplemental pay can often be used to provide sponsors who meet with students in clubs once or twice a month. The level of connectedness will increase exponentially if we can reach at-risk students early on in their schooling.

Other Ideas to Help Students Feel Connected

The following is a practitioners list of additional ways to help students feel connected to their school and thus decrease the likelihood of misbehavior and events of school violence:

- *Special awards and recognitions*: All students like to be rewarded for positive behavior and academics. This can be worked into basic structures of the schools. For example, one potential strategy is the Principal's Outstanding Worker Award (POW Award) where the teachers are asked to work with their students to decide what academic and behavioral achievements would automatically result in a POW Award. Once these are reached, the student is sent to the principal's office to receive recognition for the award: a copy of the form can be copied for the student and parent, placed on the principal's office wall, and used as a way to motivate students to be sent to the office for "good" behavior. A sample can be viewed in Fig. 12.2.
- *Recognizing students at School Council meetings*: In states and districts that have School Councils, students can be recognized at the meetings of these councils. The students can shake hands with the council members and receive a certificate of achievement. Not only does this connect the students more, it also encourages their parents to feel more connected as well.
- *Community partnerships*: Actively searching out community partners is a wonderful way to provide your students with additional resources to help them feel more connected to school. Partnerships with organizations like Big Brothers and Big Sisters need to be encouraged.
- *Student goal conferences*: Meeting with each student in third through fifth grades in order to conference with them in regard to their personal academic goals is another effective strategy to get kids connected. Assessment scores from the previous years are used to create new goals for the upcoming years. A goal contract is then completed together and monitored throughout the year. A sample can be viewed in Fig. 12.3.

Prevention with High-Risk Students: A School Psychologist's Perspective

As a school psychologist, violence among youth is an issue of urgency faced on a daily basis. This was never more poignant than the morning of Tuesday, April 17, 2007, the day after the horrific incident that reeked terror on the Virginia Technical Institute campus, leaving 22 dead, including the school shooter. By 10 A.M. on that April morning, a typical risk assessment team, in a typical American high school, had seven referrals that required a risk-for-harm assessment. In each case, an adult had overheard student comments of concern. Understanding violence is an intricate process, but on this day, the challenge was even greater than understanding violence; the challenge was assessing threats and preventing violence from happening, if possible.

Deep Springs Elementary School
1919 Brynell Dr.
Lexington, KY 40505
859-381-3069

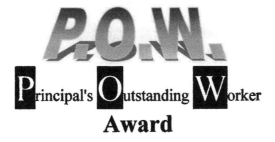

Award

Dear Parents/Guardians,

On _____, your child,

_____ was honored by the

principal for excellent work in

_____.

We are so proud of your child and we know you are too.

Please encourage your child to keep up the great work!!!

Deep Springs Elementary **Guidelines for Success**
Always Try
Be Responsible
Cooperate With Others
Do Your Best
Everyday Respect Everyone

Sincerely,

Matthew D. Thompson
Principal

Fig. 12.2 Sample Principal's Outstanding Worker (POW) award form

Although a well-established plan of "risk-for-harm assessments" is in place that includes a thorough review of the nature of the threat, information about the personality of the student, and the dynamics at school as well as family functioning, cultural issues, unsettling events, stabilizing factors for the student, previous mental health care, etc., there is often no time to complete thorough assessments on all of

My Personal Goal Sheet

Name: _____
Date: _____

Last year when I was in 3th grade, I took the KCCT test in Reading and Math. Below are my scores:

Reading:
Math:

This year in 4th grade, I will take the KCCT test in Reading, Math, Science, and Vocational Skills/Practical Living: Below are my goals for each of those areas:

Reading:
Math:
Science:
Voc. Stud/Pract.

To achieve these goals I am going to do the following:
- Monitor and graph my own open response progress.
-
-
-

Student Signature:_____

Principal Signature:_____

Fig. 12.3 Sample student goal sheet

the referrals—especially given the number generated on that horrific April day. The goal typically is not to treat all threats the same but individually evaluate the overall level of risk to prevent harm. The numbers are typically manageable and the assessments usually take up to 2 days each to complete, sometimes longer. However, there was limited time remaining on this school day when a flood of referrals was received, thus an altered plan was needed.

Meetings with administrators were immediately arranged to put a plan into action to assess the students who had made statements that evoked concern. Taking time to make a plan was critical because it aborted any knee-jerk reactions and "one size fits all" punishment for the students in question.

For each case, the team wanted to know as much about the student as possible in order to "level" the threat (O'Toole, 2007). Fortunately, the students were basically known by someone on the team so further information could be developed on each one as needed. Additionally, threatening statements were categorized ("leveled") as low (vague and indirect), medium (could be carried through but not probable), or high (direct threat and/or probable plan). Among the threats, only one clearly indicated a need for immediate attention and the administration was alerted as it potentially passed imminent threat of high priority. It was agreed that the threat assessment team would gather more information on that case later in the week as there was going to be immediate intervention from the administration. The other students would remain at school in their typical schedule and be assessed in that environment.

The threat assessment team, including the school psychologist and the school social worker in collaboration with administration, would begin work on the remaining referrals: brief interviews with each, a clinical blink (Gladwell, 2005), and background information on each from referring sources. Methodically students were to be interviewed, the school records reviewed, the teachers consulted, and the families contacted. Information about the seriousness of the threats, the mental health of the students, their level of empathy, their propensity to shift blame, their feelings of connectedness in their school and their homes, relevant cultural issues, students' level of pain, and the degree of hope they held for their future was assessed to the extent possible in the very short time allotted. By the end of the day, the identified students had been assessed to the point of knowing who needed immediate help and the type of assistance needed for them. Follow-up plans were put into place to more thoroughly review the assessment information and to prevent any possible violence toward anyone in the school. Fortunately, no one was hurt.

Philosophy

Clearly, students come to school with a variety of life experiences shaped by their own background including their own gender, family dynamics, culture, friends, geographical setting, community expectations, and religion. From this emerges the pupils' attitudes toward violence such as their response to authority, their feelings of belonging to a group, their development of self-regulation and self-concept, and their ability to cope with stress. Although there does not appear to be a single predictor of school violence or clear mechanism to predict who will act out violently, it is often the responsibility of the school psychologist and other mental health support staff, along with a team of educators, to search for behavioral indicators that suggest a student might be at risk for behaving in a manner that poses a threat at school.

From this philosophy emerges the need for schools to have a clearly defined process to assess students who may be at risk for doing harm to themselves or others in a school setting as well as intervention to address the needs of all students, not just those who act out in a potentially dangerous manner. Although there does not seem to be a standard perfect protocol for the development of a threat assessment process, based upon many years of experience, there are several issues that must be considered in the development of a school-wide threat assessment protocol.

Threat Assessment Protocol

It is important when working in any school environment to ensure that your school system has a threat assessment plan in place. It is suggested that the plan have a single point of entry so that all staff knows to whom to make a referral in the case of a potential threat. It is suggested that the staff be educated on what constitutes a referral. A multidisciplinary team should be established to field the referrals. It is suggested that the team be composed of the head administrator (typically the point of entry), a person with a background in mental health issues, any safety personnel available, and the referring person.

The primary focus of the risk assessment should be determining the likelihood that the threat will be carried out. To do this, there should be a well-defined method of responding to threats of harm to self or others that includes information about the personality and mental health status of the student, information about family dynamics, information about school functioning, past and present, as well as information about social/cultural issues that could be pertinent. This includes obtaining information about stabilizing factors in the student's life, issues that could be upsetting to the student, and information about community involvement ranging from social services, health care, community-based counseling, juvenile detention, and so on. To conclude the threat assessment, the development of a plan, noting who is going to be responsible for implementation of any recommendations, should be arranged. This must include follow up with the student.

Universal and Tailor-Made Plans

In addition to developing threat assessment plans for students who exhibit potential danger to themselves or others, it is often part of the role and function of school psychologists, counselors, and school social workers to assist in creating a school environment that is safe, civilized, and productive. One piece of this can be recommending and participating in the development of school-wide initiatives that promote safe and civil schools such as Foundations (Sprick et al., 2002). Foundations provides a venue for a team of school-based educators to discuss, develop, and implement school-wide plans that promote an educational environment that is safe, civilized, and productive at the universal level, that is, for all students.

Sprick et al. (2002) suggests that guidelines to create a successful school climate be developed and implemented, school-wide behavioral expectations be taught, and school-wide discipline plans put into place. Initiatives such as Foundations encourages school improvement based upon a data-driven process that includes review of survey results from students, teachers, staff, and parents, review of discipline, attendance, and tardy data, observational data from common areas in the school, such as the cafeteria, media center, hallways, bus loading/unloading areas, and so on. This initiative is led by a small team of key school-based personnel, often including administrators, the school psychologist as well as teachers, counselors, and other school employees and the developed plans are then endorsed by the entire school staff.

There are many school-wide initiatives to promote safe, healthy schooling environments that can be useful in addressing the behavioral needs of all students. Examples include implementation of social skills intervention programs for all students or bully prevention programs. The point is that having plans in place to meet the needs of most students will act to prevent behavioral issues that could result in violence to students or adults at school. It also helps prevent some students from moving to the next level of problems (targeted or intense), as their needs are met via universal, school-wide strategies.

School-wide, universal plans that provide behavioral expectations, supports, and consequences for all students are effective for most children and interrupt actions that would be considered inappropriate or dangerous. However, some students have issues that are not addressed by programs that are put into place for all students. For example, some students have long-standing propensities for mental health issues and behavior problems that require a more targeted approach. School psychologists, counselors, and school social workers often have an opportunity to intervene with these students in an effort to meet their needs and prevent exacerbation of problems. Assistance for targeted students may occur in the form of participation in assessment and development of individualized educational programs for students in need of special education; involvement in behavioral coaching initiatives with students who are not adjusting well to school; programs targeted to address the needs of students in transition; or the student being referred to a school-based student assistance team to plan academic or behavioral interventions specifically for an individual student. Obviously, this is a very short list of initiatives to meet the needs of students with identified needs but clearly, support staff, such as psychologists, counselors, and social workers, is critical in the process of identifying these students and planning interventions to meet their needs.

In addition to being involved in programs to assist all kids as well as those with targeted needs, there also is a small group of children who emerge with intense psychological and behavioral needs. Some students in this group have a severe propensity for violence and this cannot be ignored in order to preserve individual as well as group safety. The violence may be in the form of predatory aggression such as bringing weapons to school with the intent to harm or reactive aggression such as responding impulsively yet violently to minor stimuli.

In order to design school-based interventions that make sense for children with intense behavioral needs in a school setting, it may be worthwhile to distinguish between children who exhibit predatory aggression (e.g., children with conduct disorders) and students who exhibit biologically based impulsive dysregulation (e.g., children with attention-deficit hyperactivity disorder). Schools have traditionally intervened with short-term programming using behavioral technology for every child who exhibits disruptive behavior. Barkley (2007) notes, no one should now rationally claim that attention-deficit hyperactivity disorder arises from faulty learning or that several months of contingency management produces sustained benefits for attention-deficit hyperactivity disorder once treatment is withdrawn. He suggests that behavioral intervention, such as those implemented in school settings, is liken to a prosthetic device, a means of rearranging the environment by artificial means, to yield improved school participation. At this point, school psychologists and other school-based personnel use behavioral and cognitive behavioral interventions to address the needs of students who present with severe behavioral problems as that is the technology that is available.

Working as a multidisciplinary team with general and special educators, administrators, social workers, counselors, psychologists, nurses, parents, and community-based care providers provides perspective on children and thus emerges the most tailored and promising interventions for youth who exhibit behavior problems at school. Certainly there is no one single, straightforward, uncomplicated way to intervene with children who exhibit issues that are unregulated and potentially dangerous.

Students who exhibit the most intense behavioral challenges are often those who are involved in the threat assessment process described above. Students who act out violently at school and do not respond to typical interventions are reviewed on a case-by-case basis at school and services delivered based upon individual need. Services for these youngsters may be in the form of very restrictive programs, such as alternative school placements within the school system and/or community-based care programs.

Whatever is driving the violence at school, it is not acceptable and very troubling to educators who are working to make schools safe places where students can learn. Individualized multimodal intervention initiatives using the expertise of school-based personnel as well as health care providers in the community seem essential.

As a school psychologist interested in the mental health wellness of the students in the schools, one final note is important to make. In April, 2007, after the string of threats that had to be so rapidly evaluated, I placed a note in my desk drawer that read: "Do No Harm." There is a level of risk when we make strong recommendations for students. Do we know with any level of certainty that what we are recommending will indeed move the child to a healthier place in his/her life? Will a recommendation to return a child to the general program with support result in harm to another student? Will a referral to the principal recommending suspension or expulsion harm the child who acted out? Will a recommendation for a family to seek hospitalization create trauma for a child? Will a referral for special education create an unhealthy mindset for a student? And, the list of questions goes on. As mental health professionals in the schools, there is often a fast pace that is required including reviews of thick school files, meetings with teachers, parents and students, formal and informal assessments, and observations concluding with individualized intervention planning. Our mission is to help children, particularly who are not doing well in school behaviorally and/or academically. Our mission is not to rescue children or have low expectations for children but to be a part of a team that assists in moving children to be more responsible, healthy, happy, productive human beings … at school and in life. Ross Greene (2001) said it best when he noted that if a child can do well, he/she will and if he/she can't it is our responsibility as the adults to find out why and intervene. All school-based personnel who work with students with behavioral challenges need to get to know the children with whom they work and be thoughtful in the planning of their school-based care.

Students Who Are Valued and Know It: A Teacher's Perspective

Preventing School Violence by Creating a Community of Inclusion

Introduction

What do successful students have in common? Students who "believe" that they are genuinely valued by their families, their teachers, and their peers are highly likely to experience successes both academically and socially. Students who feel "connected" to school will engage in less disruptive, irresponsible, and violent behavior, and demonstrate more positive, responsible, civil behavior as well as increased academic performance. Being connected means feeling that adults in the school care about a student as an individual and about his/her learning as a student (Blum, 2005). The challenge of the school community is to create a culture and environment in which relationships are fostered, expectations are explicit, and structures exist which promote the value of each member of the community. The teacher and school can have a significant impact on the development of positive relationships with students which will lead to a sense of school connectedness.

Philosophy

To be successful in school, students need to feel that their school is emotionally safe and physically secure. Students should feel confident that procedures are in place to ensure their safety on a daily basis as well as during emergency situations. They need to know that the adults at school care deeply about them and their safety and are prepared in case an emergency arises. This needs to be communicated in explicit ways. While all schools are required to practice for unforeseen emergencies through fire, weather, and lockdown drills, the teacher's participation in preparing the students for such drills is critical. Students need to clearly see and hear that the significant adult is calm, sure, and definitely "in charge." The procedures for various drills need to be taught and practiced and time needs to be devoted to answering students' questions and allaying fears "prior" to the first drill.

Emotional and academic success in the classroom depends on a trusting relationship between the student and the teacher. First, teachers must recognize that each student has a strength, a gift, a passion—even if hidden—and the key is to locate that gift and connect it to what must be taught in the curriculum. The most successful teachers do this on a regular basis with all students—even with the most challenging. Teachers must believe that all of their students are capable of great things. Those great things may not be conventional and they may require some real searching on the part of the teacher, student, and parents, but believing that they exist fuels the quest and endears the student to the teacher and vice versa. The classroom environment should be inviting and engaging, one in which students can ask questions without fear of ridicule, can err with confidence that they will receive unconditional acceptance and guidance, and can risk letting their strengths shine. An important part of classroom management is teacher preparedness. The teacher who extensively plans and organizes the classroom is structuring it for success, and beginning a communication process that tells the students, "I care about you and I care about your learning." A teacher must be a master of his/her content and must be able to facilitate acquisition of knowledge along with the joy of the subject. The structures of the classroom and the instructional delivery model permit students to verbalize the goals of the course, the focus of the daily lesson, and the criteria for success in the course. At any given time, students should have a realistic understanding of their current performance level and should have access to strategies which accelerate their learning and guarantee mastery of the content.

Student–teacher relationships cannot fully exist without the teacher's understanding of the family dynamics, the experiences, the dreams, the fears, the preferred learning style, and the skill level of the student. Conversely, students should know their teachers well enough to identify their dreams, their fears, their preferred teaching style, and their strengths … and to care enough about them to accept their weaknesses. Understanding that students receive mixed messages in their everyday interactions helps teachers clarify their expectations for specific situations and encourages them to broaden their tolerance for behaviors and customs which might be different from their own. Such efforts further communicate to the students a desire to understand at a deeper, more meaningful level, which is a clear indicator of care and concern. For example, by attending different churches within the community, teachers might see behaviors that they would not consider to be appropriate in the classroom, but would see that the same behavior is most appropriate (and encouraged) during other significant times in the student's world. When a student who has been encouraged to vocalize and gesture affirmation in church does the same thing in the classroom, he often receives very different messages. This doesn't necessarily mean that a teacher must accept "church behavior" in his/her classroom but understanding that different expectations in somewhat similar environments (both church and school are considered places of respect) may be confusing for children can help the teacher clarify his/her expectations and teach those classroom expectations to all students as needed. (See "Are You a Valued Team Member?" self-assessment form (Fig. 12.4)). More importantly, such understanding would ideally influence how a teacher responds to student behavior and would influence the choice of educational activities that permit more opportunities for students to be active and fully engaged.

Are You A Valued Team Member?

Rate yourself from 0 to 3 on the following attributes:
(0 = never,   1 = sometimes,   2 = usually,   3 = always)

I, _____,
Your Name

	Aug	Jan	May
am patient and kind.			
care about others.			
explain concepts and strategies to classmates.			
encourage my team members.			
am a good listener.			
share my ideas with my team.			
can be counted on by my team; am responsible.			
respect the ideas of others.			
critique ideas, not people.			
am a positive role model.			
complete tasks and homework.			
stay focused.			
abide by the "No Put-Down Zone" rule.			
will stand up for a peer who is being treated unfairly.			
gladly work with any and all students as assigned.			
clean up after myself; put chair under table.			
take care of school materials and books.			
bring necessary supplies and books to class.			
expect and show respect.			
am willing to learn from others.			
TOTAL POINTS			

Fig. 12.4 Sample self-assessment form

Strategies for Prevention

An integral part of "knowing students" is "knowing" the family. Parents need to receive a clear message that they are valued as teammates in educating our children. That is why a teacher's first contact with parents must be positive, genuine, and engaging. The simple request to "tell me about your son/daughter" shows a desire to know our students as individuals and to consult with the "expert"—the parent. When possible, initial contact with parents should be person-to-person but other formats also work well. During the first week of the new school year, parents can be greeted through a brief letter in which the teacher introduces himself/herself, provides contact information, and asks the parents to answer a few questions pertaining to their children. Parents can be encouraged to e-mail their responses if they have access to e-mail or otherwise to return the questionnaire part of the letter. The initial responses from parents will provide correct and current e-mail addresses while also encouraging parents to introduce their children so that they might be seen through their parents' eyes. The specific questions parents may be asked to answer are typically ones that will allow better communication, such as "…most convenient time for me to contact you by phone?" but the most beneficial feedback is in response to the open-ended questions; "… tell me something that, as a teacher, I might not know about your child" and "bragging is great." Asking the parents for suggestions for "conversation starters" that will engage their children provides the teacher with a valuable resource for the year. This simple request to get to know students better pays dividends in so many ways.

There are other strategies used to help connect kids to the classroom and to their learning. These may include the following:

- *Self-assessment: "Are you a valued team member?"* This questionnaire is used to help the students begin assessing some of their strengths and weaknesses, and to help them see themselves as valued team members (see Figure 12.4 for a completed sample of the form). More importantly, the questionnaire directly states the desired classroom behaviors/expectations for small group and entire class interactions. If a teacher truly subscribes to the philosophy that what is valued is assessed, students are given a not-so-subtle message that their behavior and character skills are valued alongside their content knowledge and skills.
- *Ratio of interactions*: Behavior is corrected as needed and there are more interactions (at least three times more) with students when they are not misbehaving. Both are important and both are related to each other. Interactions take the form of contingent attention type ("catching Johnny being good"), and noncontingent attention type ("catching Johnny just being"). The ratio of 3:1 is a minimum as some students require more. There are many creative ways to increase that ratio in a positive direction: greet students as they enter the classroom, say good-bye as they leave the classroom, before/after-school activities, hallway hellos and how are you?, cafeteria talk, conferences, notes on papers and note cards home, e-mail messages, and phone calls. It should be noted that corrections are made as needed in a most professional manner: positive tone, low volume, as private as possible, no sarcasm, and never with an intent to embarrass the student. All of the latter is half of the key to having effective corrections; the other half is the high positive ratio. Why? Because whatever you attend to the most is what you will get the most of. Attention is powerful and it needs to be used most often when our students are not misbehaving. It is also a way of developing strong, positive relationships with the students as it communicates care, concern, and commitment to them as individuals and as students. Attention is so powerful and considered such a basic need for kids in school that kids frequently will take whatever type they can get—positive or negative (an adolescent counselor once summarized this concern by indicating that many students felt that it was better to be wanted by the law than not wanted at all!). The adults in the school

have control over the type of attention given to students. It needs to be used more often and frequently when our students are not misbehaving.

- *Project-based, problem-solving activities and units that promote active, engaged learning by all of the students*: The more rigorous and high-level the activity, the more engaged students seem to become. The blank stares seem to diminish as they actively participate and explore learning opportunities. One of the best behavior interventions and ways to engage students in school is to ensure that what they do is meaningful, active, and challenging. Recently, a group of high school dropouts was interviewed to assess their perspectives as to why they dropped out of school (see The Silent Epidemic, March 2006). And while there is no single reason reported for dropping out of school, almost half (47%) indicated that a major reason for leaving was that the classes were not interesting. Almost 70% stated that they were neither inspired nor motivated to work hard. Project-based, problem-solving teaching and learning helps to change that.
- *Clear rules and expectations for all of key activities and transitions*: The rules and expectations must be taught explicitly as needed. They are reviewed before and after breaks and whenever some "additional structure" is needed in the classroom. There needs to be well-defined classroom procedures for critical areas of concern for all students: grades, late or missing assignments, make up work after an absence, homework, class projects, and other student work-related areas. The procedures need to be taught explicitly as well, as they are needed and implemented in the classroom that is structured for success. Organizational skills and tools to help in this area are over emphasized—a real safety net for the students at a time when organization and structure do not come naturally.
- *A classroom environment that is neat, organized, physically attractive, comfortable, and accessible*: The teacher needs to have close proximity with each and every student, which is often times needed to communicate effectively and to encourage motivating behavior from them. The teacher cannot just stand in one place. Rather, the teacher needs to move around to enhance student attention and focus, and to communicate care for the student and belief in the student. (Individual care and care of learning combine to make up the definition of feeling "connected.")
- *SLANT*: All teachers need to teach a research-based focus/attention strategy that will increase comprehension if implemented consistently. SLANT, an acronym in which each letter is a reminder to the student to become physically engaged (resulting in cognitive engagement), is an example:

  ○ S – "sit up straight"
  ○ L – "lean forward slightly"
  ○ A – "activate your learning by asking questions and acting interested"
  ○ N – "nod and note key points"
  ○ T – "track the teacher or the speaker or the materials being used"

What about those students who are "on the fringe" or excluded from peer groups? The teacher plays a critical role in facilitating a student's acceptance into peer groups and often has more influence than (s)he might realize. The management system should allow the teacher opportunities to share and shape the desired behaviors of the entire group. More importantly though, it should allow the teacher to influence how students perceive one another, especially the "disconnected" or "devalued" students.

Consider the following examples of how to connect kids even more strongly to school:

- Devote an entire bulletin board to the listing of examples of behaviors "from the heart." Refer to this listing often by pairing an action from the classroom to a behavior from the bulletin board:

  - Expect respect
  - Come to class prepared with homework, materials, and a willing attitude
  - Be a good listener
  - Respect people and ideas; critique ideas, not people
  - Care for materials; clean up after self
  - Share ideas
  - Care for each other; encourage one another
  - Be responsible so that teammates know you can be counted on
  - Respond accordingly to the "No Put-Down Zone" that is our classroom

- Demonstrate what is valued by what is rewarded.

For example, when a teacher catches an entire team writing down an assignment from the board upon entering the classroom, the team is given (has earned) a foam cut-out heart. In seconds, the rest of the class will follow suit. This is a fairly easy way to shape behaviors that are not only helpful to students but also keep the classroom running smoothly. The most powerful characteristic of this type of management system is the potential to reach the disenfranchised students and to enhance their value as perceived by their classmates. The teacher can intentionally look for opportunities to recognize a specific student, and reward that student with a heart while the entire team receives credit for the heart. The rewarded student is recognized because of his or her contribution to the group, and (s)he is viewed with potential that might have previously been overlooked. As simple as this sounds, it has repeatedly worked effectively at drawing kids into the group and of assigning value to those tough to reach students.

Following is a summary for implementation of the above strategy. In accordance with the "heart theme," teams can earn hearts when the group or an individual displays "heart behaviors." Teams select a member to be the "Heart-Keeper" and often learn the hard way that this should be a "responsible" person who keeps the hearts in a safe place such as the pencil case inside his/her notebook. A heart earned by one is credited to the entire team. The team heart-keeper collects hearts until the day that new teams are assigned. At that time, the heart-keeper determines the number of hearts earned by the team and that number is credited into the individual student accounts (while the actual foam hearts are returned to the teacher). The management of this can be extremely simple. A Heart Notebook can be kept with rosters from each class. On collection days, the "heart-keepers" bring the hearts to the teacher's desk, tell the number earned, and state the last names of their teammates. The teacher writes down that number by each of the four members of the team. Students are then assigned to new teams and the process starts over. How the hearts are "cashed in" varies by the personality of the class, although nothing seems to be as reinforcing as the moment a heart is handed to the team or student. One option is to request that students bring in items from home for end-of-year auction. (Suggest that they clean their rooms and look for items which have been enjoyable for them and still could be enjoyed by someone else, such as a book, a pen, a trinket.) The teacher may want to invite a real auctioneer to class to auction off the items as the students use their earned hearts as capital.

In situations where the students need more frequent reinforcement, weekly "cash-ins" for a "Let's Make a Deal" opportunity can be used. The variations are endless (only limited by the teacher and students' creativity). At the end of the week, heart-keepers are asked to return their hearts to the teacher. Nothing is recorded. The team with the most hearts for the week draws an activity from the heart box to determine their reward. For each class a transparency is made of all of the potential rewards, and as one is drawn, it is marked off the list. The rewards can be quick and easy and can range from a 30s early dismissal to dancing the "Chicken Dance" for the rest of the class.

Another strategy for reaching the disenfranchised student is to match the student's skills/interests to an authentic job in the school or classroom. A powerful example that was recently observed involved a middle school student who defiantly wandered the school rather than reporting to the bus room and repeatedly missed his bus. The bus monitor worked on establishing a relationship with this young man and when she felt the time was right, she asked him to help her out. She explained that she was having difficulty in multitasking; watching for the buses to arrive, making sure that students heard the bus numbers being called, dealing with bus driver complaints, etc. She asked the young man to help her with the younger students by checking the roster and leading the students to the bus. He was given a clipboard and introduced to the younger students as "Mr. Steve." Not only has this truly helped the bus monitor but the targeted student is also the first to arrive to the bus room to pick up his clipboard. Other than the first day, when he was so engaged in his job and forgot to listen for his own bus, he has not missed the bus. He has received the unconditional affirmation and dependence of the younger students. Most importantly, he told the monitor that he would help her out next year when he attends the high school next door because he could tell that she couldn't do it all without him!

Take Home Messages for Teachers

School violence is a terrible thing. It comes in all shapes and sizes and impacts a variety of students and teachers. It can be prevented by all concerned working together to reach and touch each and every student in each and every school. Teachers can be very effective at helping to lessen the chances of school violence. How? By doing the following:

- Caring deeply about each student's personal well-being and their learning.
- Establishing well-organized and planned learning environments with clear procedures for students to follow.
- Engaging students in active, relevant learning tasks.

- Providing a variety of classroom structures and strategies that "insist" upon success for each and every student. Establishing as a motto: "attendance is mandatory in my classroom and so is learning!"
- Interacting with each student more often when he or she is being good or just being than when he or she is misbehaving.
- Teaching behavior via classroom rules, expectations for classroom activities, expectations for transitions, and all key classroom procedures that are critical for student success.
- Using numerous encouragement procedures in the classroom to prompt positive, motivated, and responsible behavior from each student.
- Providing extra help to any student who needs it.
- Modeling respectful behavior via positive, professional interactions with all.
- Reaching out to the student who appears lonely, frightened, or unsuccessful.
- Communicating care, concern, and commitment to each student's well-being.
- Communicating high expectations and developing structures to support each student's progress toward meeting those expectations.
- Providing a safe haven in the classroom where respect is taught, expected, practiced, and modeled.
- Developing student relationships beyond the classroom walls.

These are a few of the lessons learned and things that effective teachers do already that will help prevent future occurrences of school violence. We can become more intentional and we can make school violence even less of an event in our schools if we work together and focus on each individual student. It is what good teaching is really all about. It is quite simply what we are called to do.

References

Barkley, R. (2007). School interventions for attention deficit hyperactivity disorder: Where to from here? *School Psychology Review*, 36(2), 279–286.

Blum, R. W. (2005). A case for school connectedness. *Educational Leadership*, 62(7), 16–20.

Center for Effective Collaboration and Practice of the American Institutes for Research (1998). *Early Warning, Timely Response: A Guide to Safe Schools*. U.S. Department of Education.

Educational Resources Information Center (2000). *How Can We Prevent Violence in Our Schools*? U.S. Department of Education.

Gladwell, M. (2005). *Blink: The Power of Thinking Without Thinking*. New York: Little, Brown and Company.

Greene, R. W. (2001). *The Explosive Child*. New York: HarperCollins Publishers, Inc.

O'Toole, M. E. & The Critical Incident Response Group (2007). *The School Shooter: A Threat Assessment Perspective*. Quantico, Virginia: National Center for the Analysis of Violent Crimes.

Pogrow, S. (2005). HOTS revisited: A thinking development approach to reducing the learning gap after grade 3. *Phi Delta Kappan*, 87(1), 64–75.

Sprick, R., et al. (2002). *Foundations: Establishing Positive Discipline Policies*. Pacific North West Publishing Company. Eugene, Oregon.

The Silent Epidemic, March 2006: A Report on High School Dropouts by Civic Enterprises. www.gatesfoundation.org

Chapter 13
The Role of Teachers in School Violence and Bullying Prevention

Jina S. Yoon and Elizabeth Barton

A variety of aggressive behaviors among students seems to manifest in different forms ranging from extreme cases of school shootings and physical attacks to verbal threats and social exclusion. Empirical studies have also documented that these different types of conflicts are observed across developmental stages (see Dodge et al., 2006, for review). With a consistent finding that both perpetrators and victims of aggressive behaviors exhibit concurrent and future maladjustment, a lot of efforts have been geared toward a better understanding of individual markers of perpetrators and victims. Social cognitive characteristics, social skills deficits, emotional dysregulation, and peer acceptance have been heavily investigated (see Hinshaw & Lee, 2003, for review). Obviously, a clear understanding of complex interactions among these characteristics associated with different types of aggressive behaviors is an important step toward effective prevention efforts as well as an early identification of students who are likely to engage in aggressive behaviors.

Another important direction in the literature is an acknowledgment that many different contextual variables make significant contributions to the development and maintenance of aggressive behaviors. Bullying and victimization have been conceptualized as an outcome of an interaction among bullies, victims, and their environments (Swearer & Doll, 2001). Espelage (2004) defined bullying as "… an ecological phenomenon that is established and perpetrated over time as a result of the complex interplay between the individual child, their family, peer group, school and community as well as their culture" (p. 4). Consistent with this conceptualization of bullying and victimization, studies have provided evidence that different aspects of these contexts are at work in the social experiences of bullies and victims such as family characteristics, peer association, and school characteristics. Peers take various parts in a bullying incident as "assistants" who join the bullying, "reinforcers" who provide verbal encouragement, "outsiders" who ignore the bullying, or "defenders" who take action to stop the bullying (Salmivalli et al., 1996). The types and quality of peer relationships also seem to make a difference. Both the number of a child's friends and the friends' ability to defend and protect the child moderated the relation between maladjustment (internalizing and externalizing problems) and victimization (Hodges et al., 1997). Having a close friend also appears to reduce a repeated victimization (Pellegrini et al., 1999). In terms of family

T. W. Miller (ed.), *School Violence and Primary Prevention.*
© Springer 2008

contexts, low cohesion and high hostility within the family have been noted for bullies (Bowers et al., 1992). Parenting practices of bullies have been characterized with inconsistent discipline/monitoring, less autonomy, lack of structure, low warmth, and rules/interactions that reinforce aggression (Oliver et al., 1994; Rican et al., 1993; Schwartz et al., 1997).

Meanwhile, school environment has been examined as a direct influence on aggressive behavior, including the physical characteristics of the school, school polices regarding aggressive behaviors, levels of enforcement, and overall social climate (Mayer & Leone, 1999; Reinke & Herman, 2002; Skiba & Peterson, 2000). Given that peer conflicts and victimization frequently take place in school, social contexts in which these interactions take place may be particularly critical in our analysis of school environment and planning of prevention efforts. The purpose of this chapter is to examine the characteristics of school environments as a critical area of prevention with a special emphasis on critical roles of teachers in the prevention efforts of aggressive behaviors and victimization. Although there is a consensus in the literature about the characteristics of effective school environment, less explored is the role of teachers in prevention and maintenance of students' aggressive behaviors. Brophy (1996) proposes that teachers play four different roles in dealing with problem students: (1) instruction, (2) classroom management, (3) disciplinary interventions, and (4) student socialization. Although the degree to which teachers are involved in these different roles may vary depending on grade levels (elementary vs. secondary) and teachers' attitudes and expectations, it is clear that teachers exert significant influences on students' school experiences and their roles should be closely examined in prevention efforts. This chapter reviews current literature in positive school characteristics and explores the role of teachers in school violence and bullying prevention. A brief review of different school-based programs that addresses teacher contribution is also provided.

School Characteristics

The school environment is a significant part of a child's socialization experiences and has significant impact on a variety of developmental outcomes (Caldas & Bankston, 1999; Esposito, 1999; Haynes et al., 1998; Yoon, 2003). School has long been recognized as a socializing agent. Shaffer (1999) argues that schools not only provide experiences for academic competence and cognitive growth but also socialize children with informal curriculum through which they adopt school-related values (i.e., respect, cooperation, and compliance) and learn to become more socially competent individuals.

On the basis of a comprehensive literature review, Haynes et al. (1997) identified 15 ingredients of a healthy, supportive school: achievement motivation, collaborative decision making, equity and fairness, general school climate, order and discipline, parental involvement, school–community relations, staff dedication to student learning, staff expectation, leadership, school building, sharing resources, caring and sensitivity, student interpersonal relations, and student–teacher relations. As this long list of school characteristics suggests, building a school environment that promotes desirable student outcomes is not an easy task, requiring much collaboration among parents, teachers, administrators, and students in many different areas of school experiences. More importantly, studies have suggested that it should be a priority to develop and maintain a positive school environment in any prevention effort for school violence. Positive school environment is associated with reduced bullying and other aggressive behaviors (Bear, 1998; Sugai & Horner, 2002), and higher levels of perceived school connection are linked to lower levels of emotional distress and lower levels of school violence (Resnick et al., 1997).

According to Anderson (1982), school climate consists of four dimensions: school culture, organizational structure, social milieu, and ecological environments. These dimensions of school climate shape interpersonal relationships, policies and rules, social and physical climates, and formal and informal curriculum. Welsh (2000) argues that these school climate dimensions define "the parameters of acceptable behaviors among students, teachers, and administrators and assign some degree of institutional responsibilities for school safety" (p. 248). In fact, certain aspects of school environments appear to reinforce social behaviors and to deter aggressive behaviors whereas others may maintain or perpetuate aggressive behaviors and victimization. For example, areas within school seem to matter in student reports of bullying and aggressive behaviors, often related to the level of supervision and adult presence. Playgrounds, halls, and cafeterias are more prone for peer conflicts and victimization to take place (Craig & Pepler, 1997). In the playgrounds, more victimization is reported when older and younger students are put together. Also, more aggressive behaviors are reported when high numbers of students are in a limited amount of space (Welsh et al., 2000). As school size increases, reports of school crime and discipline problems also increase (DeVoe et al., 2004).

Another important area of prevention efforts is an examination of core values that schools promote and disseminate (Curwin & Mendler, 1997). Orpinas and Horne (2006) proposed three important values to be promoted in school-based bullying prevention: (1) all children can learn, (2) all people should be treated with dignity and respect, and (3) there is no place for violence in the school. They argued that these values should be clearly communicated and promoted in all interactions among students, teachers, and staff. Similarly, Barton (2003) recommends that school-based programs address "belief systems and teach tolerance, acceptance, and respect through effective communication and constructive resolution" (p. 108). Core values should be adopted by the entire school community and should be used as a framework in decision making that guides the development of school rules and policies. A mechanism to engage in continuing discussions of core values and to monitor organizational responses to these values is also required. In the level of implementation of rules and policies, the core values should be widely communicated and reinforced in classroom-wide discussions by integrating them into regular curriculum and school-wide discussions such as regular assembly. Many researchers have argued that school-based interventions are most effective in reducing aggressive behaviors when the entire school community is involved (Olweus, 1993; Song & Swearer, 2002)

It is clear that all members of the school community including administrators, parents, teachers, and students should be involved in creating a positive school climate and in preventing aggressive behaviors. We believe that teachers play particularly important roles in this process. There is widespread recognition that teachers have influence on students' academic and social adjustments. Different approaches have been used to explain how teacher influences might occur: to name a few, teaching practices (Grolnick & Ryan, 1987; Skinner & Belmont, 1993; Wentzel, 2002); classroom management (Kounin, 1970; Emmer & Stough, 2001); and teacher relationship with students (Baker, 2006; Birch & Ladd, 1996; Pianta & Steinberg, 1992). Consistent with these theoretical frameworks, a number of studies have provided support for teacher influences in student outcomes: school and behavioral adjustment (Baker et al., 1997), positive school affect and attitude (Skinner & Belmont, 1993), academic achievement (Birch & Ladd, 1998), and motivation (Connell & Wellborn, 1991).

Particularly relevant in the discussion of school climate and school violence prevention is the model of socialization (Wentzel, 2002). In this model, similar to how parents socialize and influence children (Grusec & Goodnow, 1994), teachers' modeling and caregiving styles are considered to communicate goals and values that promote students' school adjustment. In their daily interaction with students through instruction, discipline, classroom management, and other school activities, teachers are involved in socializing students toward academic goals and socially acceptable behaviors, creating social environments in which students learn to regulate their behaviors, engage in learning processes, and interact with other students.

Consistent with the notion of teachers as socializing agents, we argue that teachers could make a significant contribution to school violence prevention efforts by (1) promoting academic success for all children, (2) building a prosocial, non-aggressive environment where caring relationships are fostered in all levels of relationships, (3) promoting tolerance of and sensitivity to individual indifference, and (4) implementing appropriate management of aggressive behaviors.

Promoting Academic Success for All Children

Lower academic grades and learning difficulties have been consistently associated with aggressive behaviors (Campbell et al., 2006; Ledingham & Schwartzman, 1984), and school failure predicts violence among adolescents and adults (Walker et al., 2004). Although a direct causal relation between aggressive behaviors and learning difficulties is not clear and the underlying mechanism for this association may not be uniform for different types of aggressive children (Hinshaw, 1992), researchers argued that some children show patterns of aggressive, hostile behaviors accompanied with frustration over learning tasks in class, consequently avoiding the tasks and defying teachers. It has also been suggested that attention problems often associated with aggressive behaviors are responsible for academic failure (Shinn et al., 1987). Regardless, these children are frequently removed from instructional processes for discipline due to aggressive and/or defiant, disruptive behaviors (e.g., time-out, referral to office), and a task of overcoming academic difficulties and increasing academic competencies is particularly challenging. These children get further behind in academic skills and continue to struggle throughout their schooling with increasingly negative attitudes toward school as academic demands increase in higher grades. Yet, academic needs of aggressive, violent children have been largely ignored and few studies have addressed them in intervention (e.g., Gorman-Smith et al., 2007).

Academic remediation has to be an important area of school violence prevention, particularly in early experiences of schooling when children acquire basic academic skills that are so critical in building a solid foundation for later academic success. The U.S. Department of Health and Human Services (2001) identified increasing academic success as a primary way of preventing school violence. In this report, two specific strategies were recommended: continuous progress programs and cooperative learning.

A few studies have demonstrated the importance of early screening of students who are at risk for low academic achievement (Fuchs et al., 2003; Vaughn et al., 2003) and of providing intensive intervention to these students. Torgesen (1998) and Fuchs and Fuchs (2006) strongly argue that it is also critical to continuously monitor students' responses to intervention and adjusting intervention strategies based on responses so that students' academic concerns are addressed early on. Early remediation of academic difficulties through screening and continuous monitoring increases academic competence of all children (Greenwood et al., 1993; Slavin & Madden, 2001), but may be particularly important for aggressive children whose behavioral and social characteristics may interfere with their learning processes in the classroom.

At the instructional level, the quality of instruction has to be ensured. Hawkins et al. (1998) argued that while teachers struggle to manage the behavioral challenges of aggressive children, many teachers are not able to attend to their academic needs. From many instructional approaches that promote both academic motivation and competence, Vygotsky's concept of the zone of proximal development (ZPD) is particularly relevant to teaching aggressive children. The ZPD is the difference between what a child can do on his/her own and what can be learned with assistance from someone with advanced skills such as teachers (Vygotsky, 1986). Well-designed instruction has to be aimed slightly above a student's level so that academic tasks are challenging enough, but not too difficult with the appropriate level of teacher support. In this approach, teachers use scaffolding strategies such as leading questions, hints, modeling, and feedback, and students are actively engaged in the learning process. Students experience small steps of academic success and gradually build academic competence over time. Designing academic instructions based on students' ZPD seems like a logical approach, considering it is more likely to motivate students and to increase academic engagement rather than avoiding tasks because they are just too difficult or too easy. Yet, a variety of challenges exist for many teachers to implement individualized instruction such as the number of students per class, demands of discipline, and lack of paraprofessional assistance in the class. Despite these challenges, it is so critical that academic tasks are within the ZPD and aggressive children have opportunities to experience academic success. Otherwise, aggressive children would experience repeated failure and continued frustration at the same time they are reprimanded for behavioral problems, resulting in a sense of helplessness in personal competence and pervasively negative experiences in school.

Another instructional approach to be considered is cooperative learning in which students work in small groups to help each other learn. In general, the group sizes range from two to four (Santrock, 2006). Research supports that cooperative learning promotes academic achievement when two conditions are met: group rewards are available and individual students are accountable for their contributions to the group (e.g., Slavin, 1995). Cooperative learning has been associated with increased motivation to learn (Sapon-Shevin, 1996), higher academic achievement (Johnson et al., 1995), and greater problem-solving abilities (Qin et al., 1995). Using a cooperative learning approach in the context of violence prevention should be of particular interest because the positive effects of cooperative learning on social relationships among students have been consistently shown in the studies. A primary element of cooperative learning is its ability to promote positive interdependence (working together toward a group goal), which is linked to positive peer interaction in the group (Sharan & Shaulov, 1990), connection with other students (Johnson & Johnson, 2003), and increased liking for school and greater concern for others (Battistich et al., 1993). These characteristics are more likely to help aggressive children become more engaged in the learning process and increase their sense of belonging.

With regards to specific teacher behaviors that promote academic adjustment, research has explored a number of teacher dimensions. Students who view their teachers as providing consistent and predictive responses, clearly stated expectations, instructional support, and adjustment of instructional strategies are more likely to show efforts, attention, and persistence during learning activities (Skinner & Belmont, 1993). Instructional practices that instill a mastery orientation in learning (i.e., developing competence toward a clearly defined learning outcome) among students are linked to more engagement with greater motivation and efforts (Anderman et al., 1999; Ames & Archer, 1988; Midgley et al., 1998). Teachers' high expectations and fairness in class are also known to promote mastery learning goals (Wentzel, 2002). Interestingly, teachers' instructional behaviors that promote academic success are critical in students' perception of how much teachers care about them. Students feel that teachers care about their students by making learning tasks interesting and relevant, asking when they need help, and taking time to make sure they understand (Wentzel, 1996).

Hawkins et al. (1998) postulate that opportunities to experience academic success and recognition of the success prevent aggressive behaviors in two ways: through reinforcement of positive behaviors and through increasing school bonding and commitment to the learning process. With repeated experiences of small successes in the learning process, aggressive children are more likely to increase their academic competence and develop more positive attitudes toward school, thereby preventing significant levels of poor performance and aggressive behaviors. It is clear that proactive efforts to promote early academic competence should be a part of the prevention of a wide range of aggressive behaviors including school violence, and that it warrants special attention from teachers.

Appropriate Management of Aggressive Behaviors

Teachers may or may not witness students' aggressive behaviors and victimization, but their appropriate handling of students' aggressive behaviors has significant implications for future behaviors of both perpetrators and victims. Obviously, aggressive behaviors are reinforced and further strengthened when an aggressor experiences successful outcomes instead of negative consequences from the behaviors (Huesmann & Eron, 1984). That is, unless appropriate consequences are consistently and immediately experienced, the aggressive behaviors are more likely to continue in the future, especially when there is continuing success of dominating a victim.

Despite the importance of consistent, immediate responses to aggressive behaviors, evidence suggests that some aggressive behaviors may go without teacher attention. According to Pepler et al. (1994), 85% of teachers reported intervening "always" or "often" to stop bullying. However, only 35% of students reported that teachers intervened in bullying. Holt and Keyes (2004) also found that teachers report consistently lower prevalence rates of bullying than do students. Although this discrepancy may be because some aggressive behaviors are not witnessed by teachers or reported by students, students' reports that teachers are not intervening is concerning. Another potential reason for this discrepancy is that students and teachers have different perceptions about aggressive behaviors. In fact, research has shown that teachers greatly vary in their perceptions of aggressive behaviors (What is bullying?) and their ways of responding to aggressive behaviors (What are the appropriate ways to deal with bullying behaviors?) (Yoon & Kerber, 2003). Teachers perceive covert natured, less direct aggression as less serious and are less likely to get involved (Craig et al., 2000). In terms of what is considered as bullying, physical and verbal bullying are more acknowledged and teachers are more aware of them whereas social exclusion or indirect bullying are more likely to be ignored.

Another aspect of handling aggressive behaviors is teachers' responses to victims. Teachers are often quick to respond to aggressive, violent behaviors but not to victims, and when they do, their responses seem to vastly differ among teachers

(Jordon & Yoon, 2005). Teachers also hold faulty beliefs such as helping victims makes it worse, that victims have reasons to be bullied, and that ignoring bullying is an effective response (Horne et al., 2004). Little is known as to how teachers' instructional practices and discipline approaches shape individual students' victimization experiences and coping processes. It is possible that teachers' handling of behaviors may make victims feel more vulnerable, whereas teachers' attention to victims and ongoing conversation would communicate a caring attitude and would facilitate victims' adjustment. Victims are often reluctant to come forward and report their experiences to adults out of a fear of retaliation, which perpetuates their continuing victimization and isolation. Similarly, the lack of appropriate responses would lead victims to become increasingly reluctant to report and to feel helpless about stopping aggressors. When victims of bullying perceived their plight as going unnoticed, they are less likely to feel safe in their school environment, thus possibly affecting their school experience (Casey-Cannon, Hayward, & Gowen, 2001; Yoon & Kerber, 2003). Specifically, teachers' ignoring is likely to set an expectation for students, sending an inappropriate message that the behaviors are tolerated and even permitted (Hoover & Hazler, 1994). Thus, it is likely that teachers' responses to bullying not only influence future bullying behaviors but also contribute to students' perceptions of classroom climate.

In addition, teachers may inadvertently facilitate students' bullying and victimization by modeling inappropriate, disrespectful behaviors that exemplify domineering, coercive interactions. Song and Swearer (2002) describe an alarming finding that compared to students who were not involved in bullying, those who were bullies and victims were more likely to report that teachers and other school staff bully students in their schools. It is possible that teachers' authoritarian styles of discipline and classroom management may indeed model intimidating, overpowering styles of interpersonal interactions.

In summary, teachers' responses to students' wide range of aggressive behaviors should be carefully examined and considered in prevention efforts of more serious violent behaviors. A general myth among teachers and school administrators is that some level of interpersonal aggression, or "meanness," is a normative developmental feature (Jeffrey et al., 2001) and students will "grow out of it." This sentiment may explain teachers' indifferent perceptions and attitudes toward aggression and less consistent, lenient intervention approaches. The pattern of maturation may be applied to some children given that aggressive behaviors in general decline with age (Olweus, 1993), but it is also well documented that aggressive behaviors are quite stable over time and may be a precursor for other indices of maladjustment, highlighting the importance of teachers' attention to these behaviors. Yoon and Kerber (2003) argue that increasing teachers' awareness of negative outcomes associated with bullying behaviors may change teachers' appraisal of bullying situations. In fact, Olweus (1995) documented that when teachers are more aware of bullying and more involved in bullying situations, rates of bullying decrease significantly. Both teacher preparation and continuing education programs should include discussions about specific short- and long-term consequences for aggressors and victims, and also focus on specific intervention skills to address both aggressors and victims.

Building a Prosocial, Nonaggressive Environment Where Caring Relationships Are Fostered in All Levels of Relationships

The importance of a positive social and psychological climate in school has been well demonstrated in studies of social and academic outcomes (e.g., Esposito, 1999; Haynes et al., 1997; Kasen et al., 1990; Wallace et al., 2002). The nature of such climate is developed based on the daily activities, ongoing interactions between teachers and students, and interactions among students, leading to certain social environments where students feel/experience different levels of psychological and physical safety (Baker, 1999). So far, only a few studies have examined school climate issues in aggression and victimization, and further inquiries have been recommended to better understand the processes of victimization and overall adjustment (Espelage & Swearer, 2003). Available studies indicate that students' negative perceptions of school climate are linked to disconnection from school (Kuykendall, 1992), increased levels of behavior problems (Simons-Morton et al., 1999), and higher levels of victimization (Buckley et al., 2003). Meanwhile, a perception of school as a caring community is related to decreased victimization and delinquency (Battistich & Hom, 1997), and students' perceived positive school climate appears to mediate the relationship between victimization experience and school adjustment (Yoon et al., under review).

While these findings underscore the importance of positive school climate and interpersonal connections, research findings have consistently shown that aggressive students are more likely to be disliked or rejected by classmates (Miller-Johnson et al., 2002) and less likely to report close relationships with teachers (Hughes et al., 1999). The absence of close interpersonal connections in school is concerning, given that experiences of social affiliation and a sense of belonging are believed to serve as an underlying process through which children adopt and internalize social values (Deci & Ryan, 1985) and acquire beliefs and skills necessary for success in school (Baker, 1999; Roeser et al., 1996). Lack of close relationships may further perpetuate a sense of disconnection and social alienation in school and place some students at greater risk for becoming more hostile and aggressive. In fact, perceived social rejection and isolation have been linked to aggression (Garbarino, 1999; Twenge & Baumeister, 2005), and appear to play a major role in school shooting cases (Leary et al., 2003).

It is clear that teachers play a critical role in creating a psychologically safe climate, as previously mentioned. Sutherland (1994) states that "the students' feelings of safety, respect, belonging, and ease can be realized by the efforts of the teacher to create such climate" (p. 13). We argue one of the teachers' efforts should include establishing quality relationships with students. For students who are aggressive and/or victimized, the quality of teacher–student relationship does not appear to be high, reporting low levels of teacher support. Victims report lower levels of teacher support (Furlong et al., 1995; Rigby, 2000) whereas having teacher support is more important to victims than to nonvictims (Demaray &

Malecki, 2003). Both students and teachers report that teachers' relationships with aggressive students are distant and conflictual (Meehan et al., 2003; Ladd & Burgess, 2001). Relationship difficulties are further sustained by their daily interactions that are consistently negative in nature (Hanish et al., 2004). Although incidents of aggressive behaviors warrant effective disciplines including appropriate punishment, teachers' overreliance on the use of punitive practices and lower occurrence of positive attention have been noted. For example, Van Acker and his colleagues found that aggressive children are twice as likely to be punished as nonaggressive children for the same behaviors and the only predictable teacher behavior for highly aggressive students is the use of reprimands (Van Acker et al., 1996). Although teachers' intolerance for aggressive, disruptive, and noncompliant behaviors is understandable, teacher interactions characterized as angry, punitive responses may have far reaching influences on students' aggressive behaviors: directly increasing problem behaviors, provoking violent behaviors from students, and influencing peer reputations perpetuating further social isolation. A few studies also suggest that teachers' authoritarian, domineering ways of addressing student aggression lead to aggressive, violent responses from students (Durivage, 1989).

Available evidence also suggests that teachers' attitudes toward a student affect other students' perceptions of the student, suggesting teacher influences on peer reputations (Weinstein, 1987; White, Jones, & Sherman, 1998). Similarly, Roland and Galloway (2002) found teachers' class management style predicted bullying and influenced classroom social structure and peer relations. Although students' hostile, dominant behaviors make them become more vulnerable for peer disliking and rejection, these findings indicate that teachers' attitudes and behaviors could make unique contributions to how these students are perceived by other students in class.

When students perceive their relationships with teachers as negative with increasing hostility, disconnection, mistrust, and disrespect, students exhibit academic disengagement and feel further alienated from the class community. Meanwhile, children who are committed to academic success and feel attached to teachers and other children are less likely to engage in aggressive behaviors (Hawkins et al., 1998). Better teacher relationship is also linked to less peer victimization (Van Blyderveen, 2004). Hanish et al. (2004) argued that then it may be worthwhile to help these children develop better relationships with teachers. Many successful school-based programs (e.g., Orpinas et al., 2003; Tairaiol et al., 2005) include a school-wide effort to recognize students who demonstrate prosocial behaviors so that teachers, staff, and administrators can acknowledge good behaviors with appropriate rewards.

Promoting Tolerance and Respect to Individual Differences

Teachers' efforts to facilitate and maintain positive relationships in all levels should also extend to address students' and their own beliefs and attitudes toward individual differences. Members of the community in American schools (students, teachers, and parents) make up a heterogeneous group, reflecting a wide range of diversity in races, ethnicities, social economic statuses, religions, languages, and sexual orientations. Although diverse student body could provide rich experiences, these differences may present a challenge in creating a social climate in which all members feel valued and appreciated (Bettmann & Moore, 1994). Often these differences become sources of rejection, teasing, and harassment.

It has been noted that many aspects of American schools perpetuate the isolation and segregation of students (Barton, 2003) and that schools condone bullying, teasing, and cliques by dividing and labeling students according to their academic and/or athletic abilities (Kipnis, 1999). Students who are different from the norm with respect to achievement, special education status, sexual orientation, and social economic status often become targets of victimization due to their "low" status in the school environment. Students are likely to continue these lines of separation and maintain their position within the school hierarchy. Unnecessary divisions and hostile relationships create an organizational climate that perpetuates disrespect and intolerance among students. For example, students tease other students who cannot afford designer clothing, those who belong to a minority group in their religious, cultural, or ethnic memberships, or those who have a disability, leading them to feel inferior and marginalized (Jimerson et al., 2006). An alarming rate of taunting and ostracizing has been reported among gay, lesbian, and bisexual students (Remafedi, 1988; Savin-Williams, 1996).

Students' negative attitudes and stereotypic beliefs about different ethnic and cultural groups are in part a reflection of those commonly shared in broader contexts such as family, media, and social policies. Different approaches in multicultural education are taken to change the negative attitudes toward different groups of students (Bennett, 2003; Gollnick & Chinn, 2002). A general consensus in this literature is that successful multicultural education is accomplished when different cultural values and experiences are integrated into the curriculum and rewarded by the teachers (Banks, 2002), thus highlighting the roles of teachers in the classroom.

Related to this point, an important area of further work is multicultural understanding and sensitivity among teachers and administrators. Respect for individual differences and appreciation of diversity should be fostered not only among students but also shared and expressed by teachers and administrators. While teacher preparation and continuing education programs continue to address multicultural sensitivity and learning, teachers and administrators should explore their beliefs and expectations of minority students and carefully assess their influence on the students' academic and social experiences as a part of school violence and bullying prevention efforts. A wealth of data suggests that teachers tend to have lower expectations for minority and low socioeconomic status students and communicate lower expectations in their interaction with students (Grossman, 1995; Irvine, 1990). Furthermore, biased teacher beliefs and responses are known to explain students' disengagement and academic performance (Good & Nichols, 2001; Rosenthal, 1985; Wuthrick, 1990). This pattern of teacher influences on minority and low socioeconomic status students warrants serious consideration in our current discussion of school violence and bullying prevention. Through these influences, teachers inadvertently participate in a process of marginalizing these students, perpetuating a sense of alienation and inferiority and further creating a social hierarchy among students that have the potential to promote and justify victimization. Furthermore, these students would interpret any discipline efforts to curb aggressive behaviors as aspects of injustice they receive from teachers whom they perceive to be racially and culturally biased. Unfortunately, it has been noted that ethnic minority students receive more harsh discipline and punishments for behavioral problems than Caucasian students (Cartledge & Johnson, 1997; Forness, 1988).

Orpinas and Horne (2006) suggest it is critical that schools should embrace individual differences and celebrate diversity in order to maintain a positive social climate. They further suggest that schools should facilitate the shared experiences of individual differences among students, through which the entire school community learns to accept and appreciate differences and to gain genuine respects, instead of rejecting them because they are considered "inferior or deficient." Cartledge and Johnson (1996) point out that these shared experiences would affirm minority students and their background, which leads students to become more receptive of demands in learning process. More importantly, they argue that these shared experiences also increase teachers' own cultural knowledge and understandings, and they respond to the students in more accepting ways. Similarly, Garcia (2002) found that teachers who are successful in multicultural education tend to promote students' self-esteem by including students' cultural and linguistic backgrounds in classroom materials and activities. Recently, Williams (2006) provides the following tips for teachers in culturally competent practices:

- Learn as much as possible about the cultural and linguistic background of students they teach.
- Pronounce students' names correctly and learn key phrases in their native language.
- Allow students to share their thoughts, ideas, and feelings through use of cooperative groups, role plays, dialogue journals, and other forms of active and interactive learning.
- Enhance students' self-image, motivation, and cultural pride by using culturally relevant materials and encouraging discussion and actions that honor their cultural and linguistic heritage.
- Invite parents and families to actively participate in their child's education.
- Facilitate home–school communication and collaboration.
- Beware that families from diverse linguistic or cultural backgrounds may not initiate requests for help or use in-school resources available to address mental health issues. Teachers are urged to provide orientations to inform parents and families about school resources.
- Seek help from school psychologists or other school mental health professional if students exhibit academic, behavioral, and/or mental health problems.

Teacher Components of Selected Prevention Programs

Given the current literature on school bullying and its potential relationship to school violence, teachers' attitudes on their responsibility to teaching, intervening, and preventing bullying behavior have begun to change (Barton, 2006). Various professional organizations have recommended that professionals be trained to deal with or prevent school violence and bullying (e.g., American Psychological Association and National Education Goals Panel). Elam et al. (1994) found that 92% of the public supports violence training for school personnel. Yet, professional development opportunities are limited for teachers to learn how to address bullying and other aggressive behaviors in their classrooms. Too often, teachers must seek professional development opportunities in these areas on their own and antibullying efforts are often addressed within the umbrella topic of conflict resolution education (CRE). Scant resources in school districts across the country force administration to limit professional development days and other trainings and target topics specific to advancing students' academic competency.

Many teacher training programs across the country do not cover school safety as a core course; bullying behaviors are often not addressed unless the issue is covered during a discussion of classroom management strategies. Antibullying training efforts frequently occur within the context of teaching CRE strategies, a topic also absent from most education school coursework.

Indeed, one large-scale effort to train preservice teachers occurred in 2002. The North Carolina Department of Juvenile Justice and Delinquency Prevention and The National Center to Prevent School Violence in North Carolina piloted a teacher education program to prepare preservice educators for issues concerning school safety. The Reach In, Reach Out, and Reach Over project was one of the first statewide initiatives designed to improve teachers' skills, knowledge, and attitudes toward demonstrating and teaching constructive conflict resolution strategies.

In 2004, Project CRETE (Conflict Resolution Education in Teacher Education), a collaboration between Temple University, Cleveland State University, Kent State University, and the Ohio Commission for Dispute Resolution and Conflict Management has begun to educate preservice teachers in CRE and social and emotional learning to help create constructive learning environments, increase teacher satisfaction, and improve teacher retention in urban education environments.

The CRETE project, led by Dr. Tricia Jones of Temple University, (1) works with higher education faculty involved in preservice teacher preparation to infuse CRE into their ongoing coursework, (2) delivers a curriculum for educating teacher candidates outside the higher education course delivery system (in external mini-seminar training modules), (3) provides teacher mentors, trained in CRE, to work with teacher candidates and new teachers to facilitate new teachers' abilities to apply these skills and knowledge in their classrooms, and (4) evaluates the impact of both curriculum and training processes on teachers' success in classroom management, establishing a positive classroom climate, increasing teacher satisfaction and teacher retention. Formative evaluation on this widespread initiative will be completed in 2007.

Improving teachers' knowledge of and attitudes toward preventing and intervening in bullying and school violence is essential to improving classroom climate and school safety in the future. Comprehensive school-based programs and classroom-level programs are available for addressing the critical roles of teachers and improving school climate, although few evaluated program performance on decreasing bullying and violent behaviors.

Comprehensive School-Wide Approaches

Project BASIS is a school-wide initiative designed to improve school climate as a strategy for improving school safety and reducing bullying behaviors (Gottfredson et al., 1993). The purpose of BASIS is to (1) increase clarity of school rules and consistency of rule enforcement, (2) improve classroom organization and management through teacher training, (3) increase the frequency of communication between the school and home regarding student behavior, and (4) replace punitive disciplinary strategies with positive reinforcement of appropriate behaviors. Although it is a research project, school teams of administrators, teachers, and other school personnel implement BASIS and collaborating researchers provide quarterly feedback about implementation and targeted behavioral changes. BASIS is identified as "promising" prevention program by the Center for Substance Abuse Prevention (U.S. Department of Health and Human Services, 2002). Documented outcomes of the program are teacher reports of fewer classroom disruptions, student perceptions of the fairness of school/classroom rules, and student reports of rewards and fewer punishments.

Developed by H. Jerome Freiberg, Consistency Management and Cooperative Discipline (CMCD) is a research-based classroom and school reform model that emphasizes shared responsibility for learning and classroom organization between teachers and students. The model seeks to address the needs of students, teachers, and administrative staff in schools from pre-K through 12th grade. The consistency management component concentrates on classroom instructional organization and planning arrangement by the teacher such as seating arrangements and transitional procedures. The teacher acts as an instructional leader, but the cooperative discipline component expands the leadership roles to the students by giving each student multiple leadership opportunities (e.g., passing out papers). It incorporates five themes: prevention through classroom management, a caring environment, cooperation, classroom organization, and parental and community involvement activities.

The program provides support to teachers over a 3-year period through staff development, school-based facilitators, and data collection on students and teachers perspective of school climate and discipline referrals. Teachers learn how to work with students in establishing a cooperative plan for classrooms rules, procedures, and use of time within a developing democratic structure. Research and evaluation of the program over a 10-year period in urban and inner-city schools document its effectiveness. Schools using CMCD have reported 72–78% fewer discipline referrals to the principal's office, with additional 36-minute teaching time per day resulting from fewer discipline problems and enhanced cooperation (equivalent to 3 additional weeks of instruction) (Freiberg, 1989).

Olweus Bullying Prevention (Olweus et al., 1999) is a multilevel, multicomponent school-based program designed to prevent or reduce bullying in elementary, middle, and junior high schools (students 6–15 years old). The program attempts to restructure the existing school environment to reduce opportunities and rewards for bullies. The Bullying Prevention Coordinating Committee composed of an administrator, a school counselor/psychologist, a teacher from each grade, and a parent is largely responsible for introducing and implementing the program. Within the classroom, teachers set and enforce clear rules about bullying and victimization and hold classroom-wide meetings so that students discuss their experiences with peers (i.e., bullying, victimization, and rules). Teachers are also encouraged to hold meetings with parents to discuss bullying incidents. Intensive 2-day training is available for committee members and ongoing consultation is recommended for at least 1 year (Limber, 2006). The Olweus Bullying Prevention program has shown a significant decrease in students' reports of bullying and victimization and adult observation of bullying in the cafeteria and on the playground (Black, 2003; Limber et al., 2004).

Schoolwide Positive Behavioral Supports (SWPBS) is a system-based approach to create positive, safe school environments and reduce school behavior problems (Sprague et al., 1998; Sugai & Horner, 1999). In SWPBS, a school team creates and sustains primary (school-wide), secondary (classroom), and tertiary (individual) systems of support for the youth; thus, school-wide expectations are clarified and promoted among students and staff, expected behaviors are recognized throughout the school, and problem behaviors are addressed consistently and fairly. Both the Olweus program and the SWPBS target school context, the latter has more emphasis on promoting positive behaviors and creating supportive school climate whereas the former is limited to the bullying prevention. SWPBS allows more flexibility in teacher training so that the school team or representatives are trained first and individual teachers are trained and coached by them. In evaluation studies, SWPBS has been shown to reduce antisocial (Sprague et al., 2002) and aggressive behaviors (Grossman et al., 1997), as well as increase school engagement (O'Donnell et al., 1995) and academic achievement (Kellam et al., 1998).

Classroom-Based Curriculum/Programs

Classroom-based curriculum and programs reviewed here are available for use by teachers in their classrooms. A majority of these programs offer teacher and staff training for curriculum and monitoring. Since teachers are responsible for delivering the curriculum, training issues become very critical to ensure intervention fidelity.

Rated as an exemplary program by the U.S. Department of Education, the Second Step: A Violence Prevention Curriculum has a strong emphasis on active teacher participation. The goal of the program is to use a skill building curriculum designed to reduce impulsive and aggressive behavior by teaching students Pre-K–fifth grades skills in empathy, impulse control, problem solving, and anger management. Key teaching strategies include story/starter discussions, teacher-modeling behaviors and skills, and activities/role-playing. Developed by the Committee for Children (1992), programming is available for K–ninth grade students. Training is recommended and provided by the Committee for Children as either a 1-day staff training or a 3-day training of trainers model.

The Steps to Respect Program is specifically designed to prevent bullying in elementary schools. Although not yet empirically evaluated, the program is becoming more widely used in schools across the United States. The program consists of three phases: (1) establishing a school framework for antibullying initiatives (i.e., policies and procedures), (2) training for staff and parents on handling bullying, and (3) teaching 3rd–sixth grade students to recognize, refuse, and reporting bullying. Staff training for Steps to Respect is most often provided by the Committee for Children through a 1-day professional development program and includes training on how to respond to both bullies and victims.

The Resolving Conflict Creatively Program, developed by Educators for Social Responsibility (1992), prepares teachers to deliver high-quality instruction and an effective school curriculum in conflict resolution to K–12th grade students. The purpose of the program is also to transform the culture of participating schools so that the values and principles of creative nonviolent conflict resolution are modeled. Role-playing, interviews, group dialogue, brainstorming, and other affective experiential learning strategies are used for teaching along with curriculum, videos, and other resource materials. A 24-hour introductory course is required for effective implementation of the curriculum and on-site support for the curriculum is also available to all teachers. Compared to students who did not receive Resolving Conflicts Creatively Program (RCCP) instruction from their classroom teachers, those who did reported better social cognition (perceived their social world in a less hostile way, saw violence as an unacceptable option) and showed better conflict resolution skills (Aber et al., 1998). Teacher reports also indicated that these students showed increased positive social behaviors and better emotional control. Another evaluation study reports positive results, with 64% of teachers reporting less physical violence in the classroom and 75% of teachers reporting an increase in student cooperation (Metis Associates, 1998).

The I Can Problem Solve: An Interpersonal Cognitive Problem-Solving Program (Shure, 1992) has been implemented successfully by teachers to prevent the expression of destructive behavior. The goal of this program is to teach thinking skills to help Pre-K–sixth-grade children resolve interpersonal problems and prevent antisocial behavior. Key teaching strategies used are direct instruction via lesson plans, classroom interaction, and integration into the curriculum. On-site training is available for program directors, provided by the Mental Health Association in Illinois, and 1-day or 2-day workshops with classroom visits as follow-ups are recommended. Less impulsive classroom behavior, and better problem-solving skills, more positive, prosocial behaviors, and better peer relationships have been reported following the implementation of the program (Shure, 1997; Shure & Spivack, 1988).

Aggressors, Victims, and Bystanders: Thinking and Acting to Prevent Violence (AVB) is a 12-session curriculum designed for use with youths in grades six to nine. The AVB aims to prevent or reduce violence by altering patterns of thought and action that lead individuals to become involved in violence as aggressors, victims, or bystanders. The goal of the program is to develop youths' problem-solving skills and to help youth to identify their responses to conflict. Twelve classroom sessions deal with violence among peers and the separate but interrelated roles of aggressors, victims, and bystanders that youths play in potentially violent situations. At its foundation is a four-step, think-first model of conflict resolution. The model helps students pause and keep cool, understand what is going on before jumping to conclusions, define their problems and goals in ways that will not lead to fights, and generate positive solutions. Program developers report a decrease in self-reported bystander behavior supporting violence.

Promoting Alternative Thinking Strategies (PATHS) is a comprehensive program that promotes the development of social and emotional competencies in children during the elementary school years to achieve its goal of reducing aggression and other behavior problems (Greenberg, Kusche, & Riggs, 2004). A second program goal is to enhance the classroom atmosphere to facilitate learning and internalizing prosocial values. PATHS was developed for use in a classroom setting for children just entering school to those in grade six. Teachers provide the lessons three times per week for 20–30 minutes and 131 lessons are available for implementation over a 5-year period. PATHS lessons include instructions in understanding and expressing feelings, controlling impulses, accurate processing of social cues, perspective taking, and problem-solving steps. Both verbal and nonverbal communication skills are also taught. Teachers receive training in a 2–3-day workshop and in biweekly meetings with the curriculum consultant. Identified as a model program by the U.S. Department of Justice and Delinquency Prevention, the program has been shown to increase social cognition and emotional understanding, decrease aggressive behaviors, and promote a more positive classroom climate (Conduct Problems Prevention Research Group, 1999; Greenberg et al., 1995; Kam et al., 2004)

The Think Time Strategy program (Nelson & Carr, 1999) addresses disruptive behaviors in order to reduce classroom management issues in elementary schools. Think Time Strategy program requires that two or more teachers work together and identify disruptive behaviors early. Teachers send a disruptive student to a Think Time classroom, where another teacher directs the student to a Think Time desk, which is located in an area free from distractions. That teacher initiates a debriefing process after the student has had "thinking time." The process includes a number of steps: for example, having the student fill out a form, having the teacher check the form, and returning the student to the original classroom. Rated as a promising program by the U.S. Department of Education, evaluation studies show that the average number of critical events (e.g., verbal and physical aggression) decreased by 77% weekly and the average duration of on-task time increased by 34% weekly.

Conclusion and Future Directions

We have highlighted the roles of teachers in school violence and bullying prevention efforts. Students who exhibit aggressive and disruptive behaviors in school often view teachers as disciplinarians who enforce the rules and give out punishments. Although research suggests that aggressive students would benefit from teacher support as provided through good relationships with teachers, fair and respectful discipline, and academic assistance, these students often maintain conflictual teacher–student relationships due to their behavioral presentations and ongoing negative responses from teachers. Noddings (2001) suggests that students are most likely to develop into competent individuals when they feel cared for by people who are important to them. As this chapter outlined, teachers have a great deal of influences in these students' academic, social, and emotional adjustment and play crucial roles in ongoing prevention efforts. Teachers' day-to-day interactions with students shape classroom experiences and broaden social milieu and school climate. By creating a positive climate in which teachers actively provide academic and emotional support and consistently promote expected social behaviors and respect for individual differences, bullying and other aggressive behaviors are discouraged and academic and social competence are promoted instead.

Although the importance of school climate is increasingly recognized and the social nature of school environment is targeted in many prevention efforts, teachers' abilities to develop and maintain positive relationships with aggressive students have not been thoroughly investigated. We believe that this is a critical area of further investigation. As indicated in our review of selected prevention programs, the nature and the extent of teacher training greatly differ across prevention programs. As these programs present empirical evidence for effectiveness in prevention, a vital step is to examine the impact of the programs on teacher attitudes and beliefs toward students and teachers' behaviors in classroom management, positive behavior support, and academic support. For example, many conflict resolution curriculums are delivered by teachers to instruct effective ways to resolve conflicts and problem solve, yet teachers' conflict resolution skills are rarely examined. In our experiences in schools, some teachers are observed to model behaviors exactly opposite to what has been introduced to students, escalating conflicts with and showing disrespectful attitudes toward students and other staff.

Another important issue to be considered is program fidelity in evaluating programs. Only a few studies have considered program fidelity in evaluating the effectiveness of programs (e.g., the PATHS and SWPBS). Since teachers are responsible for implementing program curriculum and integrating lessons into their classroom activities, it is vital to examine the degree to which teachers adhere to core components and facilitate the transfer of learned values and skills into other subject areas and social contexts. This may be particularly important in replicating the effects of programs and evaluating the sustainability of reported gains.

Limited information is available regarding what determines teacher implementation of the above prevention programs. Kallestad and Olweus (2003) found five teacher variables that predicated the implementation of the Olweus Bullying Prevention Program: perceived importance of teachers as changing agents, knowledge about bullying problems and response strategies, perceived level of bullying, personal experience of victimization, and emotional responses to bullies and victims. These five variables explained 53% of the variance in program implementation, suggesting that these teacher characteristics should be considered in motivating teachers to get more involved in classroom and school-wide initiatives. Other variables may have the potential to influence the level of teacher involvement such as self-efficacy, administrative support, and level of stress and need to be investigated in the future.

References

Aber, J. L., Jones, S. M., Brown, J. L., Chaudry, N., & Samples, F. (1998). Resolving conflict creatively: Evaluating the developmental effects of a school-based violence prevention program in neighborhood and classroom context. *Development and Psychopathology*, 10, 187–213.

Ames, C. & Archer, J. (1988). Achievement goals in the classroom: Students' learning strategies and motivation processes. *Journal of Educational Psychology*, 80, 260–267.

Anderman, E. M., Maehr, M. L., & Midgley, C. (1999). Declining motivation after the transition to middle school: Schools can make a difference. *Journal of Research & Development in Education,* 32(3), 131–147.

Anderson, C. S. (1982). The search for school climate: A review of the research. *Review of Educational Research,* 52(3), 368–420.

Baker, J. A. (1999). Teacher-student interaction in urban at-risk classrooms: Differential behavior, relationship quality, and student satisfaction with school. *The Elementary School Journal,* 100(1), 57–70.

Baker, J. A. (2006). Contributions of teacher-child relationships to positive school adjustment during elementary school. *Journal of School Psychology*, 44, 211–229.

Baker, J. A., Terry, T., Bridger, R., & Winsor, A. (1997). Schools as caring communities: A relational approach to school reform. *School Psychology Review,* 26(4), 586–602.

Banks, J. A. (2002). *An Introduction to Multicultural Education*, 3rd edition. Boston, MA: Allyn & Bacon.

Barton, E. A. (2003). *Bully Prevention: Tips and Strategies for School Leaders and Classroom Teachers*. Arlington Heights, IL: Pearson Professional Development:

Barton, E. A. (2006). *Bully Prevention: Tips and Strategies for School Leaders and Classroom Teachers (2nd ed.).* Thousand Oaks, CA: Corwin Press.

Battistich, V. & Hom, A. (1997). The relationship between students' sense of their school as a community and their involvement in problem behaviors. *American Journal on Public Health*, 87, 1997–2001.

Battistich, V., Solomon, D., & Delucchi, K. (1993). Interaction processes and student outcomes in cooperative learning groups. *The Elementary School Journal,* 94(1), 19–32.

Bear, G. G. (1998). School discipline in the United States: Prevention, correction, and long-term social development. *School Psychology Review*, 27, 14–23.

Bennett, C. I. (2003). *Comprehensive Multicultural Education: Theory and Practice*, 5th edition. Boston, MA: Allyn & Bacon.

Bettmann, E. H. & Moore, P. (1994). Conflict resolution programs and social justice. *Education and Urban Society*, 27, 11–21.

Birch, S. H. & Ladd, G. W. (1996). Interpersonal relationships in the school environment and children's early school adjustment: The role of teachers and peers. In J. Juvonen & K. R. Wentzel (eds.), *Social motivation: Understanding children's school adjustment. Cambridge studies in social and emotional development* (pp. 199–225). New York, NY, US: Cambridge University Press.

Birch, S. H. & Ladd, G. W. (1998). Children's interpersonal behaviors and the teacher-child relationship. *Developmental psychology,* 34(5), 934–946.

Black, A. (2003, April). An ongoing evaluation of the bullying prevention program in Philadelphia schools: Student survey and student observation data. *Paper presented at the Safety in Numbers Conference*, Atlanta, GA. Blackwell Publishers.

Bowers, L., Smith, P. K., & Binney, V. (1992). Cohesion and power in the families of children involved in bullying/victim problems at school. *Journal of Family Therapy*, 14, 371–387.

Brophy, J. E. (1996). *Teaching problem students*. New York, NY, US: Guilford Press.

Buckley, M. A., Storino, M., & Sebastiani, A. M. (August, 2003). The impact of school climate: Variation by ethnicity and gender. *A Paper Presented at Annual Meeting of American Association of Psychologist*, Toronto, Canada. (ERIC Document Reproduction Service NO. ED481671).

Caldas, S. J. & Bankston, C. L. (1999). Multilevel examination of student, school, and district-level effects on academic achievement. *Journal of Educational Research,* 93(2), 91–100.

Campbell, S. B., Spieker, S., Burchinal, M., Poe, M. D., & NICHD Early Child Care Research Network. (2006). Trajectories of aggression from toddlerhood to age 9 predict academic and social functioning through age 12. *Journal of Child Psychology and Psychiatry,* 47(8), 791–800.

Cartledge, G. & Johnson, C. T. (1997). *School violence and cultural sensitivity*. New York, NY, US: Guilford Press.

Casey-Cannon, S., Hayward, C., & Gowen, K. (2001). Middle-school girls' reports of peer victimization: Concerns, consequences, and implications. *Professional School Counseling,* 5(2), 138–147.

Committee for Children. *Second Step: A Violence Prevention Curriculum.* Seattle, WA: Authors.

Connell, J. P. & Wellborn, J. G. (1991). Competence, autonomy, and relatedness: A motivational analysis of self-system processes. In M. R. Gunnar & L. A. Sroufe (eds.), Self processes and development. The Minnesota symposia on child psychology, (pp. 43–77). Hillsdale, NJ, England: Lawrence Erlbaum Associates, Inc.

Curwin, R. & Mendler, A. N. (1997). *As tough as necessary: Countering violence, aggression, and hostility in our schools.* Alexandria, VA: Association of Supervision and Curriculum Development.

Conduct Problems Prevention Research Group (1999). Initial impact of the Fast Track prevention trial for conduct problems: II. Classroom effects. *Journal of Consulting and Clinical psychology*, 67, 648–657.

Craig, W. & Pepler, D. J. (1997). Observations of bullying and victimization on the schoolyard. *Canadian Journal of School Psychology*, 2, 41–60.

Craig, W. M., Henderson, K., & Murphy, J. G. (2000). Prospective teachers' attitudes toward bullying and victimization. *School Psychology International*, 21, 5–21.

Demaray, M. K. & Malecki, C. K. (2003). Perceptions of the frequency and importance of social support by students classified as victims, bullies, and bully/victims in an urban middle school. *School Psychology Review*, 32, 471–489.

Deci, E. L. & Ryan, R. M. (1985). The general causality orientations scale: Self-determination in personality. *Journal of Research in Personality,* 19(2), 109–134.

DeVoe, J. F., Peter, K., Kaufman, P., Miller, A., Noonan, M., Snyder, T. D., & Baum, K. (2004). *Indicators of School Crime and Safety*. Washington, DC: U.S. Departments of Education and Justice.

Dodge, K. A., Coie, J. D., & Lynam, D. (2006). Aggression and antisocial behavior in youth. In N. Eisenberg, W. Damon & R. M. Lerner (Eds.), *Handbook of Child Psychology: Vol.3, Social, Emotional and Personality Development*, 6th edition. (pp. 719–788). Wiley.

Durivage, A. (1989). Assaultive behaviour: Before it happens. *The Canadian Journal of Psychiatry*, 34(5), 393–397.

Educators for Social Responsibility (1992). The Resolving Conflict Creatively Program. Cambridge, MA: Authors.

Elam, S. M. (1994). The 26th annual phi delta Kappa/Gallup poll of the public's attitudes toward the public schools. *Phi Delta Kappan*, 76(1), 41–56.

Emmer, E. T. & Stough, L. M. (2001). Classroom management: A critical part of educational psychology, with implications for teacher education. *Educational Psychologists*, 36, 103–112.

Espelage, D. L. (2004). An ecological perspective to school-based bullying prevention. *The Prevention Researcher*, 11, 3–6.

Espelage, D. L. & Swearer, S. M. (2003). Research on school bullying and victimization: What have we learned and where do we go from here? *School Psychology Review*, 32(3), 365–383.

Esposito, C. (1999). Learning in urban blight: School climate and its effect on the school performance of urban, minority, low-income children. *School Psychology Review. Special Issue: Beginning school ready to learn: Parental involvement and effective educational programs*, 28(3), 365–377.

Forness, S. R. (1988). Planning for the needs of children with serious emotional disturbance: The National Special Education and Mental Health Coalition. *Behavioral Disorders*, 13, 127–139.

Freiberg, H. J. (1989). A Multidimensional view of school effectiveness. *Educational Research Quarterly*, 13, 35–46.

Fuchs, D. & Fuchs, L. S. (2006). Introduction to response to intervention: What, why, and how valid is it? *Reading Research Quarterly*, 41(1), 93–99.

Fuchs, D., Mock, D., Morgan, P., & Young, C. (2003). Responsiveness-to-intervention: Definitions, evidence, and implications for the learning disabilities construct. *Learning Disabilities Research & Practice*, 18, 157–171.

Furlong, M. J., Chung, A., Bates, M., & Morrison, R. L. (1995). Who are the victims of school violence? A comparison of student non-victims and multi-victims. *Education & Treatment of Children. Special Issue: Severe behavior disorders of children and youth*, 18(3), 282–298.

Garcia, E. (2002). *Student cultural diversity: Understanding and meeting the challenge (3rd ed.)*. Boston: Houghton Mifflin.

Garbarino, J. (1999). *Lost boys: Why our sons turn violent and how we can save them*. New York, NY, US: Free Press.

Gollnick, D. A. & Chinn, P. C. (2002). *Multicultural Education in a Pluralistic Society*, 6th edition. Upper Saddle River, NJ: Merrill.

Good, T. L. & Nichols, S. L. (2001). Expectancy effects in the classroom: A special focus on improving the reading performance of minority students in first-grade classrooms. *Educational Psychologist*, 36, 113–126.

Gottfredson, D. C., Gottfredson, G. D., & Hybl, L. G. (1993). Managing adolescent behavior: A multi-year, multi-school experiment. *American Educational Research Journal*, 30, 179–216.

Gorman-Smith, D., Tolan, P., Henry, D. B., Quintana, E., Lutovsky, K., & Leventhal, A. (2007). Schools and families educating children: A preventive intervention for early elementary school children. In P. Tolan, J. Szapocznik, & S. Sambrano (eds.), *Preventing youth substance abuse: Science-based programs for children and adolescents* (pp. 113–135).Washington, DC, US: American Psychological Association.

Greenberg, M. T. & Kusche, C. A. (2002). *Promoting Alternative Thinking Strategies (PATHS): Blueprints for Violence Prevention, Book Ten.* Blueprints for Violence Prevention Series. Boulder, CO: Institute of Behavioral Science, University of Colorado.

Greenberg, M. T., Kusché, C. A., & Riggs, N. (2004). The PATHS curriculum: Theory and research on neurocognitive development and school success. In J. E. Zins, R. P. Weissberg, M. C., Wang, & H. J. Walberg (eds.), Building academic success on social and emotional learning: What does the research say? (pp. 170–188). New York, NY, US: Teachers College Press.

Greenberg, M. T., Kusché, C. A., Cook, E. T., & Quamma, J. P. (1995). Promoting emotional competence in school-aged children: The effects of the PATHS Curriculum. *Development and Psychopathology, 7,* 117–136.

Greenwood, C. R., Terry, B., Utley, C. A., & Montagna, D. (1993). Achievement, placement, and services: Middle school benefits of classwide peer tutoring used at the elementary school. *School Psychology Review, 22*(3), 497–516.

Grolnick, W. S. & Ryan, R. M. (1987). Autonomy support in education: creating the facilitating environment. In N. Hastings & J. Schwieso (Eds.), *New Directions in Educational Psychology: Vol. 2 Behavior and motivation* (pp. 213–232). London: Falmer.

Grossman, H. (1995). *Special education in a diverse society.* Needham Heights, MA: Allyn & Bacon.

Grossman, D. C., Neckerman, H. J., Joepsell, T. D., Liu, P., Asher, K. N., Beland, K., Frey, K., & Rivara, F. P. (1997). Effectiveness of a violence prevention curriculum among children in elementary school. *Journal of the American Medical Association, 277,* 1605–1611.

Grusec, J. E. & Goodnow, J. J. (1994). Impact of parental discipline methods on the child's internalization of values: A reconceptualization of current points of view. *Developmental psychology, 30*(1), 4–19.

Hanish, L. D., Kochenderfer-Ladd, B., Fabes, R. A., Martin, C. L., & Denning, D. (2004). Bullying among young children: The influence of peers and teachers. In D. L. Espelage & S. M., Swearer (eds.), *Bullying in American schools: A social-ecological perspective on prevention and intervention* (pp. 141–159). Mahwah, NJ, US: Lawrence Erlbaum Associates Publishers.

Hawkins, J. D., Farrington, D. P., & Catalano, R. F. (1998). Reducing violence through the schools. In D. S. Elliott, B. A. Hamburg, & K. R. Williams (eds.), Violence in American schools: A new perspective. (pp. 188–216). New York, NY, US: Cambridge University Press.

Haynes, N. M., Emmons, C. L., & Ben-Avie, M. (1997). School climate as a factor in student adjustment and achievement. *Journal of Educational and Psychological Consultation, 8,* 321–329.

Haynes, N. M., Emmons, C. L., & Woodruff, D. W. (1998). School Development Program effects: Linking implementation to outcomes. *Journal of Education for Students Placed at Risk.* Special Issue: Changing schools for changing times: The Comer School Development Program, 3, 71–85

Hinshaw, S. P. (1992). Academic underachievement, attention deficits and aggression: Comorbidity and implications for intervention. *Journal of Consulting and Clinical Psychology, 60,* 893–903.

Hinshaw, S. P. & Lee, S. S. (2003). Conduct and oppositional defiant diorders. In E. J. Mash & R. A. Barkley (Eds.), Child Psychopathology, 2nd edition. (pp. 144–198). New York, NY: Guildford.

Hodges, E. V. E., Malone, M. J., & Perry, D. G. (1997). Individual risk and social risk as interacting determinants of victimization in the peer group. *Developmental psychology, 33*(6), 1032–1039.

Holt, M. K. & Keyes, M. A. (2004). Teachers' attitudes toward bullying. In D. L. Espelage & S. M., Swearer (eds.), *Bullying in American schools: A social-ecological perspective on prevention and intervention* (pp. 121–139). Mahwah, NJ: Lawrence Erlbaum.

Hoover, J. H. & Hazler, R. J. (1991). Bullies and victims. *Elementary School Guidance & Counseling, 25*(3), 212–219.

Horne, A. M., Orpinas, P., Newman-Carlson, D., & Bartolomucci, C. L. (2004). Elementary school bully busters program: Understanding why children bully and what to do about it. In D. L. Espelage & S. M., Swearer (eds.), *Bullying in American schools: A social-ecological perspective on prevention and intervention* (pp. 297–325). Mahwah, NJ: Lawrence Erlbaum.

Huesmann, L. R. & Eron, L. D. (1984). Cognitive processes and the persistence of aggressive behavior. *Aggressive Behavior, 10*(3), 243–251.

Hughes, J. N., Cavell, T. A., & Jackson, T. (1999). Influence of the teacher-student relationship on childhood conduct problems: A prospective study. *Journal of Clinical Child Psychology, 28*, 173–184.

Irvine, J. J. (1990). *Black Students and School Failure*. New York, NY: Greenwood Press.

Jimerson, S. R., Morrison, G. M., Pletcher, S. W., & Furlong, M. J. (2006). Youth engaged in antisocial and aggressive behaviors: Who are they? In S. R. Jimerson & M. J. Furlong (eds.), *Handbook of school violence and school safety: From research to practice* (pp. 3–19). Mahwah, NJ, US: Lawrence Erlbaum Associates Publishers.

Jordon, J. G. & Yoon, J. (2005). *Teacher Responses to Victims of Bullying.* Unpublished manuscript.

Jeffrey, L. R., Miller, D., & Linn, M. (2001). Middle school bullying as a context for the development of passive observers to the victimization of others. In R. A. Geffner, M. Loring & C. Young (eds.), *Bullying behavior: Current issues, research, and interventions.* (pp. 143–156). Binghamton, NY, US: Haworth Maltreatment and Trauma Press/The Haworth Press.

Johnson, D. W. & Johnson, R. T. (2003). Student motivation in co-operative groups: Social interdependence theory. In R. M. Gillies & A. F. Ashman (eds.), *Co-operative learning: The social and intellectual outcomes of learning in groups* (pp. 136–176). New York, NY, US: Routledge.

Johnson, D. W., Johnson, R. T., & Smith, K. A. (1995). Cooperative learning and individual student achievement in secondary schools. In J. E. Pedersen, & A. D. Digby (Eds.), *Secondary schools and cooperative learning* (pp. 3–54). New York: Garland Publishing.

Kasen, S., Johnson, J., & Cohen, P. (1990). The impact of school emotional climate on student psychopathology. *Journal of abnormal child psychology, 18*(2), 165–177.

Kallestad, J. H. & Olweus, D. (2003). Predicting teachers' and school's implementation of the Olweus Bullying Prevention Program: A multilevel study. Prevention & Treatment, 6. Available online at http://www.journals.apa.org/prevention/volume6/pre0060021a.html

Kam, C., M., Greenberg, M.T., & Kusché, C. A. (2004). Sustained effects of the PATHS curriculum on the social and psychological adjustment of children in special education. *Journal of Emotional and Behavioral Disorders, 12*, 66–78.

Kellam, S. G., Mayer, L. S., Rebok, G. W., & Hawkins, W. E., (1998). Effects of improving achievement on aggressive behavior and of improving aggressive behavior on achievement through two preventive interventions: An investigation of causal paths. In B. P. Dohrenwend (eds.), *Adversity, stress and psychopathology* (pp. 486–505). London: Oxford University Press.

Kipnis, A. (1999). *Angry young men: How parents, teachers, and counselors can help bad boys become good men.* San Francisco: Jossey-Bass Publishers.

Kounin, J. S. (1970). *Discipline and group management in classrooms.* New York, NY: Holt, Rinehart & Winston.

Kyukendall, C. (1992). *From Rage to Hope: Strategies for Reclaiming Black & Hispanic Students.* Bloomington, IL: National Educational Service.

Ladd, G. W. & Burgess, K. B. (2001). Do relational risks and protective factors moderate the linkages between childhood aggression and early psychological and school adjustment? *Child development, 72*(5), 1579–1601.

Leary, M. R., Kowalski, R. M., Smith, L., & Phillips, S. (2003). Teasing, rejection, and violence: Case studies of the school shootings. *Aggressive Behavior, 29*(3), 202–214.

Ledingham, J. E. & Schwartzman, A. E. (1984). A 3-year follow-up of aggressive and withdrawn behavior in childhood: Preliminary findings. *Journal of Abnormal Child Psychology, 12*(1), 157–168.

Limber, S. P. (2006). The Olweus bullying prevention program: An overview of its implementation and research basis. In S. R. Jimerson & M. J. Furlong (eds.), *Handbook of school violence and school safety: From research to practice* (pp. 293–307). Mahwah, NJ, US: Lawrence Erlbaum Associates Publishers.

Limber, S. P., Nation, M., Tracy, A. J., Melton, G. B., & Flerx, V. (2004). Implementation of the Olweus Bullying Prevention programme in the Southeastern United Sates. In P. K. Smith, D. Pepler, & K. Rigby (Eds.), *Bullying in Schools: How Successful Can Interventions Be?* (pp. 55–79). Cambridge, UK: Cambridge Universality Press.

Mayer, M. J. & Leone, P. E. (1999). A structural analysis of school violence and disruption: Implications for creating safer schools. *Education & Treatment of Children*, 22, 333–356.

Meehan, B. T., Hughes, J. N., & Cavell, T. A. (2003). Teacher-student relationships as compensatory resources for aggressive children. *Child Development*, 74, 1145–1157.

Metis Associates. (1998). Atlanta Public Schools: Resolving Conflict Creatively Program. *Final Evaluation Report*, 1996–1997. New York, NY: Author.

Midgley, C., Kaplan, A., Middleton, M., Maehr, M. L., Urdan, T., Anderman, L. H., et al. (1998). The development and validation of scales assessing students' achievement goal orientations. *Contemporary Education Psychology*, 23, 113–131.

Miller-Johnson, S., Coie, J. D., Maumary-Gremaud, A., Bierman, K., & Conduct problems prevention research group (2002). Peer rejection and aggression and early starter models of conduct disorder. *Journal of Abnormal Child Psychology*, 30, 217–230.

Nelson, J. R. & Carr, B. A. (1999). *The Think Time strategy for schools kit: Bringing order to the classroom*. Longmont, CO: Sopris West.

Noddings, N. (2001). The care tradition: Beyond "add women and stir." *Theory into Practice*, 40, 29–34.

O'Donnell, J., Hawkins, J., Catalano, R., Abbott, R., & Day, L. (1995). Preventing school failure, drug use, and delinquency among low-income children: Long-term intervention in elementary schools. *American Journal of Orthopsychiatry*, 65, 87–100.

Oliver, R., Oaks, I. N., & Hoover, J. H. (1994). Family issues and interventions in bully and victim relationships. *School Counselor,* 41(3), 199–202.

Olweus, D. (1993). *Bullying at School: What We Know and What We Can Do*. Oxford, England: Blackwell Publishers.

Olweus, D. (1994). Bullying at school: Long-term outcomes for the victims and an effective school-based intervention program. In L. R. Huesmann (ed.), *Aggressive behavior: Current perspectives*. Plenum series in social/clinical psychology (pp. 97–130). New York, NY, US: Plenum Press.

Olweus, D., Limber, S. P., & Mihali, S. (1999). *The Bullying Prevention Program: Blueprints for Violence Prevention Book 10*. Boulder, CO: Center for the Study and Prevention of Violence.

Orpinas, P. & Horne, A. M. (2006). *Bullies and victims: A challenge for schools*. Washington, DC, US: American Psychological Association.

Orpinas, P., Horne, A. M., & Staniszewski, D. (2003). School bullying: Changing the problem by changing the school. *School Psychology Review,* 32, 431–444.

Pellegrini, A. D., Bartini, M., & Brooks, F. (1999). School bullies, victims, and aggressive victims: Factors relating to group affiliation and victimization in early adolescence. *Journal of Educational Psychology,* 91(2), 216–224.

Pepler, D. J., Craig, W. M., Ziegler, S., & Charach, A. (1994). An evaluation of an anti-bullying intervention in Toronto schools. *Canadian Journal of Community Mental Health. Special Issue: Prevention: Focus on children and youth,* 13(2), 95–110.

Pianta, R. C. & Steinberg, M. (1992). Teacher-child relationships and the process of adjusting to school. In R. C. Pianta (ed.), *Beyond the parent: The role of other adults in children's lives.* New directions for child development, No. 57. (pp. 61–80). San Francisco, CA, US: Jossey-Bass.

Qin, Z., Johnson, D. W., & Johnson, R. T. (1995). Cooperative versus competitive efforts and problem solving. *Review of Educational Research,* 65(2), 129–143.

Reinke, W. M. & Herman, K. C. (2002). Creating school environments that deter antisocial behaviors in youth. *Psychology in Schools*, 39, 549–460.

Remafedi, G. (1988). Adolescent homosexuality: Psychosocial and medical implications. *Pediatrics*, 79, 331–337.

Resnick M. D., Bearman, P. S., Blum, R. W., Bauman, K. E., Harris, K. M., Jones, J., et al. (1997). Protecting adolescents from harm. Findings form the National Longitudinal Study on Adolescent Health. *Journal of the American Medical Association*, 278, 823–832.

Rícan, P., Klicperová, M., & Koucká, T. (1993). Families of bullies and their victims: A children's view. *Studia Psychologica, 35*(3), 261–266.

Rigby, K. (2000). Effects of peer victimization in schools and perceived social support on adolescent well-being. *Journal of Adolescence, 23*(1), 57–68.

Roeser, R. W., Midgley, C., & Urdan, T. C. (1996). Perceptions of the school psychological environment and early adolescents' psychological and behavioral functioning in school: The mediating role of goals and belonging. *Journal of Educational Psychology, 88*(3), 408–422.

Roland, E. & Galloway, D. (2002). Classroom influences on bullying. *Educational Research,* 44(3), 299–312.

Rosenthal, R. (1985). From unconscious experimenter bias to teacher expectancy effects. In J. B. Dusek (Ed.), *Teacher Expectations.* Hillsdale, NJ: Erlbaum.

Savin-Williams, R. C. (1996). Psychosocial outcomes of verbal and physical abuse among lesbian, gay, and bisexual youths. In R. C. Savin-Williams & K. M. Cohen (Eds.). *The Lives of Lesbians, Gays, and Bisexuals: Children to Adults* (pp. 181–200). Orlando, FL: Harcourt.

Salmivalli, C., Karhunen, J., & Lagerspetz, K. M. J. (1996). How do the victims respond to bullying? *Aggressive Behavior,* 22(2), 99–109.

Santrock, J. W. (2006). *Educational psychology, 2nd revised edition: Classroom update preparing for PRAXIS and the classroom.* Dallas, TX: McGraw-Hill.

Sapon-Shevin, M. (1996). Full inclusion as disclosing tablet: Revealing the flaws in our present system. *Theory into Practice,* 35(1), 35–41.

Schwartz, D., Dodge, K. A., Pettit, G. S., & Bates, J. E. (1997). The early socialization of aggressive victims of bullying. *Child development,* 68(4), 665–675.

Shaffer, D. R. (1999). Social and personality development (3rd ed.). Belmont, CA: Wadsworth.

Sharan, S. & Shaulov, A. (1990). Cooperative learning, motivation, and academic achievement. In S. Sharan (ed.), *Cooperative learning: Theory and research* (pp. 173–202). New York, NY, England: Praeger Publishers.

Shinn, M. R., Ramsey, E., Walker, H. M., & Stieber, S. (1987). Antisocial behavior in school settings: Initial differences in an at risk and normal population. *The Journal of Special Education,* 21(2), 69–84.

Shure, M. B. (1992). *I can problem solve: An interpersonal cognitive problem-solving program: Intermediate elementary grades.* Champaign, IL, US: Research Press.

Shure, M. B. (1997). Interpersonal cognitive problem solving: Primary prevention of early high-risk behaviors in the preschool and primary years. In G. Albee & T. Gullotta (Eds.), *Primary Prevention Works* (pp. 167–188). Thousand Oaks, CA: Sage Publications.

Shure, M.B. & Spivack, G. (1988). Interpersonal cognitive problem solving. In R. H. Price, E. L. Cowen, R. P. Lorion, & J. Ramos-McKay (Eds.), *14 Ounces of Prevention: A Casebook for Practitioners* (pp. 69–82). Washington, DC: American Psychological Association.

Simons-Morton, B. G., Crump, A. D., Haynie, D. L., & Saylor, K. E. (1999). Student-school bonding and adolescent problem behavior. *Health education research,* 14(1), 99–107.

Skinner, E. A. & Belmont, M. J. (1993). Motivation in the classroom: Reciprocal effects of teacher behavior and student engagement across the school year. *Journal of Educational Psychology,* 85(4), 571–581.

Slavin, R. E. & Madden, N. A. (2001). *One million children: Success for all.* Thousand Oaks, CA, US: Corwin Press.

Slavin, R. E. (1995). When and why does cooperative learning increase achievement? theoretical and empirical perspectives. In R. Hertz-Lazarowitz & N. Miller (eds.), *Interaction in cooperative groups: The theoretical anatomy of group learning* (pp. 145–173). New York, NY, US: Cambridge University Press.

Song, S. Y. & Swearer, S. M. (2002, February). An ecological analysis of bullying in middle school: Understanding school climate across the bully-victim continuum. *Paper Presented at the Annual Convention of the National Association of School Psychologists*, Chicago, IL.

Sprague, J. R., Sugai, G., & Walker, H. (1998). Antisocial behavior in schools. In T. S. Watson & F. M. Gresham (Eds.), *Handbook of Child Behavior Therapy* (pp. 451–474). New York, NY: Plenum.

Sprague, J. R., Walker, H., Golly, A., White, K., Myers, D. R., & Shannon, T. (2002). Translating research into effective practice: The effects of a universal staff and student intervention on key indicators of school safety and discipline. *Education and Treatment of Children, 24,* 495–511.

Sugai, G. & Horner, R. H. (2002). Introduction to the special series on positive behavior support in schools. *Journal of Emotional and Behavioral Disorders, 10*(3), 130–135.

Sutherland, F. (1994). *Teachers' perceptions of school climate* (Report No. ED035-699). Chicago, IL: Chicago State University. (ERIC Document Reproduction Service, No. ED379214).

Swearer, S. & Doll, B. (2001). Bullying in schools: An ecological framework. In R. A. Geffner, M. Loring, & C. Young (2001), *Bullying behavior: Current issues, research and intervention* (pp. 7–23). Binghamton, NY: The Haworth Press.

Skiba, R. J. & Peterson, R. (2000). School discipline at a crossroads: From zero tolerance to early response. *Exceptional Children, 66,* 335–346.

Sugai, G. & Horner, R. H. (1999). The evolution of discipline practices: School-wide positive behavior supports. *Child & Family Behavior Therapy, 243,* 23–50.

Tairaiol, J., Yoon, J., & Carcamo, A. (2005). A system-wide problem solving approach in bullying intervention. *Paper Presented at the Annual Meeting of the National Association of School Psychologists*, Atlanta, GA.

Torgesen, J. K. (1998). Catch them before they fall. *American Educator, 22*(1), 32–39.

Twenge, J. M. & Baumeister, R. F. (2005). Social exclusion increases aggression and self-defeating behavior while reducing intelligent thought and prosocial behavior. In D. Abrams, M. A. Hogg, & J. M. Marques (eds.), *The social psychology of inclusion and exclusion* (pp. 27–46). New York, NY: Psychology Press.

Twenge, J. M. Baumeister, R. F., Tice, D. M., & Stucke, T. S. (2001). If you can't join them, beat them: Effects of social exclusion on aggressive behavior. *Journal of Personality and Social Psychology, 81,* 1058–1069.

Van Acker, R., Grant, S. H., & Henry, D. (1996). Teacher and student behavior as a function of risk for aggression. *Education & Treatment of Children, 19,* 316–334.

Van Blyderveen, S. L. (2004). Fact Sheets: Peer victimization among British Columbia youth. The McCreary Centre Society. Retrieved October 1, 2006 from www.mcs.bc.ca.

Vaughn, S., Linan-Thompson, S., & Hickman, P. (2003). Response to instruction as a means of identifying students with learning/reading disabilities. *Exceptional Children, 69,* 391–409.

Vygotsky, L. S. (1986). *Thought and language* (A. Kozulin, Trans.). Cambridge, MA: MIT Press. (Original work published 1934)

U.S. Department of Health and Human Services (2001). *Youth violence: A report of the Surgeon General.* Rockville, MD: U.S. Department of Health and Human Services; Centers for Disease Control and Prevention, National Center for Injury Prevention; Substance Abuse and Mental Health Services Administration, Center for Mental Health Services; and National Institute of Health, National Institute of Mental Health.

U.S. Department of Health and Human Services (2002). *SAMHSA Model Programs: Effective Substance Abuse and Mental Health Programs for Every Community.* Retrieved February 2007, from http://modelprograms.samhsa.gov/promising.htm.

Wallace, T., Reschly Anderson, A., Bartholomay, T., & Hupp, S. (2002). An ecobehavioral examination of high school classrooms that include students with disabilities. *Exceptional children, 68*(3), 345–359.

Walker, H. M., Ramsey, E., & Gresham, F. (2004). *Antisocial Behavior in School: Evidence-Based Practices*, 2nd edition. Pacific Grove, CA: Brooks/Cole.

Weinstein, J. (1987). Pygmalion and the student: Age and classroom differences in children's awareness of teacher expectations. *Child Development*, 58, 1079–1093.

Welch, W. N., Stokes, R., & Greene, J. R. (2000). A macro-level model of school disorder. *Journal of Research in Crime and Delinquency*, 37, 243–283.

Wentzel, K. R. (1996). Social and academic motivation in middle school: Concurrent and long-term relations to academic effort. *Journal of Early Adolescence,* 16(4), 390–406.

Wentzel, K. R. (2002). Are effective teachers like good parents? Teaching styles and student adjustment in early adolescence. *Child Development,* 73(1), 287–301.

White, K. J., Jones, K., & Sherman, M. D. (1998). Reputation information and teacher feedback: Their influences on children's perceptions of behavior problem peers. *Journal of Social & Clinical Psychology,* 17(1), 11–37.

Williams, B. B. (2006). Culturally competent mental health services in the schools: Tips for teachers. *National Association of School Psychologists.*

Wuthrick, M. A. (1990). Blue jays win! Crows go down in defeat! *Phi Delta Kappan,* 71, 553–556.

Yoon, J. (2003). Victimization experiences, classroom climate and school adjustment. *Poster Presented at the Biennial Meeting of the Society of Research in Child Development*, Tampa, FL.

Yoon, J. & Kerber, K. (2003). Bullying: Elementary teachers' attitudes and intervention strategies. *Research in Education,* 69, 27–35.

Yoon, J., Markman, B., & Clor, J. (under review). Peer victimization and school adjustment: A mediating role of perceived school climate.

Chapter 14
Developmental Issues in the Prevention of Aggression and Violence in School

Paul Boxer, Andrew Terranova, Sarah Savoy, and Sara E. Goldstein

Generally speaking, primary prevention has been conceptualized as ontogenetically early intervention (see Cowen, 2000, for a discussion). That is, programs seeking to prevent the emergence of some problem behavior or form of psychopathology in a population typically are construed as programs that need to be provided to children as early in development as possible given the constraints imposed by their social, emotional, and cognitive capacities. From a strictly logical standpoint, this assertion makes sense especially with regard to aggressive behavior. Aggression emerges fairly early in development (Tremblay, 2000) and can lead to socially and financially costly outcomes later on (Huesmann et al., 2002; Jones et al., 2002). Thus, it seems reasonable to maintain that aggression and violence prevention programs should target children at as young an age as possible. However, primary prevention of aggression can occur throughout childhood and adolescence given the developmental underpinnings and variants of this behavior. This chapter discusses key developmental issues and concerns in the primary prevention of aggression in school-age children and adolescents.

The need for primary prevention approaches beyond early and middle childhood is particularly pressing with respect to aggressive behavior for a variety of reasons. First, aggression exhibits significant and meaningful continuity from childhood to adolescence and into adulthood (Huesmann et al., 1984, 2006; Kokko & Pulkkinen, 2005). That is, individuals who exhibit high levels of aggression in childhood are likely to maintain this position relative to their peers into adulthood. Second, aggression is both frequent and problematic among children in elementary school as well as middle and high school (Boxer et al., 2006; Centers for Disease Control and Prevention, 2006; Nansel et al., 2001). Third, aggression shows topographical variation at different developmental periods. Whereas aggressive behavior in younger children might be limited to low-impact physical and acquisitive acts (e.g., pushing, shoving, taking others' property), mild forms of verbal provocation (e.g., teasing, name-calling), and disobedience (Eron et al., 1971), aggression among older youth can be far more varied to include interpersonal violence (including dating violence and sexual aggression), delinquency, and more elaborate verbal and social provocations (e.g., socially harmful behaviors such as defamatory gossip and ostracism). Finally, recent theoretical work suggests that aggression among younger children might result from and persist in part

T. W. Miller (ed.), *School Violence and Primary Prevention.*
© Springer 2008

because of difficulties with emotional reactivity and regulation (e.g., Eisenberg et al., 1998), whereas aggression among older youth might be maintained by social-cognitive processing styles (e.g., Huesmann, 1998).

Taken together these developmental concerns underscore the fact that primary or universal approaches to preventing aggression among children and adolescents must be sensitive to a variety of factors that covary with age and developmental level. For example, social and cognitive reasoning abilities change with development (see Tisak, 1995). Further, social goals, developmental tasks, and interpersonal needs also change with development (cf. Boxer et al., 2005a). Simply put, therefore, primary prevention of aggression among young children requires intervention strategies different from those used for older children and adolescents. This chapter will discuss the role of development in primary prevention of aggression among school-age children and adolescents (i.e., elementary school through high school) with respect to three overarching concerns: (1) The multiply determined (i.e., multiple individual and contextual risk factors) nature of aggressive behavior; (2) The forms and functions of aggression across development; and (3) The mediating mechanisms accounting for the maintenance of aggression across development. We first consider current research and theory on the general developmental foundations of aggressive behavior before turning to forms and functions and mediating mechanisms. We conclude with a discussion of the implications of developmental concerns for the design and evaluation of primary/universal prevention programming.

Developmental Foundations of Aggressive Behavior

As emphasized by Boxer and Dubow (2002; also see Hunter et al., 2001) and underscored by organizations such as the Centers for Disease Control and Prevention (Thornton et al., 2000), the National Institutes of Health (2004), and the University of Colorado's Center for the Study and Prevention of Violence, school-based aggression prevention programming should be most effective when it rests on a foundation of sound research on risk factors in the development of aggressive and related antisocial behaviors. This follows the traditional model of prevention program design advocated by the Institute of Medicine in 1994 (Institute of Medicine, 1994; also see Cowen et al., 1996), which specifies the identification of risk factors for the target behavior as the first step in a process leading ultimately to program implementation. However, perhaps even more so than other typical prevention targets such as anxiety and depression, from a risk-factor standpoint aggression clearly is a multiply determined behavior (Eron, 1994). Thus, a developmentally informed effort to prevent aggression must take into account a complex variety of risk factors.

Following Frick (2006; also see Boxer & Frick, in press), there essentially are two fairly broad approaches in research on the development of aggressive behavior. A *cumulative risk* approach involves the study of individually and contextually based risk factors for their independent and additive influences in shaping the emergence and persistence of aggression over time. In this approach, specific risk factors and interactive effects are less important than the sheer number of discrete factors and the source of risk (i.e., genetic/temperamental or contextual/environmental). A *developmental pathways* approach involves recognition that within the general normal population, there are subgroups of children and adolescents who exhibit atypical patterns of aggressive behavior resulting from complex interactions and combinations of risk factors. Individual and contextual risk factors are evaluated with respect to how well they account for empirically or theoretically derived groups representing various trajectories or patterns of aggression over time.

With respect to a cumulative risk view of aggression, research indicates generally that aggression might best be conceptualized from a *developmental-ecological* perspective (also referred to as an individual-contextual or social-contextual perspective; Coie & Dodge, 1998; Conger & Simons, 1997; Dodge & Pettit, 2003; Patterson et al., 1989; Tolan et al., 1995, 2003). This view posits broadly that aggression emerges and becomes habitual through the interaction of multiple individual/personal factors and contextual/environmental factors. In terms of individual/personal factors, aggression risk is increased by temperamental predispositions toward impulsivity, thrill-seeking, irritability, and emotional lability (e.g., Eisenberg et al., 2003; Frick & Morris, 2004; Lemerise & Arsenio, 2000; Rubin et al., 2003; Shaw et al., 2001), as well as low intelligence and learning problems (e.g., Huesmann et al., 1987) and cognitive biases supporting the use of aggression (e.g., Musher-Eizenman et al., 2004). In terms of contextually based factors, aggression risk is increased by exposure to not only aggressive models in the family (e.g., Dubow et al., 2003; Frick, 1994; Mahoney et al., 2003; Patterson, 1982) but also deviant behavior in peers, in neighborhoods, and in the media (e.g., Boxer et al., 2003; Boxer et al., 2005b; Espelage et al., 2003; Guerra et al., 2003; Huesmann et al., 2003).

Although the developmental-ecological view can accommodate population-level trends in the emergence and maintenance of aggressive behavior, it might be less effective in predicting more extreme or psychopathological manifestations of aggression such as violent and chronically delinquent behavior. For example, index scores summarizing risk from various individual and environmental sources have been shown to account fairly well for problem behavior outcomes across a variety of normative and even at-risk samples (Bowen & Flora, 2002; Morales & Guerra, 2006; Sameroff et al., 2003). That is, youth with higher risk scores (i.e., risk from multiple sources) tend to exhibit higher levels of problem behavior. However, specifying causal models for atypical, very high risk groups of youth typically has necessitated analytic procedures that identify and isolate those groups within population samples and/or more elaborated models that take interactions between risk factors into account. For example, trajectory analytic modeling of longitudinal data now is used increasingly to locate chronically aggressive youth within larger study samples; risk factor analyses then consider which risk variables predict membership in the extreme group (Broidy et al., 2003; Nagin & Tremblay, 1999; NICHD Early Child Care Research Network, 2004). Studies of children exhibiting psychopathic traits have reported interactive effects, typically between parenting styles and psychopathic tendencies, in examining conduct problems and aggression in that group (e.g., Oxford et al., 2003; Wootton et al., 1997).

The essential point of this discussion on the developmental basis of aggression with regard to primary prevention is that, as noted earlier, the traditional process of prevention program design (see Institute of Medicine, 1994) might be quite difficult to follow for such a multiply determined behavior. The primary prevention model requires identification of key risk factors for modification in order to suppress the emergence of the targeted problem behavior. With a risk matrix composed of so many potential risk factors, with the capacity for cumulative as well as interactive effects, how might one select intervention targets? Further, as Tremblay (2000) has asserted, the study of aggression really can and should begin at birth—and thus the enterprise of true primary prevention of aggression might be very difficult to accomplish.

In recent years the solution to the problem of how to attend to a multiplicity of risk factors in the prevention of aggressive behavior has been a reliance on multi-level, multifaceted programming. That is, applied researchers have implemented broadly based programming targeting a variety of sources of risk simultaneously. For example, the Metropolitan Area Child Study (MACS) Research Group (2002) examined a preventive intervention model that tested the relative utility of several different intervention modes in samples of at-risk and high-risk urban elementary school children. The MACS researchers followed the general prevention research framework by selecting their target schools based on broad social-economic risk indicators. Their attempts to address multiple additional sources of risk were manifested experimentally. Elementary schools in the MACS were assigned randomly to one of four conditions: no intervention; a classroom-based universal prevention program (Level A intervention, targeting peer group process and individual social cognitive risk); the Level A program plus a small-group selected prevention program for high-risk youth (Level B, targeting peer and social cognitive risk more intensely); and the Level B configuration of programming plus a multiple-family therapy group program for high-risk youth (Level C, targeting family risk in addition to other risk factors). Other examples of multilevel prevention programming in elementary school populations include Fast Track (e.g., Conduct Problems Prevention Research Group, 1999) and Lift (e.g., Reid et al., 1999). Multisystemic Therapy (MST; e.g., Henggeler et al., 1998) represents a multilevel prevention approach to deal with aggressive behavior in older, higher-risk youth.

Although a program might target a variety of sources of individual and contextual risk in the development of aggressive behavior, program designers still are left with the question of what precise behaviors to target. Aggression is a multifaceted construct subsuming a number of different behaviors varying in type and ranging in severity from mild to severe. Despite this, most aggression or violence prevention program materials focus only on a limited set of aggressive acts. In the next section, we consider the variety of forms and functions aggression can take, and how this behavioral diversity can be addressed in prevention programming.

Forms and Functions of Aggression

As noted previously, aggression early in development is highly correlated with later aggression, indicating that children who rank high or low in aggression compared to their peers tend to rank similarly years later (e.g., Huesmann et al., 2006). Of course, correlations are not sensitive estimates of the stability of aggression over development. Correlations may remain high even though mean levels of aggression, types of aggression, and severity of aggression changes (see Loeber & Stouthamer-Loeber, 1998, for review). In fact, children tend to exhibit heterotypic continuity in the aggressive behaviors they enact, meaning that the types of aggressive behaviors youth enact change with development. For example, a habitually aggressive individual might engage in frequent teasing, pushing, and shoving of peers in early elementary school and transition to punching, beating, and criminal behavior by adulthood.

Within the fairly broad definition of aggression as any behavior intended to "injure or irritate" another (Eron, 1987), empirical research on aggression has shown that when considered developmentally, the broad construct of "aggression" includes a wide variety of behaviors, which can range from relatively mild behaviors such as teasing and pushing in childhood to very serious acts such as assault and spousal abuse in adulthood (cf. Huesmann et al., 1984, 2003). So, in order to better understand aggression and its development, some researchers subtype aggression into more homogeneous groups, with distinctions based on the form (i.e., the topography of the behavior) and function (i.e., the goals that motivate the behavior) of the aggressive behavior. In some cases, form and function are completely independent; in other cases form and function overlap considerably.

One of the more common classification schemes for aggressive behaviors distinguishes between *indirect* and *direct* dimensions of aggression based on the forms of the behaviors (Lagerspetz et al., 1988). Indirect aggression involves harmful behavior in which the identity of the aggressor is not immediately known to the target, whereas direct aggression involves harmful behavior in which the identity of the aggressor is obvious to the target (Björkqvist et al., 1992; Lagerspetz et al., 1988). Over time Lagerspetz and colleagues' initial distinction between these two forms of aggression has come to be understood as the difference between acts relying on *covert or overt social network manipulation* to cause harm (indirect aggression) and acts relying on *overt physical or verbal attacks* to cause harm (direct aggression; see Underwood et al., 2001, for a discussion of this broad distinction). Even so, it must be emphasized that within the original Lagerspetz et al. formulation, it certainly is possible to have indirect physical aggression (e.g., a child surreptitiously leaves a sharp object on a classmate's seat). This sort of behavior has been acknowledged in the typological distinction of more general covert versus overt antisocial behavior, which refers simply to whether the aggressive acts are committed in view of others or in a clandestine manner (Hinshaw et al., 1995).

Other researchers have conceptualized the distinction between socially harmful versus physically harmful constructs slightly differently. For example, Cairns,

Underwood, and others refer to *social* aggression (Cairns et al., 1989; Galen & Underwood, 1997) and Crick and colleagues refer to *relational* aggression (Crick, 1995; Crick & Grotpeter, 1995). Whereas the distinction between indirect and direct aggression (as originally conceptualized) is based on whether the identity of the perpetrator is known, social and relational aggression are defined based on the mechanism of harm (i.e., inducing harm by manipulating social relationships) and also on the goals of the behavior (i.e., to damage one's relationships). Crick and colleagues contrast relational aggression with overt aggression, which includes physical or verbal attacks or threats of such attacks.

As operationalized, it is possible to have indirect and direct types of social and relational aggression. An example of direct social/relational aggression is telling somebody that he or she is no longer a friend, whereas an example of indirect social/relational aggression is covertly spreading a slanderous rumor about somebody. Likewise, "overt" aggression theoretically can be direct (e.g., one child pushes another child) or indirect (e.g., the aforementioned example of one child discreetly placing a sharp object on another's seat). Although there are subtle differences between relational versus social aggression (e.g., social aggression can include negative facial expressions or body movements), in practice the measurement of and scholarly discussions about these forms of aggression have more or less focused on similar behaviors.

Another common classification scheme for aggressive behavior distinguishes between *reactive* and *proactive* functions of aggression (Dodge, 1991; Dodge & Coie, 1987). The distinction between reactive and proactive aggression is based on the antecedents and consequences of the behavior, rather than on the particular form of aggression enacted in the behavior. Generally speaking, reactive aggression has been conceptualized as a highly emotional and impulsive response, enacted typically in reaction to a perceived or actual provocation during social interactions. Reactive aggression thus might have a variety of functions for the individual including defense (cf. Pulkkinen, 1996), the reduction of angry or fearful arousal (e.g., Hubbard et al., 2004), or retaliation for victimization (e.g., Schwartz, 2000). In contrast, proactive aggression has been construed as a largely unemotional and unprovoked behavior enacted for some instrumental purpose. Aggression might be emitted proactively in order to establish social dominance or social standing, obtain some concrete object, or cause pain or fear in a victim.

Although much research has been conducted with the aim of identifying subgroups of youth who engage primarily in reactive or proactive aggression, many studies have yielded fairly high correlations between these two styles of responding (e.g., Dodge & Coie, 1987). For example, studies of youth classified as "bullies" or "victims" based on their tendency to enact or be victimized by aggression have explored whether bullies are characterized by proactive aggression and victims by reactive aggression or no aggression at all. What seems to be the case, however, is that both bullies and victims tend to engage in reactively aggressive responses, whereas only bullies tend to emit proactively aggressive acts (e.g., Camodeca & Goossens, 2005). Similarly, studies examining personality correlates of aggression have shown that proactive aggression seems prominent only among highly antisocial youth who exhibit traits characteristic of psychopathy (callousness, unemotionality; Frick et al., 2003; Raine et al., 2006), whereas all aggressive or antisocial youth tend to engage in reactive aggression. Both proactive and reactive aggression have been observed in children as young as 7 (e.g., Raine et al., 2006) and inferred in preschool-age children (Persson, 2005).

The study of the distinction between generally proactive (unemotional, instrumental) and reactive (emotional, hostile) aggression has a long history (Hartup, 1974; Lorenz, 1966). Still, given the frequently observed high correlations between these two styles of aggressive responding, some researchers have suggested that it might be time to "pull the plug" on this line of inquiry (Bushman & Anderson, 2001). Even so, developmental researchers have produced a body of evidence for the validity of the classification. Youth who exhibit different patterns of reactive and proactive aggression also have been shown to possess different cognitive, social, and affective characteristics (e.g., Frick et al., 2003; Poulin & Boivin, 2000; Price & Dodge, 1989; Raine et al., 2006; Schwartz et al., 1998; Vitaro et al., 2002).

Aggression also can be subtyped based on its severity. As noted, some aggressive acts might be fairly mild with respect to their consequences, such as pushing, shoving, or teasing. Other aggressive acts can be very severe and damaging, such as physical assault, weapon use, and rape. Loeber and colleagues have divided aggressive behaviors into three categories: minor aggression, fighting, and violence. Minor aggression includes annoying behaviors and bullying. Fighting includes physical fighting and gang fights, and violence includes attacking someone, forced sex, and similar acts (Loeber & Hay, 1997; Loeber & Stouthamer-Loeber, 1998; Tolan et al., 2000). Using longitudinal data, Loeber and colleagues have proposed a developmental pathway model to illustrate progressions in the expression of aggressive behavior based on escalating severity. In the *covert* pathway, youth progress from minor, secretive behaviors in early adolescence (e.g., shoplifting, lying) to more serious property crimes in mid-adolescence (e.g., vandalism, firesetting) and then to even more serious property crimes in later adolescence (e.g. burglary, fraud). In the *authority conflict* pathway, youth begin in childhood with a variety of oppositional and defiant acts and transition into truancy and serious disobedience in adolescence. In the *overt* pathway, however, youth escalate from provoking and bullying others in childhood to physical fighting in early adolescence and then to serious violence in later adolescence—including assault, rape, and "strong-arm" robberies and intimidation (Loeber & Stouthamer-Loeber, 1998). Loeber and others (e.g., Tolan & Gorman-Smith, 1998) have found that among White, African–American, and Hispanic–Latino males, the majority who engaged ultimately in violence had progressed through this overt pathway.

Beyond categorization or classification of discrete subtypes in form and function of aggression, an additional developmental issue with respect to the underlying goals or motivations of aggressive behavior is the notion of salient developmental tasks with respect to social goals and relationships (cf. Boxer et al., 2005a). Youths' social goals influence whether they act aggressively (Crick & Dodge, 1994); aggressive youth posses more domineering, hostile, and controlling social goals than nonaggressive peers (Chung & Asher, 1996; Lochman et al., 1993, Slaby & Guerra, 1988).

Because social goals change with development, changing social goals may result in corresponding changes in the types of aggressive behaviors youth enact. Consider the goal of friendship formation and maintenance. The function and meaning of friendship change throughout development (Hartup, 1992). During the preschool years, friendships are loose associations based on shared activities, potentially explaining why conflicts over objects are common occurrences during this period of development (Fabes & Eisenberg, 1992). If a child desires a toy, taking it from a friend (damaging the relationship) is probably not such a big concern, considering there are probably others with whom the child can play.

Over the next few years (middle childhood), children begin to understand that friends are people who decide to be nice to one another, and friendships are characterized by kindness and commitment (Hartup, 1992). Thus, risking a friendship over a toy would be a less attractive option. Those youth who do not develop appropriate relational goals, however, may continue exhibiting high rates of aggression or nonnormative types of aggression because they have different social goals (retaliation or dominance). Additionally, as aggression becomes less socially acceptable, the negative consequences of aggressive behaviors begin to increase. So, the goal of avoiding retaliation or punishment probably increases in salience, as does the use of indirect forms of aggression that are less easily detected (Björkqvist et al., 1992).

In adolescence, friendships also become more intimate and emotionally supportive, and romantic relationships begin to form (Berndt, 1982; Buhrmester, 1990; Richards et al., 1998). Thus, social goals related to forming and maintaining these close friendships and romantic relationships would be considered normative. There is some evidence that maintaining friendships in adolescences includes participating in shared activities (perhaps even aggressive behaviors) for boys and conversation (perhaps even rumors or gossip) for girls (McNelles & Connolly, 1999). Additionally, more proactive aggression is related to greater influence and dominance in the peer group, and adolescent girls view dominant boys as attractive (Bukowski et al., 2000; Pellegrini & Bartini, 2001; Pellegrini & Long, 2002). Adolescents also are trying to assert autonomy as they approach adulthood, and aggression could be one of the behaviors some youth chose to enact, as it goes against adult behavioral norms (Moffitt, 1993).

Given the wealth of research that has attempted to identify categories and classifications of aggression (see Little et al., 2003, for an elaborated discussion) and that has illustrated the critical social goal-based underpinnings of aggression at various developmental stages, the prevention program developer must attend to a fairly complex matrix of form and function when considering how to target aggressive behavior. Some applied researchers have addressed this issue by selecting children for programming by using multiple informants to identify children showing early signs of any forms of potentially problematic aggression as early in development as possible (e.g., kindergarten; Flanagan et al & Conduct Problems Prevention Research Group, 2003). Others have targeted "low level" or minor forms of aggression which can be fairly common at a variety of ages across development (e.g., teasing, relational aggression; Boxer et al., 2003; Leff et al., 2004; Nansel et al., 2001).

What is critical for primary prevention is to attend to the general time periods during which certain forms and functions of aggression might be most relevant. For example, it makes no sense to target "rumor spreading" in a classroom of preschoolers. Rather, prevention with preschoolers should focus on concrete relational and physical behaviors that are meaningful for youth in that age group (e.g., telling others that they cannot play, hitting a classmate to get a toy). However, during middle childhood when peer relationships begin to take on increased salience, it would be appropriate to address issues of more circuitous behaviors such as spreading rumors and writing mean notes. Also during middle and late childhood when children begin to develop knowledge about concepts such as sarcasm and mixed messages (Creusere, 1999), issues involving nonverbal aggressive behaviors such as eye rolling and dirty looks can be addressed. In addition, although adolescents acknowledge adult jurisdiction over rules governing physical aggression, they are more likely to reject adult jurisdiction over rules governing relational aggression (Goldstein & Tisak, 2006), suggesting that interventions to reduce relational aggression in adolescence need to leave room for the adolescent to perceive some degree of self-regulation over the closely related concept of friendship selection.

It might be simpler to attend to the forms of aggression when developing primary prevention approaches rather than to the functions, particularly when considering reactive and proactive aggression. First of all, proactive aggression appears to be most prominent only in fairly small segments of the population, negating the value of a primary or universal prevention approach. Second, strictly by observation alone it can be quite difficult to infer whether an act of aggression is driven by proactive or reactive motives, especially in younger populations for whom a primary approach might be most beneficial.

Thus far we have focused on risk factors in the development of aggression, and the specific forms and functions of aggression in childhood and adolescence. These issues are of concern to primary prevention because they help to clarify the mode of program delivery (contexts for programs suggested by risk models) and the targets of programming (types of aggression used to identify participants or addressed in programs). However, essential to any intervention program is the theory of change implicit in program activities. A strong theoretical grounding in factors that shape and maintain aggression is critical to the success of any program (Boxer & Dubow, 2002; Hunter et al., 2001). In the next section, we consider theoretically specified mediating mechanisms that have been shown to account for the maintenance of aggression over time and across situations through childhood and adolescence. These are the internal processes that must be modified in order to reduce or prevent aggression.

Mediating Mechanisms Accounting for Habitual Aggression

The assertion that aggressive behavior—construed broadly—is a multiply determined behavior resulting from an array of cumulative and interactive influences is treated as fairly unequivocal across different social and behavioral science disciplines;

aggression largely has defied complete explanation within a single discipline. To illustrate, even just a cursory search of social science research abstract databases or scientific journals such as *Aggressive Behavior* or *Violence and Victims* will yield a multidisciplinary bounty of empirical studies. There is substantially less agreement, however, on the internally based mediating mechanisms that connect distal and proximal risk factors to the actual emission of an aggressive act. Biological models, for example, might focus on the role of neurotransmitters such as serotonin or the functioning of the hypothalamic-pituitary-adrenal axis system (Gollan et al., 2005), whereas sociological or criminological models might emphasize the role of ongoing social or individual strain (Baron, 2006) or individual tendencies toward deviance (Gottfredson & Hirschi, 1990) in accounting for habitually aggressive behavior. With respect to the field of youth violence prevention, however, some consensus has emerged. Strategies and programs developed from a general social-cognitive information-processing model have been identified as "best practices" by agencies such as the Centers for Disease Control and Prevention (Thornton et al., 2000) and evaluation groups such as the Blueprints for Violence Prevention program of the University of Colorado (Center for the Study and Prevention of Violence, 2006).

For quite some time, the social-cognitive information-processing (SCIP) model has been the dominant theoretical framework used to explain and predict habitual aggression in childhood and adolescence (Boxer & Dubow, 2002; Crick & Dodge, 1994; Dodge, 2006; Huesmann, 1988, 1998). The SCIP perspective asserts broadly that the way youth process social information plays a central role in the emergence and subsequent persistence of aggressive behavior. According to SCIP, in any social conflict situation, the process by which a youth initially attends to and interprets environmental cues, searches for and evaluates potential behavioral responses, and then evaluates the consequences of the chosen responses is central to explaining whether the specific behavior enacted will become an enduring style of behavioral response. Within the SCIP framework, specific behavioral response patterns are represented as mental "scripts," which are cognitive structures "laying out the sequence of events that one believes are likely to happen and the behaviors that one believes are possible or appropriate for a particular situation" (Huesmann, 1998, p. 80). Developmental research has shown that aggression supporting SCIP styles—for example, believing that it is "okay" to behave aggressively—become crystallized and predict behavior reliably during the middle childhood years (e.g., ages 6–9; Huesmann & Guerra, 1997). This behavior–belief link is similar to what has been observed in other areas of behavioral research, particularly studies of the relation between achievement beliefs and educational performance (Davis-Kean et al., In Press).

Of course, the SCIP model also incorporates the notion that youth enter into social interactions with physiological and psychological predispositions (e.g. temperament, intellectual abilities, knowledge), past experiences and memories, and current emotional states. Theoretically, these individual and contextual distal and proximal factors impact the way youth actively process social information (i.e., shape social-cognitive skills) and contribute to the social schemata and scripts upon which youth rely to make decisions about behavioral responses (i.e., shape social-cognitive structures). It is these social-cognitive processing mechanisms that more directly influence youths' behaviors.

Despite the utility of the SCIP model for explicating the individual psychological processes, it must be emphasized that this model really is a subset of more general and classic social learning theory, which places great importance on observational and direct learning experiences in shaping behavior. The developmental-ecological view described earlier is a contemporary iteration of the social learning view that more explicitly acknowledges the role of individually based factors in conjunction with contextual factors in the emergence and persistence of behavior.

Related to SCIP, a second social learning approach offering a key mediational mechanism in the maintenance of habitual aggression is the emotion regulation (ER) view. In this framework, the critical determinant of behavioral styles over time is the extent to which children appropriately manage and express their emotional arousal. Eisenberg and colleagues (Eisenberg et al., 1998; Eisenberg & Morris, 2002; also see Frick & Morris, 2004) have theorized that skills for appropriately regulating emotions largely are acquired through the parental socialization of these skills. In particular, the ER view emphasizes the importance of effortful control over emotional arousal in accounting for habitual behavior. Children unable to regulate appropriately their negative arousal, and especially their angry arousal, are more prone to developing aggressive behavioral styles.

Because the management of emotional arousal becomes necessary in essence from birth onward, parents have the opportunity very early on in development to socialize appropriate regulatory strategies. From about the first year of life, when children begin to develop the capacity to exert effortful control over their arousal, parents play an important role in the socialization of emotional regulatory skills by modeling appropriate behaviors, prompting children's responses to emotional arousal, and punishing or reinforcing these responses (Eisenberg & Morris, 2002). Thus, adaptive or maladaptive emotion regulatory styles can become crystallized quite early in development, with the potential for lifelong maintenance of social behavior (Pulkkinen, 1996).

If, as noted, aggression-supporting SCIP styles become stable by middle childhood, and maladaptive ER styles stabilize by early childhood, where does that leave the preventionist? The ideal in primary prevention is to intervene prior to the emergence of a particular problem behavior, and an essential goal of any intervention program should be to modify the factors that maintain a problem behavior. The developmental theory and research on SCIP and ER with respect to aggressive behavior does not necessarily imply that those mechanisms cannot be modified by intervention—certainly there are good, published examples of programs that have produced changes in attitudes (Huesmann et al., 1983), attributional styles (Hudley & Graham, 1993), social problem-solving skills (Guerra & Slaby, 1990), and anger control skills (Feindler & Scalley, 1998). What this treatment of relevant developmental theory meant to illustrate was that these social-cognitive and emotion-regulatory factors should be seen as key targets of specific intervention activities for two key reasons. First, SCIP and ER represent mechanisms that have been identified as at least partially responsible for the persistence of aggressive responding over time. Second, SCIP and ER are contextually sensitive functions that might only persist in problematic ways under environmental circumstances that remain fairly constant. As Guerra et al (2005) suggested, for example, an aggression-supporting SCIP style might be malleable even in older children if all aggressive contextual socializers can be modified simultaneously.

Implications for Prevention Research and Practice

Throughout this chapter we have considered various implications of developmental theory and research for the design and implementation of aggression prevention programming. Research on individual and contextual risk factors in the development of aggression implies that primary prevention programs should incorporate activities targeting different sources of risk for aggression. Research on the forms and functions of aggression suggests that prevention programs should be sensitive to the salience of different types of aggression at various points in development, and to the potential ordering and escalation in the severity of aggression over time. Finally, research on theoretical mediators of the link between risk factors and aggressive behavior suggests that programs should target certain social-cognitive and emotion-regulatory skills when attempting to halt or modify the emergence or persistence of aggressive responding.

In a more overarching sense, probably the most important implication of taking a developmental perspective when designing primary prevention programming—the basic "take home" message we mean to convey—is that prevention practice and developmental research really should go hand-in-hand. Prevention in its essence relies on a fundamentally developmental issue: change over time. In the case of prevention, the goal is to change what otherwise is expected to become a problematic chain of events.

From an empirical standpoint, it will be difficult to move the field of aggression prevention forward without careful attention to the developmental issues and processes that are addressed during the course of prevention programming. For example, as Boxer and Dubow (2002) have observed, detailed and process-oriented research on modifications to SCIP styles in tandem with reductions in aggressive behavior still is needed, and the same can be said for research on ER styles. Although there is a vast array of available research evaluating the effects of aggression prevention programming over the short term (i.e., 1–2 years; e.g., Wilson et al., 2003, meta-analyzed the effects reported in over 200 short-term evaluation studies), there is comparatively little by way of studies examining whether key mediators have permanently been altered by prevention programming. In addition, there has been little systematic effort to evaluate programs targeting aggression in the context of different developmental tasks and goals, or with respect to different types of aggressive behavior. Infusing prevention practice with developmental theory and research is a key step in the direction of better prevention strategies for aggressive behavior.

References

Baron, S. W. (2006). Street youth, strain theory, and crime. *Journal of Criminal Justice*, 34, 209–223.

Berndt, T. J. (1982). The features and effects of friendship in early adolescence. *Child Development*, 53, 1447–1460.

Björkqvist, K. J., Lagerspetz, K. M. J., & Kaukiainen, A. (1992). Do girls manipulate and boys fight?: Developmental trends in regard to direct and indirect aggression. *Aggressive Behavior*, 18, 117–127.

Bowen, N. K. & Flora, D. B. (2002). When is it appropriate to focus on protection in interventions for adolescents? *American Journal of Orthopsychiatry*, 72, 526–538.

Boxer, P. & Dubow, E. F. (2002). A social-cognitive information-processing model for school-based aggression reduction and prevention programs: Issues for research and practice. *Applied and Preventive Psychology*, 10, 177–192.

Boxer, P., Edwards-Leeper, L., Goldstein, S. E., Musher-Eizenman, D., & Dubow, E. F. (2003). Exposure to "low-level" aggression in school: Associations with aggressive behavior, future expectations, and perceived safety. *Violence & Victims*, 18, 691–704.

Boxer, P. & Frick, P. (In press). *Treating conduct problems, aggression, and antisocial behavior in children and adolescents: An integrated view*. To appear in R. Steele, M. Roberts, & T.D. Elkin, *Handbook of evidence-based therapies for children and adolescents*. Sage.

Boxer, P., Goldstein, S. E., Musher-Eizenman, D., Dubow, E. F., & Heretick, D. (2005a). Developmental issues in school-based aggression prevention from a social-cognitive perspective. *Journal of Primary Prevention*, 26, 383–400.

Boxer, P., Guerra, N. G., Huesmann, L. R., & Morales, J. (2005b). Proximal peer-level effects of a small-group selected prevention on aggression in elementary school children: An investigation of the peer contagion hypothesis. *Journal of Abnormal Child Psychology*, 33, 325–338.

Boxer, P., Musher-Eizenman, D., Dubow, E. F., Danner, S., & Heretick, D. M. L. (2006). Assessing teachers' perceptions for school-based aggression prevention programs: Applying a cognitive-ecological framework. *Psychology in the Schools*, 43, 331–344.

Broidy, L. M., Nagin, D. S., Tremblay, R. E., Bates, J. E., Brame, B., & Dodge, K. A., et al. (2003). Developmental trajectories of childhood disruptive behaviors and adolescent delinquency: A six-site, cross-national study. *Developmental Psychology*, 39, 222–245.

Buhrmester, D. (1990). Intimacy of friendship, interpersonal competence, and adjustment during preadolescence and adolescence. *Child Development*, 61, 1101–1111.

Bukowski, W. M., Sipploa, L. A., & Newcomb, A. F. (2000). Variations in patterns of attraction to same-and other-sex peers during early adolescence. *Developmental Psychology*, 36, 147–154.

Bushman, B. J., & Anderson C. A. (2001). Media violence and the American public: Scientific facts versus media misinformation. *American Psychologist*, 56, 477–489.

Cairns, R. B., Cairns, B. D., Neckerman, H. J., Gariepy, J. L., & Ferguson, L. L. (1989). Growth and aggression. I. Childhood to early adolescence. *Developmental Psychology*, 25, 320–330.

Camodeca, M., & Goossens, F. A. (2005). Aggression, social cognitions, anger and sadness in bullies and victims. *Journal of Child Psychology and Psychiatry*, 46, 186–197.

Centers for Disease Control and Prevention. (2006). Youth risk behavior surveillance-United States, 2005. *Morbidity & Mortality Weekly Report*, 55, 1–108.

Center for the Study and Prevention of Violence. (2006). *Blueprints for Violence Prevention*. See http://www.colorado.edu/cspv/blueprints/index.html.

Chung, T. & Asher, S. R. (1996). Children's goals and strategies in peer conflict situations. *Merrill-Palmer Quarterly*, 42, 125–147.

Coie, J. D. & Dodge, K. A. (1998). Aggression and antisocial behavior. In W. Damon (Series Ed.), & N. Eisenberg (Ed.), *Handbook of Child Psychology: Vol. 3 Social, emotional, and personality development* (5th ed., pp. 779–862). New York: Wiley.

Conduct Problems Prevention Research Group (1999). Initial impact of the Fast Track Prevention Trial for conduct problems: II. Classroom effects. *Journal of Consulting and Clinical Psychology,* 67, 648–657.

Conger, R. D, & Simons, R. L. (1997). Life-course contingencies in the development of adolescent antisocial behavior: A Matching law approach. In T. P. Thornberry (Ed.), *Developmental theories of crime and delinquency* (pp. 55–99). New Brunswick, NJ: Transaction Publishers.

Cowen, E. L. (2000). Psychological wellness: Some hopes for the future. In D. Cicchetti, J. Rappaport, I. Sandler, & R. P. Weissberg (Eds.), *The Promotion of wellness in children and adolescents* (pp. 477–503). Washington, DC: Child Welfare League of America.

Cowen, E. L., Hightower, A. D., Pedro-Carroll, J. L., Work, W. C., Wyman, P. A., & Haffey, W. G. (1996). *School-based prevention for children at risk: The Primary Mental Health Project.* Washington, DC: American Psychological Association.

Creusere, M. A. (1999). Theories of adults understanding and use of irony and sarcasm: Applications to and evidence from research with children. *Developmental Review,* 19, 213–262.

Crick, N. R. (1995). Relational aggression: The role of intent attributions, feelings of distress, and provocation type. *Development and Psychopathology,* 7, 313–322.

Crick, N. R. & Dodge, K. A. (1994). A review and reformulation of social information-processing mechanisms in children's social adjustment. *Psychological Bulletin,* 115, 74–101.

Crick, N. R. & Grotpeter, J. K. (1995). Relational aggression, gender, and social-psychological adjustment. *Child Development,* 66, 710–722.

Davis-Kean, P. E., Huesmann, L. R., Collins, W. A., Welland, J. B., Bates, J., & Lansford, J. (2005). *Changes in the relation of beliefs and behaviors during middle childhood.* (In Press).

Dodge, K. A. (1991). The structure and function of reactive and proactive aggression. In D. J. Pepler & K. H. Rubin (Eds.), *The development and treatment of childhood aggression* (pp. 201–218). Hillsdale, NJ: Lawrence Erlbaum Associates.

Dodge, K. A. (2006). Translational science in action: Hostile attributional style and the development of aggressive behavior problems. *Development and Psychopathology,* 18, 791–814.

Dodge, K. A. & Coie, J. D. (1987). Social information-processing factors in reactive and proactive aggression in children's peer groups. *Journal of Personality and Social Psychology,* 53, 1146–1158.

Dodge, K. A. & Pettit, G. S. (2003). A biopsychosocial model of the development of chronic conduct problems in adolescence. *Developmental Psychology,* 39, 349–371.

Dubow, E. F., Huesmann, L. R., & Boxer, P. (2003). Theoretical and methodological considerations in cross-generational research on parenting and child aggressive behavior. *Journal of Abnormal Child Psychology,* 31, 185–192.

Eisenberg, N., & Morris, A. S. (2002). Children's emotion-related regulation. In R. V. Kail (Ed.), *Advances in child development and behavior* (pp. 189–229). San Diego, CA: Academic Press.

Eisenberg, N., Cumberland, A., & Spinrad, T. L. (1998). Parental socialization of emotion. *Psychological Inquiry,* 9, 241–273.

Eisenberg, N., Valiente, C., Fabes, R. A., Smith, C. L., Reiser, M., & Shepard, S. A., et al. (2003). The relations of effortful control and ego control to children's resiliency and social functioning. *Developmental Psychology,* 39, 761–776.

Eron, L. D. (1987). The development of aggressive behavior from the perspective of a developing behaviorism. *American Psychologist,* 42, 435–442.

Eron, L. D. (1994). Theories of aggression: From drives to cognitions. In L.R. Huesmann (Ed.), *Aggressive behavior: Current perspectives* (pp. 3–11). New York, NY: Plenum Press.

Eron, L. D., Walder, L. O., & Lefkowitz, M. M. (1971). *Learning of aggression in children.* Boston: Little, Brown.

Espelage, D. L., Holt, M. K., & Henkel, R. R. (2003). Examination of peer-group contextual effects on aggression during early adolescence. *Child Development,* 74, 205–220.

Fabes, R. A., & Eisenberg, N. (1992). Young children's emotional arousal and anger/aggressive behaviors. In A. Fraezek & H. Zumkley (Eds.), *Socialization and aggression* (pp. 85–102). Berlin: Springer-Verlag.

Feindler, E. L., & Scalley, M. (1998). Adolescent anger management groups for violence reduction. In K. C. Stoiber & T. R. Kratochwill (Eds.), *Handbook of group intervention for children and families* (100–119). Needham Heights, MA: Allyn & Bacon.

Flanagan, K. S., Bierman, K. L., Kam, C., & the Conduct Problems Prevention Research Group. (2003). Identifying at-risk children at school entry: The usefulness of multibehavioral problem profiles. *Journal of Clinical Child and Adolescent Psychology, 32*, 396–407.

Frick, P. J. (1994). Family dysfunction and the disruptive behavior disorders: A review of recent empirical findings. *Advances in Clinical Child Psychology, 16*, 203–226.

Frick, P. J. (2006). Developmental pathways to conduct disorder. *Child and Adolescent Psychiatric Clinics of North America, 15*, 311–331.

Frick, P. J. & Morris, A. S. (2004). Temperament and developmental pathways to conduct problems. *Journal of Clinical Child and Adolescent Psychology, 33*, 54–68.

Frick, P. J., Cornell, A. H., Barry, C. T., Bodin, S. D., & Dane, H. A. (2003). Callous unemotional traits and conduct problems in the prediction of conduct problem severity, aggression, and self-reports of delinquency. *Journal of Abnormal Child Psychology, 31*, 457–470.

Galen, B. R. & Underwood, M. K. (1997). A developmental investigation of social aggression among children. *Developmental Psychology, 33*, 589–600.

Goldstein, S. E. & Tisak, M. S. (2006). Early adolescents' conceptions of parental and friend authority over relational aggression. *Journal of Early Adolescence, 26*, 344–364.

Gollan, J. K., Lee, R., & Coccaro, E. F. (2005). Developmental psychopathology and neurobiology of aggression. *Development and Psychopathology, 17*, 1151–1171.

Gottfredson, M. R., & Hirschi, T. (1990). *A general theory of crime.* Stanford University Press.

Guerra, N. G., Slaby, R. G. (1990). Cognitive mediators of aggression in adolescent offenders: II. Intervention. *Developmental Psychology, 26*, 269–277.

Guerra, N. G., Huesmann, L. R., & Spindler, A. (2003). Community violence exposure, social cognition, and aggression among urban elementary-school children. *Child Development, 74*, 1507–1522.

Guerra, N. G., Boxer, P., & Kim, T. E. (2005). A cognitive-ecological approach to serving students with emotional and behavioral disorders: Application to aggressive behavior. *Behavioral Disorders, 30*, 277–288.

Hartup, W. W. (1974). Aggression in childhood: Developmental perspectives. *American Psychologist, 29*, 336–341.

Hartup, W. W. (1992). Friendships and their developmental significance. In H. McGurk (Ed.), *Childhood social development: Contemporary perspectives* (pp. 175–205). Hove, England: Erlbaum.

Henggeler, S. W., Schoenwald, S. K., Borduin, C. M., Rowland, M. D., & Cunningham, P. B. (1998). *Multisystemic treatment of antisocial behavior in children and adolescents.* New York: Guilford Press.

Hinshaw, S. P., Simmel, C., & Heller, T. L. (1995). Multimethod assessment of covert antisocial behavior in children: Laboratory observations, adult ratings, and child self-report. *Psychological Assessment, 7*, 209–219.

Hubbard, J. A., Parker, E. H., Ramsden, S. R., Flanagan, K. D., Relyea, N., & Dearing, K. F., et al. (2004). The relations among observational, physiological, and self-report measures of children's anger. *Social Development, 13*, 14–39.

Hudley, C. & Graham, S. (1993). An attributional intervention to reduce peer-directed aggression among African-American boys. *Child Development, 64*, 124–138.

Huesmann, L. R. (1988). An information processing model for the development of aggression. *Aggressive Behavior, 14*, 12–24.

Huesmann, L. R. (1998). The role of social information-processing and cognitive schema in the acquisition and maintenance of habitual aggressive behavior. In R. G. Green & E. Donnerstein

(Eds.), *Human aggression: Theories, research, and implications for social policy* (pp. 73–109). San Diego, CA: Academic Press.

Huesmann, L. R. & Guerra, N. G. (1997). Children's normative beliefs about aggression and aggressive behavior. *Journal of Personality and Social Psychology*, 72, 408–419.

Huesmann, L. R., Eron, L. D., Klein, R., Brice, P., & Fischer, P. (1983). Mitigating the imitation of aggressive behaviors by changing children's attitudes about media violence. *Journal of Personality and Social Psychology*, 44, 899–910.

Huesmann, L. R., Eron, L. D., Lefkowitz, M. M., & Walder, L. O. (1984). Stability of aggression over time and generations. *Developmental Psychology*, 20, 1120–1134.

Huesmann, L. R., Eron, L. D., & Yarmel, P. W. (1987). Intellectual functioning and aggression. *Journal of Personality and Social Psychology*, 52, 232–240.

Huesmann, L. R., Eron, L. D., & Dubow, E. F. (2002). Childhood predictors of adult criminality: Are all risk factors reflected in childhood aggressiveness? *Criminal Behaviour and Mental Health*, 12, 185–208.

Huesmann, L. R., Moise-Titus, J., Podolski, C., & Eron, L. D. (2003). Longitudinal relations between children's exposure to TV violence and their aggressive and violent behavior in young adulthood: 1977–1992. *Developmental Psychology*, 39, 201–221.

Huesmann, L. R., Dubow, E. F., Eron, L. D., & Boxer, P. (2006). Middle childhood family-contextual and personal factors as predictors of adult outcomes. In A. C. Huston & M. N. Ripke (Eds.), *Developmental contexts in middle childhood: Bridges to adolescence and adulthood*. (pp. 62–86). New York, NY: Cambridge University Press.

Hunter, L., Elias, M. J., & Norris, J. (2001). School based violence prevention: Challenges and lessons learned from an action research project. *Journal of School Psychology*, 39, 161–175.

Institute of Medicine (1994). *Reducing risks for mental disorders: Frontiers for preventive intervention research*. Washington, DC: National Academies Press.

Jones, D., Dodge, K. A., Foster, E. M., & Nix, R. (2002). Early identification of children at risk for costly mental health service use. *Prevention Science*, 3, 247–256.

Kokko, K. & Pulkkinen, L. (2005). Stability of aggressive behavior from childhood to middle age in women and men. *Aggressive Behavior*, 31, 485–497.

Lagerspetz, K. M. J., Björkqvist, K., & Peltonen, T. (1988). Is indirect aggression typical of females? Gender differences in aggressiveness in 11- to 12-year-old children. *Aggressive Behavior*, 14, 403–414.

Leff, S. S., Costigan, T., & Power, T. J. (2004). Using participatory research to develop a playground-based prevention program. *Journal of School Psychology*, 42, 3–21.

Lemerise, E. A. & Arsenio, W. F. (2000). An integrated model of emotion processes and cognition in social information processing. *Child Development*, 71, 107–118.

Little, T. D., Jones, S. M., Henrich, C. C., & Hawley, P. H. (2003). Disentangling the "whys" from the "whats" of aggressive behaviour. *International Journal of Behavioral Development*, 27, 122–133.

Lochman, J. E., Wayland, K. K., & White, K. J. (1993). Social goals: Relationships to adolescent adjustment and to social problem solving. *Journal of Abnormal Child Psychology*, 21, 135–151.

Loeber, R. & Hay, D. (1997). Key issues in the development of aggression and violence from childhood to early adulthood. *Annual Review of Psychology*, 48, 371–410.

Loeber, R. & Stouthamer-Loeber, M. (1998). Development of juvenile aggression and violence: Some common misconceptions and controversies. *American Psychologist*, 53, 242–259.

Lorenz, K. (1966). *On aggression*. New York: Harcourt.

Mahoney, A., Donnelly, W. O., Boxer, P., & Lewis, T. (2003). Marital and severe parent-to-adolescent physical aggression in clinic-referred families: Mother and adolescent reports on co-occurence and links to child behavior problems. *Journal of Family Psychology*, 17, 3–19.

McNelles, L. R. & Connolly, J. A. (1999). Intimacy between adolescent friends: Age and gender differences in intimate affect and intimate behaviors. *Journal of Research on Adolescence*, 9, 143–159.

Metropolitan Area Child Study Research Group. (2002). A cognitive-ecological approach to preventing aggression in urban settings: Initial outcomes for high-risk children. *Journal of Consulting & Clinical Psychology*, 70, 179–194.

Moffitt, T. E. (1993). Adolescent-limited and life-course persistent anti-social behaviors: A developmental taxonomy. *Psychological Review*, 100, 674–701.

Morales, J. R. & Guerra, N. G. (2006). Effects of multiple context and cumulative stress on urban children's adjustment in elementary school. *Child Development*, 77, 907–923.

Musher-Eizenman, D. R., Boxer, P., Danner, S., Dubow, E. F., Goldstein, S. E., & Heretick, D. M. L. (2004). Social-cognitive mediators of the relation of environmental and emotion regulation factors to children's aggression. *Aggressive Behavior*, 30, 389–408.

Nagin, D. & Tremblay, R. E. (1999). Trajectories of boys' physical aggression, opposition, and hyperactivity on the path to physically violent and nonviolent juvenile delinquency. *Child Development*, 70, 1181–1196.

Nansel, T. R., Overpeck, M., Pilla, R. S., Ruan, W. J., Simons-Morton, B., & Scheidt, P. (2001). Bullying behaviors among US youth: Prevalence and association with psychosocial adjustment. *Journal of the American Medical Association*, 285, 2094–2100.

NICHD Early Child Care Research Network. (2004). Trajectories of physical aggression from toddlerhood to middle childhood. *Monographs of the Society for Research in Child Development*, 69, (4).

Oxford, M., Cavell, T. A., & Hughes, J. N. (2003). Callous/unemotional traits moderate the relation between ineffective parenting and child externalizing problems: A Partial replication and extension. *Journal of Clinical Child and Adolescent Psychology*, 32, 577–585.

Patterson, G. R. (1982). *Coercive family process*. Eugene, OR: Castalia Press.

Patterson, G. R., DeBaryshe, B. D., & Ramsey, E. (1989). A developmental perspective on anti-social behavior. *American Psychologist*, 44, 329–335.

Pellegrini, A. D. & Bartini, M. (2001). Dominance in early adolescent boys: Affiliative and aggressive dimensions and possible functions. *Merrill-Palmer Quarterly*, 47, 142–163.

Pellegrini, A. D. & Long, J. D. (2002). A longitudinal study of bullying, dominance, and victimization during the transition from primary school through secondary school. *British Journal of Developmental Psychology*, 20, 259–280.

Persson, G. E. B. (2005). Young children's prosocial and aggressive behaviors and their experiences of being targeted for similar behaviors by peers. *Social Development*, 14, 206–228.

Poulin, F. & Boivin, M. (2000). Reactive and proactive aggression. Evidence of a two-factor model. *Psychological Assessment*, 12, 115–122.

Price, J. M. & Dodge, K. A. (1989). Reactive and proactive aggression in childhood: Relations to peer status and social context dimensions. *Journal of Abnormal Child Psychology*, 17, 455–471.

Pulkkinen, L. (1996). Proactive and reactive aggression in early adolescence as precursors to anti- and prosocial behavior in young adults. *Aggressive Behavior*, 22, 241–257.

Raine, A., Dodge, K., Loeber, R., Gatzke-Kopp, L., Lynam, D., & Reynolds, C., et al. (2006). The reactive-proactive aggression questionnaire: Differential correlates of reactive and proactive aggression in adolescent boys. *Aggressive Behavior*, 32, 159–171.

Reid, J. B., Eddy, J. M., Fetrow, R. A., & Stoolmiller, M. (1999). Description and immediate impacts of a preventive intervention for conduct problems. *American Journal of Community Psychology*, 27, 483–517.

Richards, M. H., Crowe, P. A., Larson, R., & Swarr, A. (1998). Developmental patterns and gender differences in the experience of peer companionship during adolescence. *Child Development*, 69, 154–163.

Rubin, K. H., Burgess, K. B., Dwyer, K. M., & Hastings, P. D. (2003). Predicting preschoolers' externalizing behaviors from toddler temperament, conflict, and maternal negativity. *Developmental Psychology*, 39, 164–176.

Sameroff, A., Gutman, L. M., & Peck, S. C. (2003). Adaptation among youth facing multiple risks: Prospective research findings. In S. S. Luthar (Ed.), *Resilience and vulnerability:*

Adaptation in the context of childhood adversities (pp. 364–391). New York: Cambridge University Press.

Schwartz, D. (2000). Subtypes of victims and aggressors in children's peer groups. *Journal of Abnormal Child Psychology*, 28, 181–192.

Schwartz, D., Dodge, K. A., Coie, J. D., Hubbard, J. A., Cillessen, A. H. N., & Lemerise, E. A., et al. (1998). Social-cognitive and behavioral correlates of aggression and victimization in boy's play groups. *Journal of Abnormal Child Psychology*, 26, 431–440.

Shaw, D. S., Owens, E. B., Giovannelli, J., & Winslow, E. B. (2001). Infant and toddler pathways leading to early externalizing disorders. *Journal of the American Academy of Child & Adolescent Psychiatry*, 40, 36–43.

Slaby, R. G. & Guerra, N. G. (1988). Cognitive mediators of aggresson in adolescent offenders. I. Assessment. *Developmental Psychology*, 24, 580–588.

Thornton, T. N., Craft, C. A., Dahlberg, L. L., Lynch, B. S., & Baer, K. (2000). *Best practices of youth violence prevention: A sourcebook for community action*. Atlanta, GA: Centers for Disease Control and Prevention.

Tisak, M. S. (1995). Domains of social reasoning and beyond. In R. Vasta (Ed.), *Annals of child development: Vol. 11, A research annual* (pp. 95–130). London, England: Jessica Kingsley Publishers.

Tolan, P. H., & Gorman-Smith, D. (1998). Development of serious and violent offending careers. In R. Loeber & D. P. Farrington (Eds.), *Serious & violent juvenile offenders: Risk factors and successful interventions* (pp. 68–85). Thousand Oaks, CA: Sage.

Tolan, P. H., Guerra, N. G., & Kendall, P. C. (1995). A developmental-ecological perspective on antisocial behavior in children and adolescents: Toward a unified risk and intervention framework. *Journal of Consulting & Clinical Psychology*, 63, 579–584.

Tolan, P. H., Gorman-Smith, D., & Loeber, R. (2000). Developmental timing of onsets of disruptive behaviors and later delinquency of inner-city youth. *Journal of Child and Family Studies*, 9, 203–220.

Tolan, P. H., Gorman-Smith, D., & Henry, D. B. (2003). The developmental ecology of urban males' youth violence. *Developmental Psychology*, 39, 274–291.

Tremblay, R. E. (2000). The development of aggressive behaviour during childhood: What have we learned in the past century? *International Journal of Behavioral Development*, 24, 129–141.

Underwood, M. K., Galen, B. R., & Paquette, J. A. (2001). Top ten challenges for understanding gender and aggression in children: Why can't we all just get along? *Social Development*, 10, 248–266.

Vitaro, F., Brendgen, M., & Tremblay, R. E. (2002). Reactively and proactively aggressive children: Adolescent and subsequent characteristics. *Journal of Child Psychology and Psychiatry and Allied Disciplines*, 43, 495–506.

Wilson, S. J., Lipsey, M. W., & Derzon, J. H. (2003). The effects of school-based intervention programs on aggressive behavior: A meta-analysis. *Journal of Consulting and Clinical Psychology*, 71, 136–149.

Wootton, J. M., Frick, P. J., Shelton, K. K., & Silverthorn, P. (1997). Ineffective parenting and childhood conduct problems: The moderating role of callous-unemotional traits. *Journal of Consulting and Clinical Psychology*, 65, 301–308.

Chapter 15
Bullies and Victims at School: Perspectives and Strategies for Primary Prevention

Christian Berger, Ramin Karimpour, and Philip C. Rodkin

Overview The present chapter addresses bullying and victimization from an ecological perspective. The assumption of a multilevel approach allows for identifying several layers of complexity and, consequently, different levels for intervention strategies. First we introduce bullying and victimization, addressing three main topics: a critical review of what these phenomena involve, the notions of prevention and promotion as intervention goals, and the contextualization of bullying and victimization within the emerging peer culture of early adolescence. Then, the next section presents a layered analysis identifying four levels of complexity: the individual, the dyad, the peer group, and the institution, incorporating a developmental perspective; implications for interventions at each of these levels are included. Finally, the last section presents some guidelines for intervention based on literature on implementation and our own work in school-based bullying prevention.

Introduction

Bullying and victimization has become a central concern for all participants of the educational community (Elias & Zins, 2003; Espelage & Swearer, 2004; Pellegrini, 1998). During the past three decades, beginning with the seminal work of Olweus (1978, 1993, 2001), scholars have been addressing aggressive behavior and its related factors within school contexts. However, the extremely rare yet shocking events of extreme violence that has lately occurred in schools and amplified by the sensational media coverage have made bullying a pressing societal concern. Even though there is no definitive evidence that supports a hypothetical association between extremely violent incidents and school bullying and victimization, bullying and victimization constitutes a major concern for all members of the community associated with schools. A growing body of research is trying to better understand the role that aggression plays in school environments, and particularly how violent situations and aggressive behavior can be moderated, if not eradicated, from schools.

Scholars have raised a considerable amount of evidence regarding bullying and victimization and have underscored their negative implications. Several studies

T. W. Miller (ed.), *School Violence and Primary Prevention.*
© Springer 2008

over the past decade have shown an association with negative developmental outcomes for both bullies and their victims (Graham et al., 2003; Swearer & Espelage, 2004; Swearer et al., 2004). For instance, children who are victimized are more likely to evidence both internalizing (e.g., depression, anxiety, and with-drawal) and externalizing (aggression and delinquent behaviors) problems. Victimized children also show a decrease in self-esteem and can become disliked by their peers (Hodges et al., 1999; Juvonen et al., 2001). Nansel et al. (2003) found that children involved in bullying and/or victimization demonstrated poorer school adjustment and also perceived a more negative school climate than other children. Similar negative social–psychological effects for aggressors have also been found (Werner & Crick, 1999). In a broader perspective, negative outcomes have also been observed at the group level by normalizing aggressive behaviors (Rodkin et al., 2003; Allen et al., 2005). Unchecked bullying can also establish a school culture in which aggression may become a validated mode of interpersonal relationships (Berger et al., 2001; Rodkin & Fischer, 2003).

Despite the broader consensus among scholars, teachers, educational adminis-trators, and policy makers regarding these issues, strategies have not been successful—or consistent—in trying to eradicate aggressive behaviors from schools (Salmivalli et al., 2005; Smith et al., 2003). One possible explanation for this difficulty is that there is still not a complete understanding of the phenomenon of bullying, and particularly its implications for the children and the peer culture (Rodkin & Hodges, 2003). Thus, a better understanding of bullying and victimization consti-tutes a necessary step in order to develop nurturing and healthier environments.

Definition, Assessment, and Prevalence of Bullying and Victimization

Identifying and assessing bullying and victimization is a challenging enterprise. For instance, the boundaries of what is understood as bullying and victimization are not clear and vary across studies. For example, distinctions and associations established between enmities (i.e., least-liked cross-nominations), bully–victim relationships (Abecassis, 2003), or bullying and peer sexual harassment (Rodkin & Fischer, 2003; Stein, 1995) approach the phenomenon from different perspectives. Also, different assessment methodologies have been used, such as distinctions regarding informant source, including peer-, self-, and teacher-reported measures (Leff et al., 1999; Graham & Juvonen, 1998), as well as observational reports (Pellegrini, 2001; Boulton, 1999). In the same way, different criteria to define what constitutes a bully and/or a victim have been used: self-reports of involvement in bullying or victimi-zation with specific definitions (Olweus, 1993), peer nominations as a bully or a victim (Paul & Cillessen, 2003) with or without a predefinition, distinctions between *real* victims (i.e., children who are consensually identified as a victim by peers and the self) from other types of victims (Graham et al., 2003), and finally, the consideration of subgroups of aggressive children (Estell et al., 2003;

Vaillancourt et al., 2003). Nonreporting also implies methodological challenges. Unnever and Cornell (2004) reported that among self-reported victims in middle school, 25% had not told anyone that they were bullied and 40% had not told an adult about their victimization. Cultural and developmental differences on how children understand and define bullying also play a role in assessing the problem (Smith et al., 2002). Finally, the fact that a majority of bullying episodes occur in areas with minimal or absent adult supervision and unstructured settings (Leff et al., 2003) stresses the need for reliable assessment tools that allow us to better capture this phenomenon.

How pervasive is bullying and victimization? Schwartz et al. (2001) found prevalence estimates to vary widely across studies, due in their opinion as to the influence of design-specific factors and also because of the use of arbitrary classification criteria that are not necessarily comparable. Despite these methodological difficulties, several studies have presented estimates of children involved in aggressive behaviors. For instance, Pellegrini's review of the literature found that bullies represent about 7% to 15% of the school age population; victims, on the other hand, represent around 10% of it (Pellegrini, 1998). More recently, Rodkin and Berger (in press) obtained prevalence rates through peer reports of 7.3% for bullies, 13% for victims, and 2.4% for bully/victims in fourth- and fifth- grade students; similar rates are presented by other researchers, perhaps with bullies under-identified (Olweus, 1993; Paul & Cillessen, 2003; Schwartz et al., 2001; Solberg & Olweus, 2003). In comparison, Pellegrini et al. (1999) determined bullies and victims using self-reported Olweus Senior Questionnaire scores, identifying 14% of their sample as bullies, 19% as victims, and 5% as aggressive victims.

Prevention and Promotion

Even though there is consensus about the negative impact of bullying and victimization in schools and the need for developing adequate strategies to face these problems, there is still uncertainty regarding the underlying assumptions, goals, and main features of any program aimed at this objective. Two main goals can be identified as underlying anti-bullying interventions: First, to control and eradicate bullying situations from schools, and second, to promote school environments in which all participants feel safe and valued, thus constituting nurturing and healthy environments (Aron & Milicic, 1999). The first goal refers to preventive interventions, whereas the second refers to promotional interventions. As simple as this distinction seems, it has important implications for practice.

Prevention and promotion constitute two sides of the same coin; they should coexist in any intervention program. Prevention focuses on negative outcomes (i.e., aggressive behaviors and negative attitudes) and is aimed at avoiding these occurrences by identifying both risk and protective factors and modifying them accordingly. Particularly, primary prevention works before the negative outcomes are present, trying to stop their emergence (as compared to secondary and tertiary prevention). Promotion focuses on expected or desired outcomes; instead of trying to stop the emergence of particular behaviors, it fosters their positive emergence. Promotion, thus, is the positive perspective of how schools should look like, and it is aimed at identifying those factors that may lead to an ideal school environment. These two perspectives are complementary and should be integrated in any intervention initiative (Gubbins & Berger, 2004). In order to diminish or suppress aggressive behavior, there is a need to provide alternatives through which children may get the same benefits that they are trying to achieve through involvement in aggressive behaviors. As noted by behavioral theorists, the suppression of a particular behavior is not effective unless the association between that particular behavior and the perceived outcome is suppressed; an effective way to do that is by giving other optional behaviors that can be associated with the expected outcome. For instance, Edwards et al. (2005) consider a key factor in prevention, the promotion of constructive behaviors that constitute alternatives to aggression. Malecki and Demaray (2004) also refer to this need of alternatives in order to break the rewarding nature of bullying by the peer group. As Pellegrini (1998) points out, in a bully–victim relationship there must be a balance between costs and benefits. Some positive outcomes may be found for aggressive behavior; for example, Malecki and Demaray (2004) found that bullying behavior may increase peer social support for students who exert it; for victims, the benefits are not so clear.

Bullying and Victimization within Peer Ecologies

Bullying and victimization cannot be understood as isolated phenomena; they are intertwined within the particular peer ecology that emerges, constituting social processes that serve particular functions to the individual and to the group (Rodkin, 2004; Swearer & Tam, 2003). Bullying and victimization are phenomena that emerge within the particular peer culture of children and adolescents. Therefore, better understanding needs to consider the particular features of this social context and how aggression is integrated within it.

Normalization of Aggressive Interpersonal Relations

García and Madriaza (2005) studied the meaning of school violence from the student perspective. They found that aggressive behavior within the school context acts as a "social organizer" meant to structure social relationships. More than breaking social rules, aggression can create new social rules and therefore organize the peer social group. This notion is in line with other authors who have conceptualized bullying and victimization as social phenomena involving the whole group (Boulton, 1999; Salmivalli, 2001). As Espelage et al. (2004) suggest, research on bullying should consider "the complex interaction among the need for dominance, changes in social surroundings, peer group structure, and the desire to interact with the opposite sex" (p. 22). Schäfer et al. (2005) found that the social hierarchical structure of the classroom impacts victimization by establishing a social context in which fixed social hierarchies resemble bully–victim power imbalances, therefore normalizing hierarchical interpersonal relations and weakening the social rejection of victimization as a relational pattern.

As Dishion et al. (1996) argue, friends can provide "deviancy training" when shared norms that favor aggression are established and nourished within a peer group. In the context of the peer group, aggressive behavior can be adopted as a way to fit peer norms. For instance, Allen et al. (2005) propose that if aggressive behavior, tough attitudes, and a higher position within the social hierarchy are valued among the peer group, then popular kids will be "requested" by their peers to meet these characteristics. In the authors' words, "popular adolescents would be in a position to have their behavior socialized more strongly by the broader peer culture in ways consistent with prevailing peer norms" (Allen et al., 2005, p. 748–749). Implicit in the Allen et al. (2005) study is the notion that aggressive behavior and bullying can become normalized among the peer group. Bullying and victimization may become a constitutive part of the day-to-day school experience for students (Rodkin et al., 2003). Astonishingly, as argued by Elias and Zins (2003), many in society ignore, overlook, or even consider bullying a normal developmental behavior.

Social Status, Bullying, and Victimization

Olweus (1993) established power asymmetry as a main characteristic of bully–victim relationships. Understanding power as the capacity to influence others, social status asymmetries should be clearly observed in bully–victim relationships, with bullies displaying higher popularity and social status than their victims. Recent studies have also addressed the relationship between aggression and popularity (Boulton, 1999; Cillessen & Mayeux, 2004; Paul & Cillessen, 2003; Rodkin & Berger, in press; Rose et al., 2004; Vaillancourt et al., 2003) and the co-occurrence of popularity, aggression, and prosocial behavior (Estell et al., 2003; Rodkin et al., 2000), concluding that bullies can be popular (Pellegrini, 1998; Rodkin et al., 2000) despite their social rejection. This apparent contradiction may be explained by the overlap of several dimensions of social status. Sociometry defines social status as a likability index measured by how many nominations a child receives as "most liked." Vaillancourt et al. (2003) discuss the notion of popularity and argue that it is not necessarily tied to being liked or disliked. As they point out, "sociometric liking/disliking is not necessarily synonymous with perceived popularity; being rejected is not the same as being viewed by peers as unpopular or low in status" (p. 160). In their findings, they report that many of the students identified as bullies were not marginalized and/or maladjusted; rather, bullies were considered both popular and powerful, even if they were disliked.

Swearer and Tam (2003) argue that social status is related to a developmental need of fitting into a new group; they argue that while entering middle school, "bully behaviors appear to reflect the needs of students to establish social status as they transition into a new peer group." Taking this argument further, aggressive behavior can be understood as a structural phenomenon, with a developmental functionality and concomitant benefits and costs (Hawley et al., 2007). Aggression can, thus, be considered as a way to gain social position within the peer group.

Gender, Bullying, and Victimization

During preadolescence, bullies are mostly boys but victims are both boys and girls (Olweus, 1993; Pellegrini et al., 1999; Solberg & Olweus, 2003). However, differences regarding gender go much deeper than prevalence rates. Crick and Grotpeter (1995) found that boys display more physical aggression, whereas girls display more relational aggression. Vaillancourt et al. (2003) found that female bullies are viewed by their peers as more relationally but less physically aggressive than their male counterparts; moreover, female bullies are perceived as more attractive, whereas male bullies are perceived as more athletic, which, as the authors point out, is not unexpected considering prevailing gender-role stereotypes.

Differential developmental outcomes by gender have also been found for victims (Owens et al., 2005; Tapper & Boulton, 2005). Prevalence rates of victimization are contradictory. Schwartz (2000) reported that boys are more likely than girls to be perceived by their peers as victims. Owens et al. (2005) reported a higher rate of boys identifying themselves as victimized compared to girls. However, Rodkin and Berger (in press) found that over 60% of victimized children were girls. These differences may be because of the use of different reporting sources and assessment criteria. For instance, Graham et al. (2003) reported a multivariate effect of victims' reporting source and gender: even though peer-identified victims were more likely to be boys, more girls than boys identified themselves as victims and were also peer- and self-identified as victims (what the authors called "true" victims). Regarding developmental correlates and outcomes, Paul and Cillessen (2003) found male victims to be perceived by their teachers lower on peer sociability, school competence, and prosocial behavior, whereas female victims reported more internalizing problems. Rodkin and Berger (in press) found female victims of male bullying displaying high social status, as compared to the low social status displayed by male victims of male bullies. As argued by Troop-Gordon and Ladd (2005), boys and girls may interpret victimization in different ways: girls may attribute peer victimization to their own lack of abilities to form positive social relationships, whereas boys would blame peer victimization on their peers' characteristics, as well as their own shortcomings.

Along with gender differences found regarding the type of aggression exerted by boys and girls (Crick & Grotpeter, 1995), which have been associated with gender norms and stereotypes, victimization may have completely different implications for boys and girls. For boys, being victimized may reflect a lower social position that does not fit the male stereotype of being tough (Kindlon & Thompson, 1999). For girls, the implication may relate to gaining certain recognition and attention that can accompany victimization status—as dysfunctional as this attention might be (Stein, 1999).

Especially important in entering middle school is the consideration of cross-gender relationships. Adler and Adler (1998) argued that during preadolescence, the uncertainty regarding relationships with the opposite sex within the gendered peer ecology favors hostile expressions and behaviors toward the opposite gender. Swearer and Tam (2003) consider bullying as a way to minimize risks that are involved in breaking the previous well-established norms of interaction between sexes. As argued by Rodkin et al. (2003, pp. 78–79), "sometimes, antipathy between a boy and a girl may be the only socially legitimate way to express deep feelings toward a member of the opposite sex." In this sense, aggressive behaviors would be functional as a way to manage the changing interactional sphere with the opposite sex, particularly to minimize the risks of breaking the norms of same- and cross-sex interactions (Pellegrini, 2001). Aggression can be acknowledged either as cross-gender interest or dismissed as bullying behavior that confirms the rejection of the opposite sex in front of the peer group. Some authors go further in establishing potential connections between cross-gender bullying and later sexual harassment (McMaster et al., 2002; Pellegrini, 2002; Rodkin & Fischer, 2003; Stein, 1995). Overall, there is sufficient evidence to claim that cross-gender and same-gender bullying may differ in their implications within social contexts and their psychological correlates for both bullies and victims.

Layered Environments of Bullying and Victimization: A Multilevel Approach for Interventions

Several authors have adopted an ecological perspective inspired by Bronfenbrenner's framework (Espelage & Swearer, 2004; Rodkin, 2004; Rodkin & Hodges, 2003; Salmivalli, 2001; O'Connell et al., 1999), arguing that aggressive behavior must be understood as a function of individual and social factors (Bronfenbrenner, 1979). This approach does not deny the influence of individual characteristics on aggressive behavior (Boxer et al., 2005; Crick & Dodge, 1994; Olweus, 1993) or the knowledge that such an approach has raised, but highlights the social complexity of individual behavior within peer ecologies. From an ecological perspective, several layers should be considered when approaching the social character of bullying and victimization, such as the individual, the bully–victim dyad (Coie et al., 1999; Rodkin & Berger, in press; Rodkin & Hodges, 2003; Veenstra et al., 2005), the peer group (Allen et al., 2005; O'Connell et al., 1999; Salmivalli & Voeten, 2004), and the school social environment in which bullying and victimization takes place (Bellmore et al., 2004; Nishina, 2004; Schäfer et al., 2005; Swearer & Espelage, 2004).

Individual Level

Are there individual characteristics that determine particular profiles of bullies and victims? Which individual characteristics constitute risk or protective factors of later involvement in bullying and victimization? Olweus (1993) offered a picture of bullies as *"having an aggressive reaction pattern combined* (in the case of boys) *with physical strength"* (p. 35, italics original). On the other hand, typical victims are portrayed as "more anxious and insecure ... often cautious, sensitive and quiet." Also, they were thought to display "lower self-esteem and hold negative views of themselves and their situation" (op cit., p. 32).

However, this stereotypical portrait of bullies and victims has been questioned by studies establishing great variability between both groups (Boulton, 1999; Estell et al., 2003; Goldbaum et al., 2003; Graham et al., 2003; Holt & Espelage, 2003; Rodkin, 2004; Rodkin & Berger, in press; Tapper & Boulton, 2005). The traditional picture of an unpopular, tough, and powerful bully who harasses weaker peers is getting fuzzier in the light of new research findings (Boulton, 1999; Estell et al., 2003; Rodkin et al., 2000). For instance, Vaillancourt et al. (2003) questioned the unpopularity of bullies. They measured powerfulness, popularity, likability, and other power-related characteristics such as physical competence. Their findings showed that bullies do not necessarily "fit the stereotype of a psychologically maladjusted, marginalized individual" (p.168). On the contrary, Vaillancourt et al. (2003) found that high-power bullies were considered popular by their peers, even though they were disliked overall. The authors argue that bullying behavior is associated in many cases with a higher social status position within the peer group. In the same line, Vitaro et al.'s theoretical review distinguished subtypes of aggressive children according to the form (physical or relational) and the function (reactive or proactive) of aggression (Vitaro et al., 2006).

The heterogeneity presented by bullies also holds for victims. Children who are harassed do not necessarily fit the stereotypical picture of a weeping, maladjusted, and isolated child (Graham et al., 2003; Holt & Espelage, 2003; Goldbaum et al., 2003). For example, several studies (Paul & Cillessen, 2003; Swearer & Tam, 2003; Pellegrini et al., 1999) have found victimized children who are highly aggressive (also named bully/victims or aggressive victims). Another approach is presented by Graham and Juvonen (1998) by considering the reporting source of victimization. These authors distinguished peer-reported victims (consensually considered as such by their peers) and self-reported victims (who subjectively report the experience of being victimized). They found that the negative developmental outcomes associated with victimization differed for both groups. Self-perceived victimization was a predictor for loneliness, social anxiety, and low self-worth, whereas peer-perceived victimization was a predictor of rejection and negatively related to acceptance. In other words, self-reports of victimization were associated with psychological maladjustment, whereas peer reports of victimization were associated with social maladjustment, dimensions that do not necessarily overlap. Gender also plays a role in victim differences. Prior research comparing male and female victims has found male victims to be perceived by their teachers lower on peer sociability, school competence, and prosocial behavior; female victims reported more internalizing problems (Paul & Cillessen, 2003). Other authors also reported differences between male and female victims on conflict resolution strategies (Owens et al., 2005), victims' attitudes and responses to aggressive behavior (Tapper & Boulton, 2005), and victims' beliefs regarding causes of their victimization (Troop-Gordon & Ladd, 2005).

Despite all previous findings, less is known about the antecedents of bullying and victimization. In other words, what might lead a child to display aggression, or to become a target of aggression? Paul and Cillessen (2003) found that loneliness, anxiety, and disruptive behavior during fourth and fifth grades constitute risk factors for early adolescent victimization. Rodney et al. (2005) found that exposure to violent episodes also constitute a risk factor. Earlier, Olweus (1993, p. 35) argued as possible psychological causes that can lead an individual into becoming a bully, a "strong need for power and dominance; a certain degree of hostility toward the environment; satisfaction from inflicting injury and suffering upon other individuals. ..." On the other hand, school competence, social and academic self-efficacy, and peer sociability were considered protective factors against becoming a bully (Paul & Cillessen, 2003; Rodney et al., 2005). Scholars have also considered social-cognitive processes as mediating aggressive behaviors. For example, Crick and Dodge (1994) considered that aggressive behavior would be related to impairments in social skills. Particularly, aggressive children would have difficulties in understanding others' mental states, and therefore behave in dysfunctional ways. As argued by Boxer et al. (2005), higher social-cognitive processing constitutes a personal mediating component. However, a thorough understanding of how personal characteristics interact with social factors in promoting aggression or protecting from it is still lacking.

Implications for Prevention and Promotion

There are at least three avenues that should be addressed at the individual intervention level. First, there is a need for supporting children who are already victimized by their peers. These children should be provided with coping strategies and tools to ameliorate the negative outcomes of victimization (Nishina, 2004). Findings by Unnever and Cornell (2004) regarding victims' reporting of harassment directly underscore this. In other words, there is a silencing phenomenon that may reinforce all developmental risks that are related to victimization, and any intervention program should acknowledge this and offer appropriate channels for overcoming this silencing cycle. Also, because of the social nature of bullying (Salmivalli, 2001; Salmivalli et al., 2005), negative outcomes for all other children—bullies included—who are part of the peer culture should also be taken into account.

Second, following Crick and Dodge's hypothesis of a lack of social skills involved in bullying behavior, the answer is straightforward (Crick & Dodge,

1994). In the light of Boxer et al.'s findings of social-cognitive processes as mediating aggressive behaviors, social skills training seems to be a crucial dimension of intervention (Boxer et al., 2005). Programs that foster social-cognitive skills, such as perspective taking, emotional intelligence, and alternative problem-solving strategies, together with moral reasoning and meta-cognitive skills, constitute effective ways to reduce or stop aggressive behaviors.

Third, it is necessary to take into account what the expectations are regarding children's behavioral modifications and their implications. Usually, children tend to like other children who display similar characteristics, and dislike children with opposite profiles; this is known as homophily (Kupersmidt et al., 1995). In this sense, any attempt to modify individual characteristics or behaviors (i.e., aggressive behavior) would imply for children to modify their social profiles and even behave dissimilarly, that is, behave as children who they may even dislike (Nangle et al., 2004). The challenge, then, is how to make available for students alternative social behavioral patterns that exclude aggressive behaviors but at the same time fit their expectancies and the benefits they think they are gaining through bullying (Edwards et al., 2005).

Furthermore, any intervention targeted at the individual level needs to consider the heterogeneity among bullies and victims. Assuming homogeneity in their characteristics or their response, any action aimed to prevent the occurrence of aggressive situations might weaken intervention efficacy, and can even worsen the situation in particular cases. Interventions at the individual level should take into account risk and protective factors, but at the same time should address the variability and diversity of aggressive and victimized children, tailoring individual interventions to the particularities of each student in any given situation.

Dyadic Level

Factors influencing bullying and victimization can also be found at the interpersonal level. At this layer, the question about who bullies whom constitutes a central issue to better understand bullying and victimization (Rodkin & Berger, in press; Veenstra et al., 2005). However, to date few studies have included a dyadic approach. Coie et al. (1999) found differences between mutually aggressive dyads compared to asymmetric ones. More recently, Rodkin and Berger (in press) showed that bully–victim dyads differed depending on the gender of the victim. Boys who bullied other boys were portrayed as tough and popular and their victims as weak and displaying low social status, whereas in cross-gender bullying, bullies were rejected maladjusted boys harassing popular girls with adaptive social profiles.

The role that friends play regarding victimization has been the focus of several studies (Hamm & Faircloth, 2005; Hodges & Perry, 1999; Hodges et al., 1999, Hartup, 1996). For instance, Hodges et al. (1999) reported that having friends acts as a moderator of the victimization experience. Hodges et al. (1997) found a negative correlation between the number of friends that a child has and victimization. Moreover, they found that adjustment problems onset by victimization diminished as the number of friends increased. However, having friends per se does not constitute a protective factor against victimization. As Hartup (1996) warns, the friend's identity (his or her personal characteristics) and the friendship's quality are crucial factors that determine the degree to which friends can provide protection against victimization. Hodges et al. (1999) go further by concluding that "… having a friend characterized by high protection eliminated the relation of internalizing behaviors to changes in victimization, whereas having a friend characterized by low protection exacerbated this relation" (p. 98).

Regarding research on enmities, Abecassis (2003) hypothesized that enemies might constitute a developmental need. She argues, "the need for enemies may be most deeply tied to an individual's need to develop an integrated sense of self. Perhaps the most important function of enemies is to help children (and adults) deal with unacceptable parts of the self" (p. 19). Cross-gender enmities are interesting, in particular, because of their emergence during the middle childhood years in the context of a gender segregated peer culture in which positive behavior and attitudes toward the opposite gender are not sanctioned (Adler & Adler, 1998; Maccoby, 1998). In this context, cross-gender antipathies may be the only way legitimized by the peer group to express deep feelings toward members of the opposite sex in order to avoid peer censure (Rodkin et al., 2003).

The boundaries between cross-gender enmities and sexual harassment are unclear, but associations can be easily observed. Stein (1995) claimed that peer sexual harassment among children and adolescents is frequent, dangerous, and too often dismissed as romantic interest rather than bullying. As stated by the American Association of University Women Educational Foundation (2001), 81% of secondary students reported experiencing sexual harassment before sixth grade. Even though both boys and girls (79% and 83%, respectively) reported being sexually harassed at school, "girls reported being harassed more frequently, experiencing more severe types of harassment, and having more negative emotional reactions to harassment than boys" (Young & Raffaele Mendez, 2003, p. 13). Two important features of sexual harassment are highlighted by Young and Raffaele Mendez (2003). First, the occurrence of sexual harassment is determined by the impact of the behavior rather than the intent of it; in other words, sexual harassment is determined by its consequences for the victim, rather than by the intentions of the aggressor(s). Second, aggressors and their victims usually have different perspectives on how they perceive the harassing behavior; harassers may perceive their behavior as harmless teasing or flattering, while for the victim it may constitute an unpleasant, awkward, and humiliating situation. Unfortunately, the gendered cultures that arise in middle childhood may constitute fertile soil for the occurrence of sexual harassment (Duncan, 1999).

Implications for intervention at this level are discussed together with the next layer, the peer group and the classroom.

Peer Group/Classroom Level

The group nature of bullying has been stressed by many authors (Boulton, 1999; Malecki & Demaray, 2004; Nishina, 2004; Salmivalli et al., 2005). The participant role approach (Salmivalli & Voeten, 2004) understands bullying and victimization as a group phenomenon in which children play different roles: as bully, victim, assistant, reinforcer, defender, and outsider. From this perspective, all children are involved in bullying situations and their behavior either promotes or hinders bullying, therefore playing a social role within the group.

Peer norms play a central role in the social function of aggression (Chang, 2004; Salmivalli et al., 2005). Espelage et al. (2003) found that peer group bullying (understood as aggregated scores of group members) was a significant predictor of individual bullying at a later time, even after controlling for previous individual bullying behavior. In other words, despite the stability of individual bullying behavior, the group influence still explained a significant portion of its variance over and above individual aggression baseline scores after a 6-month period, which is in line with research on homophily. In the same line, Nesdale et al. (2005) found that exclusion group norms fostered a negative attitude and dislike toward out-group members, as compared to inclusion group norms. Moreover, regardless of the in-group norms of inclusion, children expressed dislike when the out-group threatened their group. Social structure also plays an important role in bullying and victimization. Schäfer et al. (2005) addressed the impact of fixed social hierarchical structures over the shift from primary to secondary school on bullies and victims among German students. Their study tested the hypothesis that differences in the social dynamics between primary—displaying power symmetry—and secondary—featuring a hierarchical structure based on power differentials in status—student peer cultures modulates the stability of bullying and victimization. They found that elementary classrooms that presented an earlier hierarchical structure promoted victimization by establishing fixed social positions, and therefore making victimization more stable. However, peer hierarchical structures did not mediate stability for bullies. As Schäfer et al. (2005, p. 333) point out, "showing aggression towards an already disliked (low-status) individual virtually manipulates social norms as aggression directed towards the victim appears more 'in line' with negative attitudes, thus probably less 'non-normative'." Seemingly, Allen et al. (2005) found that popularity can also be a risk factor in terms of the need of popular adolescents to match the expectancies of their peers regarding those behaviors that are approved within the peer group, which can easily be dysfunctional or even delinquent.

Implications for Prevention and Promotion

One difficulty for interventions at this level is that the peer culture is not accessible to adults who want to intervene; therefore, indirect intervention methods need to be explored. The first step is to gain a better knowledge of the peer culture and how aggressive behaviors are embedded within it. As argued by Nishina (2004), peer aggression may serve the social function of establishing a hierarchy that allows some social stability. Following this argument, one could think that bullying is a constitutive part of the social structure of peer groups. But, as Nishina (2004) points out, this is a dangerous and misleading assumption. The challenge is to find different methods that lead to positive outcomes and social structuring without validating abusive and damaging interpersonal relationships. A privileged sphere to do this is that of peer norms.

Salmivalli and Voeten (2004) found that group norms associated with bullying explain in part how children behave regarding bullying. Accordingly, Salmivalli et al. (2005) stress the group level as the key dimension to target any anti-bullying intervention. Their perspective is based on a participant role approach, understanding bullying and victimization as group phenomena in which all children are involved through different roles (see also Malecki & Demaray, 2004). Their intervention approach follows a three-step path: First is raising awareness. Even though most students have negative attitudes toward bullying, in actual bullying situations they do not behave accordingly and may even encourage the bully; negative attitudes toward bullying do not necessarily translate into positive intervening behaviors (Salmivalli et al., 2005). In this sense, this first step is aimed at raising awareness of children regarding feelings, behaviors, and attitudes toward bullying. Consistently, O'Moore and Minton (2005) argue that raising awareness of bullying behavior may by itself lead to an increase in the levels of reporting such behavior. The second step encourages self-reflection; following the participating roles in bullying, students can reflect on their own behavior. Finally, the third step involves a commitment to suppressing bullying behaviors, as well as modifying the role that other students play in any aggressive situation.

Quality of interpersonal relationships among group members should be another focus of anti-bullying interventions. Poor quality friendships may lead to an increase in victimization, whereas quality friendships are associated with positive developmental processes even if victimization occurs (Bukowski & Sippola, 2005). As argued by Garandeau and Cillessen (2006), a socially skilled bully operating in an environment with low interpersonal quality friendships could lead to an increase in the likelihood of victimization. Interpersonal relationships between students and also between students and teachers were found to be relevant factors by Leff et al. (2003). Different approaches have been proposed to foster positive interpersonal relationships. For example, particular activities such as after-school programs have been associated with the emergence of quality friendships (Hansen et al., 2003). Also, Espelage et al. (2004) note that promoting empathy is associated with decreases in bullying behavior. Other scholars advocate for prosocial classroom practices as important factors for anti-bullying interventions. For instance, Doll et al. (2004) argued that classroom routines and practices such as inclusive methodologies might protect students against bullying. Fostering and promoting positive student–teacher relationships have also been proposed as a key factor to prevent bullying (Aron & Milicic, 1999). Birch and Ladd (1997) proposed three dimensions of the student–teacher relationship that should be taken into account: closeness, dependency, and conflict. Close, independent, and nonconflict relations were described as most effective in fostering overall positive school adjustment.

Institutional Level

Several school characteristics have been associated with the occurrence of bullying and victimization. For example, Olweus (1993) reported higher bullying rates in middle and elementary schools compared to high schools. However, school size and/or class size, school location, and socioeconomic status seem not to directly influence bullying and victimization. Payne and Gottfredson (2004) argue that bullying promotes a climate of fear and intimidation throughout a school, where students feel unhappy and unwelcome. Seemingly, through their structure and climate, schools may reinforce fixed hierarchies through social stratification (Nishina, 2004), which, in turn, may reinforce bullying behaviors. Leff et al. (2003) identified four particularly relevant school/bullying components: the general school climate, order and discipline, student interpersonal relations, and student–teacher relations. Another main feature of school climate is the attitudes and beliefs that all school members have regarding certain topics and the concomitant relational pattern (Aron & Milicic, 1999). Payne and Gottfredson (2004, p. 163) found that teachers' attitudes related to bullying are directly associated with its occurrence. As they argue, "Schools in which teachers are more likely to discuss bullying with students, recognize bullying behavior, are interested in stopping bullying, and actually intervene in bullying incidents are less likely to have a bullying problem" (Payne & Gottfredson, 2004, p. 163). Students' negative attitudes toward bullying are also correlated with less bullying. However, as mentioned earlier, caution is that anti-bullying attitudes do not necessarily translate into intervening behavior, such as telling an adult or actually trying to stop the situation (Salmivalli et al., 2005). At a broader level, O'Moore and Minton (2005) highlight the importance of having all the school staff involved in policy development in order to improve the effectiveness of an anti-bullying program. As found by Salmivalli et al. (2005), and discussed later, there is, not surprisingly, a positive association between the degree of implementation of an anti-bullying program and its positive outcomes.

Teachers, who because of their position in the school social environment constitute the "firewall" to assess and intervene in bullying situations, are considered to play a central role in any intervention program. However, research has found that they are overwhelmed and lack adequate tools to identify and intervene in bullying situations (Aron & Milicic, 1999; Holt & Keyes, 2004). For instance, Leff et al. (1999) found that teachers were able to identify less than half of peer-reported bullies and victims, and that this mismatch between teacher and peer perceptions increased through middle and high school. However, the authors found that the accuracy of teachers in identifying bullies and victims increased when combining general education teacher reports with multiple art teacher reports. In other words, a consensus among staff members enhanced the ability of teachers to identify bullies and victims. Another hypothesis is that teachers may not recognize bullying episodes as a problem (Holt & Keyes, 2004), or may experience a feeling of having no power to make a difference in the peer group or the ability to deal with a bullying situation (Boulton, 1997). Consensually, several authors conclude that effective staff training is critical for any intervention program (Holt & Kayes, 2004; Olweus, 1993; Salmivalli et al., 2005).

Implications for Prevention and Promotion

Implications for interventions at the school level point to two main directions: school climate and staff training. Fixed hierarchies are reinforced by the school climate and structure; this stratification may be regarding age, grade, gender, or also more subtle factors such as particular areas or interests (e.g., sports) that are more valued and therefore possess a higher status within the school culture. The ways in which the school staff relate to each other or to the community is an important factor in school climate (Nishina, 2004; Thompson & Kyle, 2005). Actions to foster nurturing environments can be taken on three levels regarding school climate: the individual level, which includes self-concept, beliefs, attitudes, attributions, and expectancies of all participants in the school experience; the classroom level, interpersonal relationships and practices; and the institutional level, which can include administrative style, norms and regulations, and how all participants of the educational community are functionally integrated (Cornejo & Redondo, 2001). Intra-individual intervention activities might include raising aware- ness of negative attitudes and how they may be connected to negative behavioral outcomes (Salmivalli et al., 2005). Classroom level interventions might strive to develop inclusive methodologies that foster positive relationships and empathy among students such as cooperative work, role-playing, and quality circles (Doll et al., 2004; O'Moore & Minton, 2005). Institutional level interventions can include employing democratic administrative styles combined with shared and known school regulations (Aron & Milicic, 1999; Verhoek-Miller et al., 2002) as well as fostering meaningful partnerships between families and school staff (Sheridan et al., 2004), and the integration of extracurricular activities and culturally relevant experiences for youth (Rodney et al., 2005).

The other dimension of school level interventions involves teacher and school staff training. As argued by Salmivalli et al. (2005), a key factor for effective intervention is the degree of implementation of an intervention program, which is driven by teachers and school staff. Teacher accuracy in identifying and assessing bullying and victimization is a critical factor. Unfortunately, different studies have found that teachers do not accurately identify bullies and victims, as compared to student peer perceptions (Holt & Keyes, 2004; Leff et al., 1999). Lack of teacher skills in identifying bullies and victims is particularly troubling, considering that generally bullying is more likely to occur in areas with minimal or absent adult supervision and on unstructured settings, particularly the playground and lunchroom

(Leff et al., 2003). More broadly, the work of Little (2005) and Infantino and Little (2005) showed inconsistency between teachers' and students' perceptions of what constitutes problematic behavior. Teacher training should also include methodological issues on how to raise awareness among students, and how to lead group dynamics that foster an anti-bullying social climate.

Developmental Trajectories of Bullies and Victims

Are bullying and victimization stable over time? Olweus's review of several longitudinal studies found high stability coefficients for physical aggression (Olweus, 1978). More recently, Cillessen and Mayeux (2004) assessed the stability of physical and relational aggression by gender from fifth through ninth grade, finding all correlations to be significant (ranging from 0.33 to 0.87) and higher across shorter intervals and in later grades. Moderate to high stability coefficients for victimization have also been reported. Paul and Cillessen (2003) found victimization stability to be equally high in elementary ($r = 0.70$) and middle school ($r = 0.68$), and even across the transition ($r = 0.62$). Victimization stability correlates ranging between 0.60 and 0.91 from fourth to sixth grade were found by Troop-Gordon and Ladd (2005). Rodkin and Berger (in press) found that more than half of fourth graders identified as bullies and victims remained as such over a 6-month period. Moreover, as argued by Hodges and Perry (1999), victimization may become more stable over the course of development especially in early adolescence.

What are the developmental trajectories that accompany bullying and victimization? Paul and Cillessen's findings suggest an effect of victimization on later negative outcomes (Paul & Cillessen, 2003). These authors found negative short-term effects of victimization for girls, displaying higher levels of depression, anxiety, negative social self-perception, and self-reported disruptive behavior. Troop-Gordon and Ladd (2005) found that peer victimization is more related to internalizing than to externalizing problems. Particularly for boys, increases in peer victimization predicted significant decline in positive perception by their peers.

However, developmental correlates have also been found regarding adaptive characteristics, particularly social status (Boulton, 1999; Rodkin et al., 2000). As several studies point out, aggression has been associated with social centrality and prominence (LaFontana & Cillessen, 2002; Rodkin et al., 2000), but at the same time it has been associated with peer rejection (Parkhurst & Hopmeyer, 1998). Cillessen and Mayeux (2004) found that the correlation between the two forms of social status (i.e., social prominence and likability) declined steadily over time. Their analyses showed that physical aggression was decreasingly predictive of perceived popularity but increasingly less disliked, and relational aggression was increasingly predictive of perceived popularity but decreasingly predictive of liking. The authors conclude, "although physical aggression is increasingly less censured in the peer group, relational aggression is increasingly reinforced" (p. 159). In the same way, Rose et al. (2004) assessed the distinctive prospective relations between overt and relational aggression and popularity (as distinguished from social preference). The authors found relational aggression to be predictive of perceived popularity for girls—but not for boys—after controlling for overt aggression. In addition, perceived popularity was a significant predictor of later relational aggression for both boys and girls. These findings are in line with those of Bukowski et al. (2000), who found that adolescents show more attraction to aggressive peers than do young children. In other words, the attractive character of aggressive peers seems to rise during adolescence.

Implications for Prevention and Promotion

Adopting a developmental perspective requires that all layers identified previously are viewed not as static but rather in constant dynamic interaction (what Bronfenbrenner, 1979, called the *chronosystem*). In this sense, both developmental factors of the students and of the institution play a central role in the occurrence and severity of bullying and victimization. Therefore, it is reasonable to think that differing interventions should target different grade levels. For instance, Salmivalli et al. (2005) found positive results for their anti-bullying intervention program in fourth grade, whereas in fifth grade the effects, even though in the same direction, were not as significant.

Time is also a critical factor for schools; the implementation of any program needs a certain amount of time to be absorbed by the school culture, and this may depend on several organizational factors that determine how it is integrated into the school system. Specific interventions focused on particular situations and administered by outsiders may not get integrated into the school culture and remain as an "outsider" program. In this sense, the stability of the outcomes is not assured. On the other hand, interventions that become embedded in the curriculum and in the organizational system may be more effective in improving the school climate and therefore have long-term positive effects (Limber, 2004; Salmivalli et al., 2005). As argued by Orpinas et al. (2003, p. 441), "Bullying prevention programs are more likely to be incorporated into sustained practice when teachers and administrators have played a key role in the development and implementation of the program."

Steps to Intervention

There is consistency among scholars that multilevel approaches are the most effective way in developing and implementing anti-bullying interventions (Aron & Milicic, 1999; Espelage & Swearer, 2004; Limber, 2004; Nishina, 2004; O'Moore & Minton, 2005; Olweus, 1993; Payne & Gottfredson, 2004; Salmivalli et al., 2005; Smith et al., 2003; Thompson & Kyle, 2005). However, a perfect prepackaged program to prevent school violence does not exist since effective interventions should be local programs that fit the school culture and idiosyncrasy addressing a school's particular weaknesses and strengths (Edwards et al., 2005).

Smith et al. (2003), in their meta-analysis of intervention programs against bullying, identified several factors common to successful interventions. Among the success factors were the type of intervention (multilevel interventions were found more effective), the length of the program (better results were found for longer programs), the support of researchers, the time and effort invested by schools, the age of students (better results were found with elementary school students, maybe because they are more willing to accept teacher authority and curriculum activities), the program comprehensiveness (interventions that were part of more comprehensive programs were found to be more effective), and student gender (girls were found to be more receptive to interventions). Along the same lines, Leff et al. (2001) identified as key factors for any intervention program the need for designing comprehensive programs combining universal prevention with specific selective interventions, including an adequate monitoring process and empirical evaluation. They also point out the need for providing services within naturalistic settings; in other words, the efforts to prevent aggression should move beyond the classroom setting to other arenas where bullying is likely to occur. Moreover, to be more effective, anti-bullying interventions should become part of the institutional culture, and not just constitute specific cross-sectional interventions (Aron & Milicic, 1999; Olweus, 1993).

There is a growing scientific consensus on effective research-based prevention programs. However, there is decidedly a lack of research concerning the implementation of bullying prevention programs in schools. In one study, Durlak (1997) analyzed over 1,200 prevention studies and noted only ~5% provided any data on implementation. While there are valid quantitative methods to study the impact of a given program in an individual school, Durlak (1998) states accurately that without attention to the variability in program implementation, all statistical conclusions based on comparisons between programs are suspect since no internal, external, or construct validity can be claimed. Since bullying prevention programs are best implemented through local design, there will always be significant variation between schools. The difficulty in quantitative analysis of bullying prevention programs can be overcome with qualitative attention to program implementation factors that can be identified and analyzed. Fagan and Mihalic (2003) and Elliot and Mihalic (2004) through work done by the University of Colorado at Boulder's Center for the Study and Prevention of Violence identify some key implementation factors. Fagan and Elliot and Mihalic identify such factors as school readiness, the presence of a local champion of the program, the enthusiastic support of administrators and staff, quality training, and integration of the program into the school curriculum and community. These factors are also what we have found to be decisive factors in the success of implementing bullying prevention programs that we engage in as consultants to schools.

Schools must be ready to accept the complex and long-term process of whole school bullying prevention. Some key elements in a school's readiness for intervention are a local champion of the program, administrative support and buy-in, as well as staff support and buy-in (Elliot & Mihalic, 2004). Attention should be paid to distinct differences between school staff members championing a bullying prevention program versus the role of the outside consultant. In many cases, lack of funding, coupled with increases in caseloads of counselors, social workers, and school psychologists, means that the work of implementing a comprehensive research-based bullying prevention program falls to outside consultants. An outside consultant can only begin work in conjunction with a resident champion of the prevention program. This member is the key to the consultant gaining admission and acceptance into the school building (Fagan & Mihalic, 2003). In our work, we are very much aware that the program is to be created in close partnership with the initial individual who requested our consulting services. It is the building champion that is the face and coordinator of the entire project. We strive to develop and reinforce the leadership of the local champion in the schools for which we consult.

Any project must have the full and unconditional support of the school administrators. It is the administrators who will provide the authority, coordination, and funding for any program (Orpinas & Horne, 2006). In Fagan and Mihalic's study, success was directly related to administrative support in program adoption, integration of the program into the curriculum, and actively ensuring that modules are taught in the classroom (Fagan & Mihalic, 2003). Limber (2004) associates the principal's support in actively ensuring programs were implemented in the classroom as important to the overall adoption of the program. In our work, we meet with the local champion first and the principal second. We do not proceed without the explicit and strong support of the building principal. We make it clear that we are consulting and are agents of first and foremost the building administration. In schools, no decisions can be made further along in a program without the express consent and support of the principal. We strive to keep the school administration informed of all decisions at all times.

At this point, before moving on to faculty and staff buy-in, it is imperative to note that a baseline survey should be administered before any dialogue with additional building personnel or students. Initiating even a preliminary discussion of bullying within the school risks confounding the baseline survey.

As noted, any prevention program requires teachers as principal implementers. High quality prevention programs are related to high teacher involvement in planning and implementation (Gottfredson & Gottredson, 2002). Without the buy-in, support, and motivation of teachers, a comprehensive school-wide program cannot be effective (Fagan & Mihalic, 2003; Hunter et al., 2001). In our prevention programs, we make no program decisions without an initial presentation to the teachers usually in the context of a staff meeting. For us, the purpose of this meeting is threefold. The first purpose is to share the results of the baseline survey and to discuss the results if they point to an actual problem within the school. If it is agreed that there is a problem, the second purpose of the staff meeting presentation is to present a brief overview of bullying and its negative developmental consequences and to present an example of a comprehensive solution to preventing and dealing with bullying. The third purpose is to recruit a cadre of the most interested teachers to join in the process of creating a comprehensive bullying prevention program for the school. It is critical to us that there is an understanding that no decisions have been made without teacher awareness and input and that faculty contribution is needed from the outset of the program. The process of an initial presentation is ideally repeated to all members of the school staff, including office, maintenance, transportation, and food personnel.

It is essential to engage the whole school community in dialogue in order to consensually establish the groundwork in developing a building-based committee to develop and coordinate the bullying prevention program. It is the work of this committee that will ultimately shape and run the program suited to the particular school (Limber, 2004; Olweus et al., 1999).

In our programs, the school committee, once established, is given extensive education on scientific findings on bullying and bullying prevention strategies. This allows the committee to create a research-based prevention program. Once committee members have studied the problem, the process of program design can begin. Two main goals should be pursued: First, the overarching program philosophy and goals must be articulated in order to guide in designing the intervention (Orpinas & Horne, 2006). Particular activities to articulate goals can include a questionnaire given to all members of the school community (students, school staff, and parents), observational and action-research methodologies. As stated previously, the best bullying prevention programs maintain a philosophy and goals that emphasize values of warmth and caring to which the entire school should adhere.

We believe that care must be taken by those charged with initiating an intervention program to work with all participants in order to gain consensus and maintain an impartial position and not to take sides between differing school staff. Even though the team in charge of the intervention may have some insights and ideas to contribute, it is essential that the entire school community own the program. In the long run, the program needs to remain effective even after the committee disbands and the outside consulting team leaves. This longevity requires the school culture to integrate and internalize the intervention program (Fagan & Mihalic, 2003). The design of the program should take particular care in considering the characteristics of the school environment, including opportunities (e.g., community efforts and activities available in contributing to a positive development) and menaces (e.g., the presence of gangs and high teacher rotation).

Two dimensions should be included in the design of the program: A whole-school policy on bullying, including general measures (i.e., a discipline code, adequate opportunity for children to share their feelings about bullying, staff training, decision on particular anti-bullying materials to be used, and adequate opportunity for expressing the consensual ideal toward which the school community is working), and specific activities and measures tailored for the particular setting (i.e., in-class activities, after-school activities, playground improvements, and staff supervision). Decisions should be made regarding how the program will be implemented on different levels such as individual, classroom, and school. Care must be taken to plan differentially according to the age of the students in order to make the intervention developmentally relevant.

We begin the implementation phase at the start of a new academic year. The entire staff receives as extensive a training on the locally adapted bullying prevention program as can be arranged. The training is done as part of teacher orientation for the new academic year. While there are a myriad of competing topic sessions for new and returning teachers, the enthusiastic support of the principal can translate into sufficient time to train teachers in the specifics of their new bullying prevention program.

Once school officially begins and students enter the building, an all-student assembly is a crucial step in communicating the behavioral expectations of the new program to the students. This step requires the cooperation of the entire staff. The assembly also forces the school to publicly announce its bullying prevention program and articulate the behavioral goals of the program as well as the associated discipline policy. This is the final step in creating universal buy-in from the members of the building, which most importantly now includes the students.

Beyond the school, our programs also include training for parents and so there is a unified message from the school to home regarding bullying prevention guidelines. Details must not be overlooked in planning for parent meetings. Care must be taken to listen and incorporate the felt needs of the parents into the program. Parents must also have buy-in and their views must be solicited and when possible incorporated into the program. Both day and evening sessions are a must to obtain the widest participation from parents. Through experience we have found that when scheduling an evening session food and childcare are desirable components to achieving a well-attended parent session.

Limber (2004) addresses the need to broaden anti-bullying efforts to include the surrounding community. Limber discusses three key components of community involvement. She stresses the primary need to inform residents of the local community of the school's bullying prevention programs using community meetings and the media. She suggests involving the local community by volunteer opportunities for supervision of students as well as asking local business owners for material donations to the program. She also advocates that bullying prevention efforts should be encouraged to move beyond the school and into after-school programs, summer camps, as well as community and religious organizations. In our work, we add an additional layer of education and training by inviting key members of the community to informational sessions, including religious and civic leaders as well as law enforcement, in order to amplify the central goals of the prevention program into the community setting. Local media plays an important role for us in disseminating the program's goals and expectations to the larger community.

Once a program has been in implementation, troubleshooting is required. Researchers have identified many obstacles to the successful implementation of prevention programs. Limber (2004) cites the resistance of staff and students in accepting that bullying is a problem and not just a rite of passage. While certainly this attitude is waning in society with each passing violent episode in the schools, the attitude is still evident in some schools. Coupled with dismissal of bullying as a problem is denial by school staff that their particular building has a problem.

Drake et al. (2004) report that of 378 principals responding to their survey, only 2 (0.5%) felt that the level of bullying in their schools was worse than the average in US elementary schools. The overwhelming majority felt that their schools fell below the national average. Some schools that feel they have a bullying problem attempt homegrown anti-bullying efforts. Some principals and teachers feel that they have done enough and that there is no need for comprehensive research-based programs. Limber (2004) cites the tendency for schools to seek short-term and simple solutions to bullying problems. In our work, we observe the strong tendency of teachers to seek more punitive measures by administrators. This is akin to the desire of the patrolman for lengthy prison sentences handed down by judges for their arrestees. Administrators cannot punish every act of transgression, and there is enough evidence that strict policies such as "zero tolerance" may be detrimental to controlling bullying. Mulvey and Cauffman (2001) argue that harsh punitive measures may decrease bullying reports from students and staff. Another troubling aspect bullying prevention efforts is reported by Fagan and Mihalic (2003) in their study of 70 sites involved in the Life Skills Training Program for violence prevention. The authors cite one of the main barriers to program implementation as the perception of teachers and administrators that intervention programs take time away from "core" academic subjects.

Successful implementation will depend mainly on the design and the particular activities that each school defines as desirable. However, the need of a good monitoring process should be stressed. The committee should plan regular meetings in order to monitor the implementation of the program and discuss any difficulties or adjustments that should be made. Instruments should be developed to keep records of the implementation and any other relevant feature.

Finally, the Evaluation phase of the program should establish objective measures regarding the effectiveness of the intervention. Results should be considered in light of the baseline bullying level (determined during the diagnosis phase). Seeking comparison with control schools is ideal. The evaluation should consider as indicators of success those items that were considered by the school community as features of the consensually derived expectation for positive outcomes. Feedback should be provided to all members of the school community, tailored to their roles within the school. Shortcomings of the program should be pointed out, and the committee should discuss ways to keep the program functioning as an integral and sustained part of the school curriculum. Caution is in order to not look at program success on a monthly or annual basis. There must be a realization that in the real world of schools, effectiveness of any program will not be linear but rather some years will be better than others (Berger, 2007). It is only with this long-term multiyear view that bullying prevention programs can be accurately evaluated.

References

Abecassis, M. (2003). I hate you just the way you are: Exploring the formation, maintenance and need for enemies. *New Directions for Child and Adolescent Development*, 102, 5–22.

Adler, P. A. & Adler, P. (1998). *Peer Power. Preadolescent Culture and Identity.* New Jersey: Rutgers University Press.

Allen, J., Porter, M., McFarland, F., Marsh, P., & McElhaney, K. (2005). The two faces of adolescents' success with peers: Adolescent popularity, social adaptation, and deviant behavior. *Child Development*, 76, 747–760.

American Association of University Women Educational Foundation (2001). *Hostile Hallways: Bullying, Teasing, and Sexual Harassment in School.* Washington, DC: American Association of University Women.

Aron, A. & Milicic, N. (1999). *Clima social escolar y desarrollo personal: Un programa de mejoramiento.* Santiago: Andres Bello.

Bellmore, A., Witkow, M., Graham, S., & Juvonen, J. (2004). Beyond the individual: The impact of ethnic context and classroom behavioral norms on victims' adjustment. *Developmental Psychology*, 40, 1159–1172.

Berger, C., Milicic, N., Alcalay, L., & Torretti, A. (2001). Adolescencia y Género: la voz y la fuerza de esta etapa vital. *Revista Sociotam*, 11, 9–42.

Berger, S. K. (2007) Update on bullying at school: Science forgotten? *Developmental Review*, 27, 90–126.

Birch, S. & Ladd, G. (1997). The teacher-child relationship and children's early school adjustment. *Journal of School Psychology*, 35, 61–79.

Boulton, M. J. (1997). Teachers' views on bullying: Definitions, attitudes and ability to cope. *British Journal of Educational Psychology*, 67, 223–233.

Boulton, M. J. (1999). Concurrent and longitudinal relations between children's playground behavior and social preference, victimization, and bullying. *Child Development*, 70, 944–954.

Boxer, P., Goldstein, S., Musher-Eizenman, D., Dubow, E., & Heretick, D. (2005). Developmental issues in school-based aggression prevention from a social-cognitive perspective. *The Journal of Primary Prevention*, 26, 383–400.

Bronfenbrenner, U. (1979). *The Ecology of Human Development.* Cambridge, MA: Harvard University Press.

Bukowski, W. & Sippola, L. (2005). Friendship and development: Putting the most human relationship in its place. In L. Jensen & R. Larson (Eds.), *New Horizons in Developmental Theory and Research* (pp. 91–98). San Francisco: Jossey-Bass.

Bukowski, W. M., Sippola, L. K., & Newcomb, A. F. (2000). Variations in patterns of attraction to same- and other-sex peers during early adolescence. *Developmental Psychology*, 36, 147–154.

Chang, L. (2004). The role of classroom norms in contextualizing the relations of children's social behaviors to peer acceptance. *Developmental Psychology*, 40, 691–702.

Cillessen, A. H. N. & Mayeux, L. (2004). From censure to reinforcement: Developmental changes in the association between aggression and social status. *Child Development*, 75, 147–163.

Coie, J., Cillessen, A., Dodge, K., Hubbard, J., Schwartz, D., Lemerise, E., & Bateman, H. (1999). It takes two to fight: A test of relational factors and a method for assessing aggressive dyads. *Developmental Psychology*, 35, 1179–1188.

Cornejo, R. & Redondo, J. (2001). El clima escolar percibido por los alumnos de ensenanza media. *Ultima Decada*, 15, 11–52.

Crick, N. & Dodge, K. (1994). A review and reformulation of social information-processing mechanisms in children's social adjustment. *Psychological Bulletin*, 115, 74–101.

Crick, N. & Grotpeter, J. K. (1995). Relational aggression, gender, and social-psychological adjustment. *Child Development*, 66, 710–722.

Dishion, T. J., Spracklen, K. M., Andrews, D. W., & Patterson, G. R. (1996). Deviancy training in male adolescent friendships. *Behavior Therapy*, 27, 373–390.

Doll, B., Song, S., & Siemers, E. (2004). Classroom ecologies that support or discourage bullying. In D. Espelage & S. Swearer (Eds.), *Bullying in American Schools: A Social-Ecological Perspective on Prevention and Intervention* (pp. 161–183). Mahwah, NJ: Lawrence Erlbaum Associates.

Drake, J. A., Price, J. H., Telljohann, S. K., & Funk, J. B. (2004) Principals' perceptions and practices of school bullying prevention activities. *Health Education & Behavior*, 31, 372–387.

Duncan, N. (1999). *Sexual Bullying: Gender Conflict and Pupil Culture in Secondary Schools*. New York: Routledge.

Durlak, J. A. (1997). *Successful Prevention Programs for Children and Adolescents*. New York: Plenum.

Durlak, J. A. (1998). Why program implementation is important. *Journal of Prevention and Intervention in the Community*, 17, 5–18.

Edwards, D., Hunt, M., Meyers, J., Grogg, K., & Jarrett, O. (2005). Acceptability and student outcomes of a violence prevention curriculum. *The Journal of Primary Prevention*, 26, 401–418.

Elias, M. & Zins, J. (2003). Bullying, other forms of peer harassment, and victimization in schools: Issues for school psychology research and practice. *Journal of Applied School Psychology*, 19, 1–6.

Elliot, D. & Mihalic, S. (2004). Issues in disseminating and replicating effective prevention programs. *Prevention Science*, 5, 47–53.

Espelage, D. & Swearer, S. (Eds.). (2004). *Bullying in American Schools. A Social-Ecological Perspective on Prevention and Intervention*. Mahwah, NJ: Lawrence Erlbaum Associates.

Espelage, D., Holt, M., & Henkel, R. (2003). Examination of peer-group contextual effects on aggression during early adolescence. *Child Development*, 74, 205–220.

Espelage, D., Mebane, S., & Swearer, S (2004). Gender differences in bullying: Moving beyond mean level differences. In D. Espelage & S. Swearer (Eds.), *Bullying in American Schools: A Social-Ecological Perspective on Prevention and Intervention* (pp. 15–35). Mahwah, NJ: Lawrence Erlbaum Associates.

Estell, D., Farmer, T., Pearl, R., Van Acker, R., & Rodkin, P. C. (2003). Heterogeneity in the relationship between popularity and aggression: Individual, group, and classroom influences. *New Directions for Child and Adolescent Development*, 101, 75–85.

Fagan, A. & Mihalic, S. (2003). Strategies for enhancing the adoption of school-based prevention programs: Lessons learned from the blueprints for violence prevention replications of the life skills training program. *Journal of Community Psychology*, 31, 235–253.

Garandeau, C. & Cillessen, A. (2006). From indirect to invisible aggression: A conceptual view on bullying and peer group manipulation. *Aggression and Violent Behavior*, 11, 641–654.

García, M. & Madriaza, P. (2005). Sentido y sinsentido de la violencia escolar: Análisis cualitativo del discurso de estudiantes chilenos. *Psykhe*, 14, 165–180.

Goldbaum, S., Craig, W., Pepler, D., & Connolly, J. (2003). Developmental trajectories of victimization: Identifying risk and protective factors. *Journal of Applied School Psychology*, 19, 139–156.

Gottfredson, G. D. & Gottredson, D. C. (2002). Quality of school-based prevention programs: Results from a national survey. *Journal of Research in Crime and Delinquency*, 39, 3–35.

Graham, S. & Juvonen, J. (1998). Self-blame and peer victimization in middle school: An attributional analysis. *Developmental Psychology*, 34, 587–599.

Graham, S., Bellmore, A., & Juvonen, J. (2003). Peer victimization in Middle school: When self- and peer views diverge. *Journal of Applied School Psychology*, 19, 117–138.

Gubbins, V. & Berger, C. (2004). Bases, conceptos y estrategias: una reflexión desde la perspectiva del desarrollo familiar. In V. Gubbins & C. Berger (Eds.), *Pensar el Desarrollo Familiar: una Perspectiva Transdisciplinaria*. Santiago: Lom Ediciones.

Hamm, J. & Faircloth, B. (2005). The role of friendship in adolescents' sense of school belonging. *New Directions for Child and Adolescent Development*, 107, 61–78.

Hansen, D., Larson, R., & Dworkin, J. (2003). What adolescents learn in organized youth activities: A survey of self-reported developmental experiences. *Journal of Research on Adolescence*, 13, 25–55.

Hartup, W. (1996). The company they keep: Friendships and their developmental significance. *Child Development*, 67, 1–13.

Hawley, P. H., Little, T. D., & Rodkin, P. C. (Eds.). (2007). *Aggression and Adaptation: The Bright Side to Bad Behavior*. Mahwah, NJ: Lawrence Erlbaum Associates.

Hodges, E., Malone, M., & Perry, D. (1997). Individual risk and social risk as interacting determinants of victimization in the peer group. *Developmental Psychology*, 33, 1032–1039.

Hodges, E. & Perry, D. (1999). Personal and interpersonal antecedents and consequences of victimization by peers. *Journal of Personality and Social Psychology*, 76, 677–685.

Hodges, E., Boivin, M., Vitaro, F., & Bukowski, W. (1999). The power of friendship: Protection against an escalating cycle of peer victimization. *Developmental Psychology*, 35, 94–101.

Holt, M. & Espelage, D. (2003). A cluster analytic investigation of victimization among high school students: Are profiles differentially associated with psychological symptoms and school belonging? *Journal of Applied School Psychology*, 19, 81–98.

Holt, M. & Keyes, M. (2004). Teachers' attitudes toward bullying. In D. Espelage & S. Swearer (Eds.), *Bullying in American Schools: A Social-Ecological Perspective on Prevention and Intervention* (pp. 121–139). Mahwah, NJ: Lawrence Erlbaum Associates.

Hunter, L., Elias, M. J., & Norris J. (2001). School-based violence prevention: Challenges and lessons learned from an action research project. *Journal of School Psychology*, 39, 161–175.

Infantino, J. & Little, E. (2005). Students' perceptions of classroom behaviour problems and the effectiveness of different disciplinary methods. *Educational Psychology*, 25, 491–508.

Juvonen, J., Nishina, A., & Graham, S. (2001). Self-views versus peer perceptions of victim status among early adolescents. In J. Juvonen & S. Graham (Eds.), *Peer Harassment in School: The Plight of the Vulnerable and Victimized* (pp. 105–124). New York: Guilford.

Kindlon, D. & Thompson, M. (1999). *Raising Cain: Protecting the Emotional Life of Boys*. New York: Ballantine.

Kupersmidt, J. B., DeRossier, M., & Patterson, C. P. (1995). Similarity as the basis for children's friendships: The roles of sociometric status, aggressive and withdrawn behavior, academic achievement, and demographic characteristics. *Journal of Social and Personal Relationships*, 12, 439–452.

LaFontana, K. M. & Cillessen, A. H. N. (2002). Children's perceptions of popular and unpopular peers: A multi-method assessment. *Developmental Psychology*, 38, 635–647.

Leff, S., Power, T., Costigan, T., & Manz, P. (2003). Assessing the climate of the playground and lunchroom: Implications for bullying prevention programming. *School Psychology Review*, 32, 418–430.

Leff, S., Power, T., Manz, P., Costigan, T., & Nabors, L. (2001). School based aggression prevention programs for young children: Current status and implications for violence prevention. *School Psychology Review*, 30, 344–362.

Leff, S., Kupersmidt, J., Patterson, C., & Power, T. (1999). Factors influencing teacher identification of peer bullies and victims. *School Psychology Review*, 28, 505–517.

Limber, S. (2004). Implementation of the Olweus Bullying Prevention Program in American schools: Lessons learned from the field. In D. Espelage & S. Swearer (Eds.), *Bullying in American Schools: A Social-Ecological Perspective on Prevention and Intervention* (pp. 351–363). Mahwah, NJ: Lawrence Erlbaum Associates.

Little, E. (2005). Secondary school teachers' perceptions of students' problem behaviours. *Educational Psychology*, 25(4), 369–377.

Maccoby, E. E. (1998). *The Two Sexes: Growing up Apart, Coming Together*. Cambridge, MA: Harvard University Press.

Malecki, C. & Demaray, M. (2004). The role of social support in the lives of bullies, victims, and bully-victims. In D. Espelage & S. Swearer (Eds.), *Bullying in American Schools: A Social-Ecological Perspective on Prevention and Intervention* (pp. 211–225). Mahwah, NJ: Lawrence Erlbaum Associates.

McMaster, L. E., Connolly, J., Pepler, D., & Craig, W. M. (2002). Peer to peer sexual harassment in early adolescence: A developmental perspective. *Development and Psychopathology*, 14, 91–105.

Mulvey, E. P. & Cauffman, E. (2001). The inherent limits of predicting school violence. *American Psychologist*, 56, 797–802.

Nangle, D., Erdley, C., Zeff, K., Stanchfield, L., & Gold, J. (2004). Opposites do not attract: Social status and behavior-style concordances and discordances among children and the peers who like or dislike them. *Journal of Abnormal Child Psychology*, 32, 425–434.

Nansel, T., Haynie, D., & Simons-Morton, B. (2003). The association of bullying and victimization with middle school adjustment. *Journal of Applied School Psychology*, 19, 45–62.

Nesdale, D., Maass, A., Durkin, K., & Griffiths, J. (2005). Group norms, threat, and children's racial prejudice. *Child Development*, 76, 652–663.

Nishina, A. (2004). A theoretical review of bullying: Can it be eliminated? In C. Sanders & G. Phye (Eds.), *Bullying: Implications for the Classroom* (pp. 36–62). San Diego: Elsevier Academic Press.

O'Connell, P., Pepler, D., & Craig, W. (1999). Peer involvement in bullying: Insights and challenges for intervention. *Journal of Adolescence*, 22, 437–452.

Olweus, D. (1978). *Aggression in the Schools: Bullies and Whipping Boys*. Washington, DC: Hemisphere Press.

Olweus, D. (1993). *Bullying at School*. Oxford: Blackwell Publishers.

Olweus, D. (2001). Peer harassment: A critical analysis and some important issues. In J. Juvonen & S. Graham (Eds.), *Peer Harassment in School: The Plight of the Vulnerable and Victimized* (pp. 1–20). New York: Guilford.

Olweus, D., Limber, S., & Mihalic, S. (1999). *The Bullying-Prevention Program: Blueprints for Violence Prevention*. Boulder, CO: Center for the Study and Prevention of Violence.

O'Moore, A. & Minton, S. (2005). Evaluation of the effectiveness of an anti-bullying programme in primary schools. *Aggressive Behavior*, 31, 609–622.

Orpinas, P. & Horne, A. (2006). *Bullying Prevention: Creating a Positive School Climate and Developing Social Competence*. Washington, DC: American Psychological Association.

Orpinas, P., Horne, A., & Staniszewski, D. (2003). School bullying: Changing the problem by changing the school. *School Psychology Review*, 32, 431–444.

Owens, L., Daly, A., & Slee, P. (2005). Sex and age differences in victimization and conflict resolution among adolescents in a south Australian school. *Aggressive Behavior*, 31, 1–12.

Parkhurst, J. T. & Hopmeyer, A. (1998). Sociometric popularity and peer-perceived popularity: Two distinct dimensions of peer status. *Journal of Early Adolescence*, 18, 125–144.

Paul, J. & Cillessen, T. (2003). Dynamics of peer victimization in early adolescence: Results from a four-year longitudinal study. *Journal of Applied School Psychology*, 19, 25–44.

Payne, A. & Gottfredson, D. (2004). Schools and bullying: School factors related to bullying and school based bullying interventions. In C. Sanders & G. Phye (Eds.), *Bullying: Implications for the Classroom* (pp. 159–176). San Francisco: Elsevier Academic Press.

Pellegrini, A. D. (1998). Bullies and victims in school: A review and call for papers. *Journal of Applied Developmental Psychology*, 19, 165–176.

Pellegrini, A. D. (2001). A longitudinal study of heterosexual relationships, aggression, and sexual harassment during the transition from primary school through middle school. Applied *Developmental Psychology*, 22, 119–133.

Pellegrini, A. D. (2002). Bullying and victimization in middle school: A dominance relations perspective. *Educational Psychologist*, 37, 151–163.

Pellegrini, A. D., Bartini, M., & Brooks, F. (1999). School bullies, victims, and aggressive victims: Factors relating to group affiliation and victimization in early adolescence. *Journal of Educational Psychology*, 91, 216–224.

Rodkin, P. C. (2004). Peer ecologies of aggression and bullying. In D. Espelage & S. Swearer (Eds.), *Bullying in American Schools: A Social-Ecological Perspective on Prevention and Intervention* (pp. 87–106). Mahwah, NJ: Lawrence Erlbaum Associates.

Rodkin, P. C. & Berger, C. (in press). Who bullies whom? Social asymmetries by victim gender. *International Journal of Behavioral Development*.

Rodkin, P. C. & Fischer, K. (2003). Sexual harassment and the cultures of childhood: Developmental, domestic violence, and legal perspectives. *Journal of Applied School Psychology*, 19, 177–196.

Rodkin, P. C. & Hodges, E. (2003). Bullies and victims in the peer ecology: Four questions for psychologists and school professionals. *School Psychology Review*, 32, 384–400.

Rodkin, P. C., Farmer, T. W., Pearl, R., & Van Acker, R. (2000). Heterogeneity of popular boys: Antisocial and prosocial configurations. *Developmental Psychology*, 36, 14–24.

Rodkin, P. C., Pearl, R., Farmer, T. W., & Van Acker, R. (2003). Enemies in the gendered societies of middle childhood: Prevalence, stability, associations with social status, and aggression. *New Directions for Child and Adolescent Development*, 102, 73–88.

Rodney, L., Johnson, D., & Srivastava, R. (2005). The impact of culturally relevant violence prevention models on school-age youth. *The Journal of Primary Prevention*, 26, 439–454.

Rose, A. J., Swenson, L. P., & Waller, E. M. (2004). Overt and relational aggression and perceived popularity: Developmental differences in concurrent and prospective relations. *Developmental Psychology*, 40, 378–387.

Salmivalli, C. (2001).Group view on victimization: Empirical findings and their implications. In J. Juvonen & S. Graham (Eds.), *Peer Harassment in School: The Plight of the Vulnerable and the Victimized* (pp. 398–419). New York: Guilford.

Salmivalli, C. & Voeten, M. (2004). Connections between attitudes, group norms, and behaviors associated with bullying in schools. *International Journal of Behavioral Development*, 28, 246–258.

Salmivalli, C., Kaukiainen, A., & Voeten, M. (2005). Anti-bullying intervention: Implementation and outcome. *British Journal of Educational Psychology*, 75, 465–487.

Schäfer, M., Korn, S., Brodbeck, F., Wolke, D., & Schulz, H. (2005). Bullying roles in changing contexts: The stability of victim and bully roles from primary to secondary school. *International Journal of Behavioral Development*, 29, 323–335.

Schwartz, D. (2000). Subtypes of victims and aggressors in children's peer groups. *Journal of Abnormal Child Psychology*, 28, 181–192.

Schwartz, D., Proctor, L. J., & Chien, D. H. (2001). The aggressive victim of bullying: Emotional and behavioral dysregulation as a pathway to victimization by peers. In J. Juvonen & S. Graham (Eds.), *Peer Harassment in School: The Plight of the Vulnerable and Victimized* (pp. 145–174). New York: Guilford.

Sheridan, S., Warnes, E., & Dowd, S. (2004). Home-School collaboration and bullying: An ecological approach to increase social competence in children and youth. In D. Espelage & S. Swearer (Eds.), *Bullying in American Schools: A Social-Ecological Perspective on Prevention and Intervention* (pp. 245–267). Mahwah, NJ: Lawrence Erlbaum Associates.

Smith, P. K., Cowie, H., Olafsson, R. F., & Liefooghe, A. P. (2002). Definitions of bullying: A comparison of terms used, and age and gender differences, in a fourteen-country international comparison. *Child Development*, 73, 1119–1133.

Smith, P. K., Ananiadou, K., & Cowie, H. (2003). Interventions to reduce school bullying. *Canadian Journal of Psychiatry*, 48, 591–599.

Solberg, M. E. & Olweus, D. (2003). Prevalence estimation of school bullying with the Olweus bully/victim questionnaire. *Aggressive Behavior*, 29, 239–268.

Stein, N. (1995). Sexual harassment in schools: The public performance of gendered violence. *Harvard Educational Review*, 65, 145–162.

Stein, N. (1999). *Classrooms and Courtrooms: Facing Sexual Harassment in K-12 Schools*. New York: Teachers College Press.

Swearer, S. & Espelage, D. (2004). A Social-ecological framework of bullying among youth. In D. Espelage & S. Swearer (Eds.), *Bullying in American Schools: A Social-Ecological Perspective on Prevention and Intervention* (pp. 1–15). Mahwah, NJ: Lawrence Erlbaum Associates.

Swearer, S. & Tam, P. (2003). Perceptions and attitudes toward bullying in middle school youth: A developmental examination across the bully/victim continuum. *Journal of Applied School Psychology*, 19, 63–79.

Swearer, S., Grills, A., Haye, K., & Cary, P. (2004). Internalizing problems in students involved in bullying and victimization: Implications for intervention. In D. Espelage & S. Swearer (Eds.), *Bullying in American Schools: A Social-Ecological Perspective on Prevention and Intervention* (pp. 63–83). Mahwah, NJ: Lawrence Erlbaum Associates.

Tapper, K. & Boulton, M. (2005). Victim and peer group responses to different forms of aggression among primary school children. *Aggressive Behavior*, 31, 238–253.

Thompson, S. & Kyle, K. (2005). Understanding mass school shootings: Links between personhood and power in the competitive school environment. *The Journal of Primary Prevention*, 26, 419–438.

Troop-Gordon, W. & Ladd, G. W. (2005). Trajectories of peer victimization and perceptions of the self and schoolmates: Precursors to internalizing and externalizing problems. *Child Development*, 76, 1072–1091.

Unnever, J. & Cornell, D. (2004). Middle school victims of bullying: Who reports being bullied? *Aggressive Behavior*, 30, 373–388.

Vaillancourt, T., Hymel, S., & McDougall, P. (2003). Bullying is power: Implications for school-based intervention strategies. *Journal of Applied School Psychology*, 19, 157–176.

Veenstra, R., Lindenberg, S., Oldehinkel, A., de Winter, A., Verhulst, F., & Ormel, J. (2005). Bullying and victimization in elementary schools: A comparison of bullies, victims, bully/victims, and uninvolved preadolescents. *Developmental Psychology*, 41, 672–682.

Verhoek-Miller, N., Miller, D. I., Shirachi, M., & Hoda, N. (2002). Dimensions of school climate: Teachers or principals power styles and subjects propensities to be climate vigilant as related to students perceptions of satisfaction and of peers abusive behavior. *Psychological Reports*, 91, 257–262.

Vitaro, F., Brendgen, M., & Barker, E. (2006). Subtypes of aggressive behaviors: A developmental perspective. *International Journal of Behavioral Development*, 30, 12–19.

Werner, N. & Crick, N. (1999). Relational aggression and social-psychological adjustment in a college sample. *Journal of Abnormal Psychology*, 108, 615–623.

Young, E. & Raffaele Mendez, L. (2003). The mental health professional's role in understanding, preventing, and responding to student sexual harassment. *Journal of Applied School Psychology*, 19, 7–23.

Chapter 16
The Psychiatrist's Role After a School Shooting: The Emergency Room and Beyond

Elissa P. Benedek and Praveen Kambam

Introduction

In recent years, our society has witnessed a sharp increase in abusive, violent, and sexually aggressive behavior by our youth. Violent crime by youth decreased for a period in the last few years of 1990s but, once again, is on the upswing. The violent crimes committed by these children and adolescents have been a consistent social problem despite targeted prevention programs and juvenile school-specific interventions becoming increasingly popular around the country. Violent crimes have increased 2.3% from 2004 to 2005 (U.S. Federal Bureau of Investigation, 2006). The Bureau of Justice Statistics (BJS), investigating murders committed during the years 1974 through 2004, found that almost half of the offenders were under the age of 25 years, and 11% were under the age of 18 years. In 1994, FBI national self-report studies indicated that the highest risk for initiation of serious violent behavior occurred between the ages of 15 and 16, and the risk of initiating violent behavior after age 20 was much lower (Elliott, 1994).

Between 8 and 10% of US high school students carried guns to school each day. In a typical middle-size city, 35–50 cases of school violence were reported daily and in half of these cases, guns were involved (Shaffi & Shaffi, 2001).

Everyday in the USA, 12–13 children and adolescents die of violent death, either from homicide or from suicide (Shaffi & Shaffi, 2001). An additional number of physical injuries at schools occur from gunshot wounds. The spread of endemic school violence from urban settings to suburban and smaller communities has brought this major public health problem to national attention. In the decade between 1990 and 2000, the incidence of tragic school shootings increased across the country. There were school shootings in Pearl, Mississippi, Paducah, Kentucky, Springfield, Oregon, Jonesboro, Little Rock, Colorado, Conyers, Georgia, and Fort Gibson, Oklahoma. Other authors have examined the factors contributing to the increase in school violence, described the changed school environment and the contemporary school community, detailed biological and social causes of school violence, and profiled children and adolescents who may be violent offenders in school systems. In this chapter, after presenting a hypothetical case example, we

T. W. Miller (ed.), *School Violence and Primary Prevention.*
© Springer 2008

will discuss the multifaceted role of the emergency room psychiatrist in the aftermath of a school violence incident (Elliott et al., 1998).

Case Example

JM, a 14-year-old boy, brought a duffle bag of weapons to a suburban school on a Monday morning. He brought the loaded duffel bag into a school assembly, attended by sixth, seventh, and eighth graders. In a seemingly random fashion, he began shooting. Tragically, he killed four young students and wounded seven others. His actions terrified the adolescents in the suburban high school, their parents, and the community at large.

JM was seized by the school principal and subdued. School administrators called local police, who brought JM to a midsize hospital emergency room in hand-cuffs. In the days and weeks that followed this tragedy, other adolescents were seen by the emergency room doctor—some physically wounded and others emotionally traumatized. They were followed by a group of concerned parents, administrators, and the media. The emergency room child psychiatrist played an important role in this traumatic situation.

Evaluation

Confidentiality

In the acute emergency situation, it is important for the emergency room physician to assess the issues of confidentiality which may be confronted in an evaluation of the perpetrator. The emergency room psychiatrist must provide a clear explanation of the purpose of the assessment. Limits of confidentiality need to be discussed before any information is sought from the victim, family members, or other adolescents. Students and their families need to know what information will be disclosed to other interested parties, such as police and media. They need to know about the psychiatrist's legal obligations under state law and mandatory reporting, such as duty to warn in the event that additional violence is intended (Schetky, 2002).

During the assessment process, the perpetrator may disclose significant information and then ask that it be withheld from the police and other law enforcement officials. Such information may be related to the violence itself, other psychiatric problems of the youth in question, such as substance abuse and prior family violence, or other issues.

Adolescents, their families, child witnesses, and school officials must understand from the onset the limits of confidentiality, which include the duty to warn (Simon, 2001). The emergency room psychiatrist must also recognize that his or her treatment record of the interview may be subpoenaed and become a legal document, open to the public, and not protected by the law. The press and law enforcement understand issues of confidentiality intellectually, but they may unwittingly or wittingly attempt to elicit confidential information.

Assessment and Management of the Violent Youth

In assessing a youngster brought in after an incident of violent behavior, the clinician's first concern must be for personal safety, staff safety, and safety of the individual child. The emergency room clinician must decide the best setting in which to interview the violent youngster. Usually it is best to see a youngster alone in a room with an open door. Clinicians should sit between the patient and the open door, in case escape is necessary. Unfortunately, after a violent act, the youth may repress the incident in question, and if the emergency room doctor confronts the youngster about the act in question, the youngster may recall it vividly and react. During the confrontation, the youngster's response may be defensiveness or increased violence. The physician or staff member may be attacked. The clinician should not feel omnipotent, despite the feeling that many staff members have that a psychiatrist has magical powers and is able to calm all patients and reduce aggression (Schetky, 2002).

The emergency room doctor's task is to obtain a history of the recent event from the adolescent patient as quickly as possible. A calm, nonprovocative, nonjudgmental, and nonconfrontational approach is best. Initial contact with a violent youngster which is confrontational may result in argument and violence. The psychiatrist must first listen to the patient's story, with an ear toward potential for additional violence to himself or herself as well as to others. The emergency room psychiatrist's role is to obtain the patient's view of the incident in question and decide on an emergent treatment plan, which may include in-patient hospitalization or simply the return of the violent youngster to the attending law enforcement officers with a recommendation for psychopharmacology (Schetky, 2002; Tardiff, 1999).

Youth Witnesses

In the midst of the trauma of the emergency room situation, it is easy to forget the adolescents who have witnessed the violent act and may follow the patient into the emergency room or be seen at a later date for psychological or general medical symptoms. Youngsters who have observed a violent act feel threatened themselves (Al-Mateen, 2002). As described earlier in the hypothetical case, many of the adolescents in the assembly auditorium were in danger had the youthful gunman turned on them. Other adolescents who observed the violent acts felt at risk. They reported what they had witnessed to the authorities. Some youngsters had discussed the violent plans of the young man in question with him before the acts occurred. All of these youngsters, if they present to the emergency room, must be assessed for acute and eventual chronic stress problems. The emergency room psychiatrist's role is also to listen to their stories in a noncritical and nonjudgmental fashion, evaluate the symptoms they describe, and suggest future treatment plans. Such treatment may include psychopharmacology, mental health care from a school health counselor, or simply an attempt to educate the adolescent about symptoms of acute stress and adoption of a watchful attitude.

Family

The emergency room psychiatrist may also have the role of interviewing the family of the youthful perpetrator at the emergency room. It is important to assess the family as a unit and to attempt to predict how the family members will respond to this crisis. Will they be able to provide support to the child or adolescent or will their response be one of rejection, anger, anxiety, or depression? The emergency room psychiatrist may choose to delegate this role to a social worker or another mental health worker. After assessing the parents, a decision about emergency treatment, be it psychopharmacology or referral, is critical. The assessment is always also an initiation of treatment and is received as such by parents.

School and Community

In the aftermath of the Columbine school shootings, uncertainty gripped the school community about how such a terrible event could have occurred. There were fears that many other high schools in the community would be at risk of violence. There were fears that there were other disturbed kids in the community who were not identified by parents, teachers, and administrators. In the days that followed the tragic event, a community consultation was needed in response to this community tragedy.

The psychiatrist has a role in evaluating and managing acute distress and shock that follow the initial response of school personnel to a violent incident. The emergency room psychiatrist may be the first person to discuss the acute grief of administrators and school officials. In addition, a psychiatrist can provide information to school personnel about how to talk with the children and adolescents about what happened and to help children cope with fears for their own safety. The very school personnel whom students rely upon to help normalize the return to school may themselves be badly traumatized and grieving (Rowan, 2001). Rather than just providing psychoeducation to teachers on how to assist students, it is critical for the emergency room doctor to provide school personnel with adequate support and attention to their own experiences, losses, ongoing distress, and reactivity to reminders of the trauma. They must have adequate guarantees of confidentiality so that they can take advantage of treatment offered in the emergency room, without having to worry that their teaching careers will be adversely affected by seeking help. It is only when they have this assurance that they can help traumatized students and families.

Media

The Case for "Copycat" Suicides

There is evidence to suggest significant impacts of media on suicide, especially in adolescents. In many European states, Goethe's 1774 novel *The Sorrows of Young Werther* was banned because of impressions that it triggered an increase in suicides. Today, the "Werther effect" describes the occurrence of imitative "copycat" suicides after media coverage. The level of impact seems to follow a "dose–response" relationship (Etzersdorfer et al., 2001) where the distribution and prevalence of media coverage after a suicide is positively related to the rate of increase in subsequent imitative suicides. An imitative effect was 14.3 times more likely to be found in studies examining effects of a celebrity suicide than those that did not (Stack, 2000), suggesting a prominence effect as well. Furthermore, the impact of media coverage on suicide rates has been documented internationally, from Western countries to East Asian countries (Gould et al., 2003) and shows a temporal relationship between coverage and suicide rates. In fact, the Surgeon General's 1999 report on Mental Health concluded that evidence supports suicide can be facilitated in vulnerable teens by exposure to real or fictional accounts of suicide (Surgeon General of the United States, 1999).

The Case for "Copycat" School Violence

Although less studied, we believe a substantive case can be made for imitative school violence. To date, the best evidence of imitation related to school shootings comes from a study of threats of school violence after media coverage of the Columbine school shootings in Pennsylvania, one of the few states with centralized records (Kostinsky et al., 2001). From day 2 to 50 after the Columbine shootings, 354 threats of school violence were reported to the Pennsylvania Emergency Management Agency—a staggering increase from the typical rate of 1 or 2 threats per year. The overall trend demonstrates a crescendo–decrescendo pattern with an increase to day 10 (particularly on days 8 through 10) followed by an exponential decline. The crescendo pattern was interrupted by weekends and the decrescendo pattern was accelerated by days off from school. The study's findings are consistent with anecdotal evidence, media opinions, and professional opinions of an imitative process occurring after the Columbine shootings.

This crescendo–decrescendo pattern is similar to the pattern documented in imitative suicides following media coverage (Phillips & Carstensen, 1986; Bollen & Phillips, 1982). The later peak and longer duration may be attributed to the increased media attention as coverage of the Columbine shootings was the third most closely watched news story of the 1990s (Kas, 1999). Further evidence that a common etiological explanation may account for the imitative effects is the statistical phenomenon of temporal clustering of suicides among teenagers and young adults, accounting for 1–5% of all teenage suicides (Gould et al., 1989, 1990a, b).

Theoretical Underpinnings

Several theoretical perspectives can be used to explain an imitative school violence phenomenon. Common explanations rely on the learning of behaviors through observation and modeling and stem from social learning theory (Bandura, 1973, 1977). Moreover, media or public attention may serve as an inadvertent reward associated with the observed behavior. A particularly close fitting theoretical explanation views imitative school violence in the context of behavioral contagion theory (Wheeler, 1966). Here, a similar behavior spreads spontaneously and rapidly throughout a group and factors may serve to modulate an approach–avoidance conflict for a particular behavior. Media coverage may, in this manner, make imitative school violence more likely by reducing the avoidance gradient.

Role of the Psychiatrist

Although there is limited data on imitative school shootings, more easily modifiable risk factors for imitative violence should be focused upon. One such factor would include modifying media coverage after an incident. Attempted and completed suicides on the Viennese underground railway were significantly reduced after the media were given guidelines for reporting suicide, including recommendations to write shorter, nonsensational pieces that generally were not placed on the front page (Etzerdorfer et al., 1992). Although there were 9 suicides on the underground railway in 1980–1984, 13 suicides occurred in 1986 and 9 in the first half of 1987. After the media guidelines were introduced, the numbers fell to 3 in 1989 and 4 in 1990.

The psychiatrist has a potentially powerful role in educating the media regarding responsible coverage after a school shooting. We do not know of clearly established guidelines for media reporting for minimization of imitative school shootings; however, several guidelines for the reporting of suicide in the media exist (Centers for Disease Control and Prevention et al., 2001; World Health Organization, 2000). These may help guide the psychiatrist advising the media after a violent incident in a school. The initial goal would be to educate the media on the potential for imitative violence and the imperatives to minimize such risk, especially in the immediate period of high prominence and frequency of coverage of an incident. Attempts should be made to highlight the negative outcomes and to minimize possible interpretation of the individuals committing the violence as countercultural heroes. Emphasis on treatable precursors and resources for assistance should occur, possibly in a sidebar format. Detailed descriptions of the method and site of the crime should not be included in a news story. Sensational headlines and coverage should be avoided. Avoiding prominent placement in the newspapers or television news broadcasts is also recommended.

Forensic Assessments

The process of emergency management of a traumatic incident does not end after the first emergency room evaluation. The emergency room psychiatrist may be asked to conduct a further evaluation or a forensic evaluation. It is always tempting to acquiesce. However, the clinician must be aware that the role of the treating psychiatrist (emergency room psychiatrist) and the evaluating psychiatrist differ. Before deciding to agree, it is important for the physician to remember the risks of wearing these two hats.

The emergency room psychiatrist will have at his disposal confidential information that is not necessary, appropriate, or relevant to the forensic evaluation. Information that may be disclosed in the initial emergency situation is confidential and cannot be used by the emergency room doctor in a subsequent evaluation. Additionally, there are ethical constraints preventing the treating physician from acting as an expert.

There may also be occasions when an emergency room doctor may be asked to evaluate a youngster, after the initial consultation in the emergency room, for the question of future risk assessment. In that regard, a more complete evaluation and risk assessment for violence is indicated. A more extensive evaluation would include questions focusing on history of violence toward self, others, and fire setting. It would include an evaluation of the severity, frequency, and chronicity of past violence as well as an evaluation of the youngster's violent thoughts, plans, and fantasies about family, friends, or peers. Questions may focus around future dispositional options and assess whether current violent ideation, threats, or acting-out behaviors need to be managed in a detention center or an in-patient psychiatric facility (Schetky, 2002).

If the emergency room physician is asked to do a more complete forensic evaluation, it is generally advisable to decline, even though attorneys, courts, and family attempt to sway the doctor, suggesting that the emergency room doctor knows the youngster, has seen him or her in an acute situation, and is familiar with all the actors in this drama.

In many situations, the emergency room doctor will be asked to testify in future court hearings. It is advisable to discuss the extent and limitations of testimony the attorney requests, the testimony, and the actual time of testimony (Benedek, 2002). The emergency room doctor may be able to answer some questions even if he or she has not completed a forensic evaluation. Beware that it is always tempting to hypothesize and to offer opinions outside of one's area of expertise and knowledge. Attorneys are adept at persuasion, and they may overtly or covertly attempt to coerce or seduce a clinician into an expression of opinions for which there is no medically based evidence.

The Aftermath

The role of the emergency room psychiatrist is not limited to evaluation, treatment, and referral in the emergency room. The psychiatrist has a long-term role in the community. That role may include long-term consultations to schools, community agencies, and parent groups.

Schools

With regard to schools, the psychiatrist can consult with the school system and share information about how trauma in the school affects classrooms and school systems (i.e., does it lead to classroom togetherness or classroom disintegration and does it lead to closer liaisons with law enforcement?). The normal psychiatric/psychological response to trauma is not a part of a teacher's usual curriculum or advanced training. The difference between normal emotional reaction to stress, that is, coping, and a psychiatric or psychological disorder is not intuitive. Most children do well emotionally and do not develop mental illness or emotional disorders after a crisis. Most children do continue to have painful memories of the stressful situation. In some instances, teachers may need to help students contact professional resources.

Teachers also need to know that techniques that they are already familiar with work well in classrooms. Such techniques as empathic listening, validation of feelings, dispelling unrealistic fears and concerns about violence, and instilling hope are useful in traumatic situations. Classroom debriefings seem to be helpful. They may offer students opportunities for sharing information and talking about their fears, worries, and concerns in a safe setting. Teachers need to know that while demonstrating empathy and understanding is helpful, they must not fall apart or demonstrate excessive emotion as it may send inadvertent messages to children that they cannot be trusted with information that students may give them. Teachers must understand that they must give students reliable information and if they are unsure about their information, it is acceptable to say "I'm not sure. I will find out for you." Teachers should be educated that despite the temptation to withdraw from students because of their own trauma, withdrawal creates problematic role models for the child. When a child or adolescent has faced a violent situation, it is most important for him or her to have empathic, supportive, normalizing, and affirmative contact with adult role models.

Community

With regard to the community at large after a violent incident, the community members who are not directly involved in the trauma often request consultations from mental health professionals in an attempt to understand and deal with their own feelings and reactions after a tragic event. This consultation may be in the form of a request for an office visit, a lecture, or for written educational materials. Again, it is important for the psychiatrist to normalize the reactions to a trauma, including sleep, appetite, and energy disturbances, as well as brief problems with memory, cognition, and sadness. Educating the community helps to allay fears that these normal behaviors are "crazy" or signs of impending mental illness.

The psychiatrist will likely be called upon to speak at community or school meetings. These forums should be viewed as opportunities to convey support, psychoeducation, normalization of common reactions, and warnings about indications of more problematic reactions. Medical information about more problematic reactions, such as posttraumatic stress disorder, may be inquired about and it may serve the psychiatrist well to have patient education documents available to be circulated. Online resources from organizational Web sites, such as the American Academy of Child & Adolescent Psychiatry's (www.aacap.org) "Facts for Families," can be conveniently downloaded and printed.

The psychiatrist should include a discussion of factors associated with greater risk of posttraumatic stress disorder after a school shooting. Nader et al. (1990) reported a 14-month follow-up of a longitudinal study of children exposed to a sniper attack on a playground. Key factors associated with increased posttraumatic stress symptoms included greater proximity to the violence, a higher degree of life threat, and greater acquaintance with the victim(s). The psychiatrist should recommend schools and families to identify youth with these risk factors and monitor them, as identification of youth exposed to the violence is one of the greatest challenges in providing services (Saltzman et al., 2001). Interestingly, in the Nader et al. (1990) study, a previous history of trauma was not associated with an increase in symptoms specific to the current incident but did seem to renew symptoms from previous trauma. We agree with the authors' recommendations that guilt and bereavement, separate from posttraumatic stress disorder symptoms, should be addressed. Additionally, co-occurring disorders, such as depression and substance abuse, need to be monitored.

Detailed treatment of trauma is beyond the scope of this chapter; however, trauma-focused group psychotherapy interventions, such as the University of California Los Angeles Trauma Psychiatry school-based therapy program (focusing on traumatic experiences, posttraumatic reactions, bereavement, and developmental disruptions), have successfully treated violence-exposed and victimized youth (Layne et al., 2001; Saltzman et al., 2001). Targets addressed by such programs may indicate that additional attention should be paid to youth who suffer with physical reminders, for example, scars from the incident, and have life goals and developmental trajectory significantly disrupted. Unfortunately, such trauma-focused group psychotherapy interventions are rare and the psychiatrist can be an advocate for creation of such resources.

Media

The psychiatrist should continue to follow the recommendations for dealing with the media in the immediate period after an incident. Further emphasis upon the negative consequences of the incident, treatable precursors, and resources for assistance should occur. The psychiatrist should also discuss with the media that continual news coverage may not only prolong the risk of imitative violence but also greatly impact the healing process of the community. The aftermath of an incident may be an opportune time to solidify the message and education of the media with respect to imitative violence and potentially could encourage collaboration with the media to balance motivations for reporting to gain as many consumers as possible with recommendations for minimizing impacts on imitative violence. The psychiatrist may want to prepare or have available a brief summary of guidelines to offer the media. Lastly, in educating the media regarding the risks of imitative violence, the psychiatrist should acknowledge the limitations of available data, but emphasize that several theoretical reasons as well as empirical evidence in similar behaviors point to a strong case for imitative violence after a school shooting, demanding focus on more easily modifiable risk factors such as media coverage.

Conclusion

After a school shooting, an emergency psychiatrist may be asked to fulfill an array of diagnostic, assessment, treatment, and educational roles for an array of audiences including the perpetrator(s), witnesses, community, and media. These demands may require skills and knowledge not routinely used by an emergency room psychiatrist and may therefore be anxiety provoking. The clinician would be served well to become familiar with the special implications beyond the routine emergency room case, from confidentiality to potential media impacts, and to understand his or her limitations with respect to the demands that may be imposed.

References

Al-Mateen, C. (2002). Effects of witnessing violence on children and adolescents. In D. Schetky & E. P. Benedek (Eds.), *Principles and Practice of Child and Adolescent Forensic Psychiatry* (pp. 213–224). Washington, D.C.: American Psychiatric Publishing.

Bandura, A. (1973). *Aggression: A Social Learning Analysis*. Englewood Cliffs, NJ: Prentice-Hall.

Bandura, A. (1977). *Social Learning Theory*. New York: General Learning Press.

Benedek, E. P. (2002). Testifying: The expert witness in court. In D. Schetky & E. P. Benedek (Eds.), *Principles and Practice of Child and Adolescent Forensic Psychiatry* (pp. 33–34). Washington, D.C.: American Psychiatric Publishing.

Bollen, K. A. & Phillips, D. P. (1982). Imitative suicides: A national study of the effects of television new stories. *American Sociological Review* 47, 802–809.

Centers for Disease Control and Prevention, National Institute of Mental Health, Substance Abuse and Mental Health Services Administration, Office of the Surgeon General, American Foundation for Suicide Prevention, American Association of Suicidology, Annenberg Public Policy Center (2001). *Reporting on suicide: Recommendations for the media.*

Elliott, D. S. (1994). Youth violence: An overview. *Congressional Program: Children and Violence*, 15–20.

Elliott, D. S., Hamburg, B. A., & Williams, K. R. (1998). *Violence in American Schools.* Melbourne: Cambridge University Press.

Etzerdorfer, E., Sonneck, G., & Nagel-Kuess, S. (1992). Newspaper reports and suicide. *New England Journal of Medicine*, 327, 507–508.

Etzersdorfer, E., Voracek, M., & Sonneck, G. (2001). A dose-response relationship of imitational suicides with newspaper distribution. *Australian & New Zealand Journal of Psychiatry*, 35, 251.

Gould, M. S., Wallenstein, S., & Davidson, L. (1989). Suicide clusters: A critical review. *Suicide & Life-Threatening Behavior*, 19, 17–29.

Gould, M. S., Wallenstein, S., & Kleinman, M. H. (1990a). Time-space clustering of teenage suicide. *American Journal of Epidemiology*, 131, 71–78.

Gould, M. S., Wallenstein, S., & Kleinman, M. H. (1990b). Suicide clusters: An examination of age-specific effects. *American Journal of Public Health*, 80, 211–212.

Gould, M., Jamieson, P., & Romer, D. (2003). Media contagion and suicide among the young. *American Behavioral Scientist*, 46, 1269–1284.

Kas, J. (1999). The loud echo of Littleton's gunfire. *US News and World Report*, 126, 24.

Kostinsky, S., Bixler, E. O., & Kettl, P. A. (2001). Threats of school violence in Pennsylvania after media coverage of the Columbine High School Massacre. *Archives of Pediatrics & Adolescent Medicine*, 155, 994–1001.

Layne, C. M., Pynoos, R. S., & Cardenas, J. (2001). Wounded adolescence: School-based group psychotherapy for adolescents who sustained or witnessed violent injury. In M. Shafii & S. Shafii (Eds.), *School Violence: Contributing Factors, Management, and Prevention* (pp. 163–186). Washington, D.C.: American Psychiatric Press.

Nader, K., Pynoos, R., Fairbanks, L., & Frederick, C. (1990). Children's PTSD reactions one year after a sniper attack at their school. *The American Journal of Psychology*, 147(11), 1526–1530.

Phillips, D. P., & Carstensen, L. L. (1986). Clustering of teenage suicides after television news stories about suicide. *The New England Journal of Medicine*, 315, 685–689.

Rowan, B. (2001). Coping With School Violence: An Eyewitness Account. In Shaffi, M. & Shaffi, S. (Eds.). *School Violence Assessment, Management, Prevention* (pp. 117–128) Washington, D.C.: American Psychiatric Press.

Saltzman, W. R., Pynoos, R. S., & Layne, C. M. (2001). Trauma and grief-focused intervention for adolescents exposed to community violence. Results of a school based screening and group treatment protocol. *Group Dynamics: Theory, Research, and Practice*, 5(4), 291–303.

Schetky, D. (2002). Risk assessment of violence in youths. In D. Schetky & E.P. Benedek (Eds.), *Principles and Practice of Child and Adolescent Forensic Psychiatry* (pp. 231–246). Washington, D.C.: American Psychiatric Publishing.

Shaffi, M. & Shaffi, S. (2001). *School Violence Assessment, Management, Prevention.* Washington, D.C.: American Psychiatric Press.

Simon, R. I. (2001). Duty to foresee, forewarn, and protect against violent behavior. In M. Shaffi & S. Shaffi (Eds.), *School Violence Assessment, Management, Prevention* (pp. 201–215). Washington, D.C.: American Psychiatric Press.

Stack, S. (2000). Media impacts on suicide: A quantitative review of 293 findings. *Social Science Quarterly*, 81, 957–971.

Surgeon General of the United States (1999). Mental health: A report by the Surgeon General (Chap. 3).

Tardiff, K. T. (1999). Psychopharmacological and neurobiological issues in the treatment of violent youth. In D. J. Flannery & R. C. Huff (Eds.), *Youth Violence Prevention, Intervention, and Social Policy*. Washington, D.C.: American Psychiatric Press.

U.S. Federal Bureau of Investigation. (2005). *Uniform Crime Report*. Washington D.C. www.fbi. gov/ucr/uscius/offenses/violent_crime/index.html

Wheeler, L. (1966). Toward a theory of behavioral contagion. *Psychological Review*, 73, 179–192.

World Health Organization (2000). Preventing suicide: A resource for media professionals. www.who.int/mental_health/media/en/426.pdf

Chapter 17
Current Perspectives on Linking School Bullying Research to Effective Prevention Strategies

Dorothy L. Espelage and Susan M. Swearer

Primary, Secondary, and Tertiary Prevention Strategies for Bullying

In the prevention literature, the terms "primary," "secondary," and "tertiary" refer to specific prevention and intervention strategies designed to reduce problem behavior in youth. Perhaps the most widely recognized model that embraces this three-tiered model is Positive Behavior Supports (PBS; Sprague & Golly, 2004; Sprague & Walker, 2005). PBS is a systems-based, behaviorally focused prevention and intervention set of strategies designed to improve educational outcomes and social development for all students. PBS models illustrate that approximately 80% of students will need primary prevention strategies, 15% will need secondary prevention strategies, and 5% will need tertiary prevention strategies. Applied to the problem of bullying, the goal of primary prevention is to reduce the number of new cases of bullying. The idea is that through whole-school and classroom-wide strategies, new incidents of bullying can be curtailed. Fifteen percent of students will need secondary prevention strategies designed to reduce engagement in bullying. These might be the students who are involved in bullying as a bystander or students who are involved in bullying less frequently or less severely. Finally, tertiary prevention strategies are designed for the 5% of students who are involved in frequent and intense bullying behaviors. These are the students who might have concomitant psychological problems (i.e., depression and anxiety) as a result of their involvement in bullying behaviors (Craig, 1998; Kaltiala-Heino et al., 2000; Kumpulainen et al., 2001; Swearer et al., 2001). The goal of tertiary prevention is to reduce complications, severity, and frequency of bullying behaviors. While not an exhaustive list, Figure 17.1 outlines three bullying prevention and intervention initiatives that illustrate the three PBS tiers. A description of these three initiatives will be provided in the next section of this chapter.

T. W. Miller (ed.), *School Violence and Primary Prevention.*
© Springer 2008

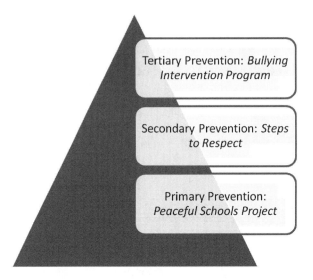

Fig. 17.1 Bullying Prevention and Intervention: Examples of primary, secondary, and tertiary prevention school-based efforts

An example of Primary Prevention for Bullying Behaviors—The Peaceful Schools Projects

The *Peaceful Schools Project* (Twemlow, Fonagy, & Sacco, 2001) was developed in 2000 (www.backoffbully.com). The defining feature of the *Peaceful Schools Project* is that it is a "philosophy rather than a program" (Twemlow, Fonagy, & Sacco, 2005, p. 296). As such, the *Peaceful Schools Project* is an excellent example of primary prevention for bullying behaviors. The goal is to focus on developing healthy relationships between all stakeholders in the educational setting. Related to primary prevention, the main goal of the *Peaceful Schools Project* is to alter the school climate in permanent and meaningful ways. In a school community where the *Peaceful Schools* philosophy is lived, bullying would cease to exist.

The *Peaceful Schools Project* includes five main components (Twemlow et al., 2005). First, schools embark upon a positive climate campaign that includes counselor-led discussions and the creation of posters that help alter the language and the thinking of everyone in the school (i.e., "back off bullies!" or "stop bullying now"). All stakeholders in the school are flooded with an awareness of the bullying dynamic. Understanding bullying from this primary prevention perspective requires an understanding that bullying is a social relationship problem. Second, teachers are fully supported in classroom management techniques and are taught specific techniques to diffuse disruptive behavior from a relational perspective rather than from a punishment perspective. Third, peer and adult mentors are used to help everyone in the school resolve problems without blame. These adult mentors are particularly important during times when adult supervision might be minimal (i.e., in hallways and on the playground). The fourth component is called the "gentle warrior physical education program." The component uses a combination of roleplaying, relaxation, and defensive martial arts techniques to help students develop strategies to protect themselves and others. These are essentially confidence-building skills that support positive coping skills. Fifth, reflection time is included in the school schedule each day. Teachers and students talk for at least 10 min at the end of the day about bully, victim, and bystander behaviors. By engaging in this important dialogue, language and thinking about bullying behaviors can be subtly altered (Twemlow et al., 2005). The *Peaceful Schools Project* is a holistic philosophy that attempts to alter negative social relationships in schools, which, in turn, will reduce or eliminate bullying behaviors. In a recent study, it was found that elementary students whose schools participated in the the *Peaceful Schools Project* had higher achievement scores than did students from schools without the program (Fonagy et al., 2005).

An Example of Secondary Prevention for Bullying Behaviors—Steps to Respect

Steps to Respect: A Bullying Prevention Program was developed and evaluated by the Committee for Children (www.cfchildren.org). This is a school-wide bullying prevention and intervention program with strong empirical support in peer-reviewed journals (Frey et al., 2005; Hirschstein & Frey, 2006). The mission of *Steps to Respect* includes creating a "safe, caring, and respectful" culture and increasing adult intervention in bullying episodes. As such, this program falls under both primary and secondary levels of intervention. This program is designed for students in grades three through six and encompasses three phases. Phases 1 and 2 are primary prevention phases designed to increase school-wide awareness. The curriculum guide outlines the role of the administrator as a supportive leader of implementation and program evaluator. An antibullying committee is formed to facilitate this process, which should include teachers, administrators, bus drivers, nurses, secretaries, social workers, parents, and other persons who work with the students. All staff are trained in bullying awareness (e.g., teachers, administrators, playground aides), and staff who will be coaching children (coined, "coaching training") are trained in the *Steps to Respect* curriculum for classroom teachers. Coaching training includes affirming the child's feelings, asking questions, assessing the child's safety, and proactive responding. Coaches are taught to define and recognize bullying, establish consistent bullying reporting, and create and maintain a positive school climate. Formats include large group presentation, small and group discussions, video segments, worksheets, and roleplays.

Phase 3 falls under secondary prevention and includes the curriculum for classroom lessons and the coaching training curriculum kits include a comprehensive teacher's guide and skill lessons, literature units, copy of each of the books, six posters, and a classroom video. Skills sets that are taught include learning to recognize bullying, learning bullying-refusal skills, learning to seek help and help someone else who is being bullied, practicing friendship-making skills, and developing bullying-reporting skills. Research has found the effects of *Steps to Respect* were strongest when teachers actively coached students involved in bullying (Edstrom et al., 2004). Thus, direct involvement on the part of adults can help reduce engagement in bullying others or responding to being bullied.

An Example of Tertiary Prevention for Bullying Behaviors—Bullying Intervention Program

The *Bullying Intervention Program* (BIP; Swearer & Givens, 2006) is an individual cognitive–behavioral intervention for use with students who bully others. The guiding premise behind BIP is twofold. First, we are guided by the reality that the social-cognitive perceptions of students involved in bullying interactions are as critical as are the aggressive behaviors, because the perceptions and cognitions of the participants serve to underlie, perpetuate, and escalate bullying interactions (Doll & Swearer, 2005; Swearer & Cary, 2003). Second, there is compelling research that suggests that homogeneous group interventions are not helpful for aggressive youth and in fact, may be damaging (Dishion et al., 1999). Based on these two underlying premises, the BIP was developed as a mechanism for school counselors and school psychologists to work directly with students who bully others.

The BIP is in part based upon a decade of research on school bullying under the research project, "Target Bullying: Ecologically-Based Prevention and Intervention for Schools." Target Bullying is a participatory research project whereby university researchers and school personnel and families work together to understand the bullying phenomenon. BIP was developed by the request of a middle school principal who experienced the fact that in-school suspension, suspension, and expulsion were ineffective strategies for reducing bullying behaviors. Research has also found that zero tolerance policies are not effective in curbing aggressive behaviors (Casella, 2003) and that expulsion is equally ineffective in reducing aggressive behavior (Gordon, 2001). Thus, the interventions typically employed in school settings (group treatment, zero tolerance, and expulsion) are ineffective in dealing with bullying behaviors.

The BIP is an alternative to in-school suspension for bullying behaviors that is being implement in a large middle school ($N = 725$). When a student is referred for bullying behaviors, the typical protocol is that the student is sent to in-school suspension. In BIP, parents are given a choice: in-school suspension or the BIP. In all cases ($n = 15$) since the program's inception (2005), parents have chosen BIP. In order to participate in BIP, active parental consent and student assent are obtained. Then, the BIP is scheduled according to the same policies and procedures that the school uses to schedule in-school suspension.

The BIP is a 3 hour one-on-one cognitive–behavioral intervention session with a masters-level student-therapist under the supervision of a licensed psychologist. There are three components to the BIP: (1) assessment, (2) psychoeducation, and (3) feedback. The assessment component consists of widely used measures to assess experiences with bullying, depression, anxiety, cognitive distortions, school climate, and self-concept. The assessment component lasts ~1 hour. The psychoeducation component lasts about 2 hour and consists of the student-therapist presenting an engaging and youth-friendly PowerPoint presentation about bullying behaviors. The presentation is followed by a short quiz to assess for understanding. This is followed by several worksheet activities about bullying behavior that are used from Bully Busters (Newman et al., 2000). Finally, the student-therapist and the referred student watch a video about bullying that Music Television (MTV) produced. The session ends with a debriefing component where the referred student talks about his or her experiences with bullying and impressions of BIP. Based on the assessment data and the interactions with the referred student, a bullying intervention treatment report is written. Recommendations are based on the data collected. The treatment report is reviewed with the parents, student, and school personnel during a face-to-face solution-oriented meeting.

Since mid-fall 2005 there have been 15 participants in grades sixth through eighth. The mean age was 12.27 years (range: 11–14 years old). Ninety-three percent of participants have been European-American, which is consistent with the demographic makeup of the middle school where BIP is taking place. In terms of self-reporting engagement in bullying, 46.7% of participants reported they both bullied others and were bullied (bully-victims); 20% reported they bullied others (bully); 13.3% reported they observed bullying (bystander); 13.3% reported they were victimized only (victim); and 6.7% reported that they were not involved at all in bullying. In terms of psychosocial functioning, two participants endorsed clinical levels of depression and two participants endorsed clinical levels of anxiety. Interestingly, most participants held positive perceptions of their school climate and most endorsed average to above average self-concept. Participants endorsed a range of cognitive distortions and behavioral problems. The variety of presenting problems acknowledged by the participants suggests that homogeneous group interventions for students who bully others are likely to be ineffective. At the tertiary level, it appears that individually focused interventions for bullying are likely to be more efficacious than group forms of treatment (Dishion et al., 1999).

Linking School Bullying Research to Explanatory Theoretical Paradigms

Not only is it important to understand how primary, secondary, and tertiary prevention and intervention can be utilized to reduce bullying, but it is also important to understand explanatory theoretical paradigms that guide bullying research. Some of the more prominent theories are social-ecological theory, social-information processing theory, theory of mind, dominance theory, and attraction theory. They will be briefly reviewed here.

Solid theoretical underpinnings are invaluable to understanding human behavior. *Webster's New World Dictionary* defines theory as "a formulation of apparent relationships or underlying principles of certain observed phenomena which has been verified to some degree." While no one theory describes most human phenomenon, there are several theories that have particular applicability to bullying behaviors and will be reviewed briefly here.

Social-ecological theory (Bronfenbrenner, 1979) is perhaps the most all-encompassing theory of human behavior that posits a reciprocal interplay between the individual, peer group, family, school, community, and culture. Each system impacts the other. Social-ecological theory has been used to explain students' engagement in bullying behaviors (Garbarino & deLara, 2002; Newman et al., 2000; Olweus, 1993; Swearer & Doll, 2001; Swearer & Espelage, 2004). Thus, based on this theory, it is impossible to understand bullying behaviors without also understanding the many environments, the relation between the individual and these environments, and the interaction between multiple settings that all influence engagement in (or not) bullying behaviors.

Social cognitive theory is a cognitive theory that explains the complex interplay between an individual's cognitions and his or her behaviors (Bandura, 1986). Relatedly, the social-information processing model (Crick & Dodge, 1994; Dodge & Coie, 1987) provides a useful heuristic to understanding engagement in bullying behaviors. Essentially, the model and underlying theory purport that individuals engage in a series of cognitive processes that result in behavioral enactment. How an individual responds to a given situation is based on his or her prior experiences and his or her cognitive interpretation of the situation. Thus, engagement in bullying behaviors is based, in part, on the individual's prior experiences with bullying and his or her cognitive construction of those experiences.

Theory of mind (Leslie, 1987) describes the phenomena of being able to "put yourself in another's shoes." Theory of mind asserts that some individuals are very adept at attributing mental states to others. This notion challenges the prevailing belief that students who bully others do so because of social and cognitive deficits. In fact, proponents of theory of mind (Sutton et al., 1999) suggest that some students bully others because they can determine who is weaker, who can be picked on, and who is unlikely to be able to defend himself or herself. Thus, the findings that some students who bully others are in the "cool" crowd (Garbarino & deLara, 2002; Rodkin, 2004) can be, in part, explained by theory of mind.

Linking School Bullying Research to Effective Assessment

Operationalization

Initial research endeavors focused on bullying emerged in Scandinavia where Olweus (1978) spearheaded a nationwide campaign against bullying. This initiative, which began in the 1970s, set forth the following definition of bullying which remains current today: "A student is being bullied or victimized when he or she is exposed, repeatedly and over time, to negative actions on the part of one or more students" (Olweus, 2001). The preceding definition highlights the aggressive component of bullying and the associated inherent power imbalance and repetitive nature (Olweus, 2001). In recent years, scholars have recognized the wide range of behaviors consistent with bullying, including both physical and relational manifestations.

> ### Defining Bullying
> A student is being bullied or picked on when another student says nasty and unpleasant things to him or her. It is also bullying when a student is hit, kicked, threatened, locked inside a room, sent nasty notes and when no one ever talks to him. (Smith & Sharp, 1994, p. 1)

Dodge (1991) conceptualized bullying as proactive aggression because bullies carefully seek and choose vulnerable victims, who are generally disliked by their peers, initiate aggression themselves, and use it for their own benefit.

In the literature, bullying and peer harassment are often used interchangeably and include negative actions on the part of one or more students inflicted upon or directed toward another student repeatedly and over time (Olweus, 2001). At its core, peer harassment involves behaviors that hurt someone, whether through verbal teasing, physical harm, social exclusion, or lies and rumors. Recently, some researchers have made a distinction between peer harassment and bullying by conceptualizing bullying as a subset of peer harassment that involves only verbal teasing and threatening behaviors that have the potential to cause harm (Espelage & Holt, 2001). This definition eliminates the component of direct aggression causing physical harm, and is done so for two reasons. First, especially with regard to middle school populations, ethnographic analysis has shown that teasing occurs with considerably more frequency than physical aggression (Eder, 1995). Second, aggressive conflicts, such as fistfights, that could potentially cause physical harm can occur between two students but would not be considered bullying. Because the focus of this study was on the middle school population, bullying was defined and assessed as chronic (determined by frequency) verbal teasing and threatening behaviors that have the potential to cause harm, and bullying did not include behaviors of overt physical aggression. The term "chronic" distinguishes bullying from normal daily conflict between students that could be expected in a middle school setting.

Assessment

A wide range of self-report surveys is available to assess the prevalence of bullying perpetration and victimization, locations where the bullying happens, attitudes students' hold toward bullying, and willingness to intervene. In some cases, students are provided with a definition of bullying (Olweus, 1991; Swearer, 2001) and then asked a series of questions related to their perceptions, attitudes, and behaviors. In contrast, some surveys do not provide the students with a definition (Espelage & Holt, 2001; Reynolds, 2003); rather they are just asked to indicate how often they have engaged in specific behaviors (e.g., I called other student names) or whether certain things had happened to them (e.g., I was called names). Often times, these surveys are then supplemented with measures of potential correlates of bullying in order to determine the protective factors (e.g., empathy, caring, parental support) and risk factors associated with bullying perpetration and victimization. A small percentage of these surveys include peer nomination tasks that ask students to identify who teases others often and who gets teased often (Espelage & Holt, 2001). It is recommended that these items are asked separately for boys and girls because when students are asked in general to identify students who are bullies boys are nominated most often. Rodkin and colleagues (2005) have developed their *Who Bullies Whom?* questionnaire in order to identify more specifically who gets bullied by whom.

Behavioral Observations

Direct behavioral observations of children and adolescents in the natural school setting is an ideal manner of collecting data on bullying frequency and the role of all students (Craig & Pepler, 1997; Salmivalli et al., 1996). For example, Craig and Pepler (1997) videotaped aggressive and socially competent Canadian children in grades one through six on the playground; peers were involved in bullying in an astounding 85% of bully episodes. Among other things, this involvement consisted of active participation in the episode (30%), observing the interaction (23%), and intervening (12%). Furthermore, peers were coded as being respectful to the bully in 74% of the episodes, but respectful to the victim in only 23% of the episodes. Observational methods provide invaluable data about how students interact; however, observations need to be conducted across a long period and in a variety of settings (e.g., gym, lunchtime, different classrooms) to assess the situational and contextual variables that contribute to bullying (Pellegrini, 2002a).

Linking School Bullying Research to Understanding the Dynamics Behind Bullying

The bully/victim continuum is used to conceptualize bullying as a dynamic phenomenon where individuals can move in and out of different roles depending upon the social ecology that might promote or inhibit bullying behaviors. There is a huge need to move beyond static labels (i.e., "bully" and "victim") and "debunk this dyadic bias" (Espelage & Swearer, 2003, p. 370). In recent years, more researchers are identifying that involvement in bullying might not be fixed over time and that individuals involved in bullying might do so as both bullying others and being bullied (i.e., "bully-victims"). Thus, there is greater recognition of the diversity of experiences along the bully/victim continuum.

There are many individual influences that might support or discourage engagement in bullying behaviors. While it is generally accepted that boys engage in bullying behaviors to a greater degree and frequency than do girls, teasing out engagement in overt versus covert forms of bullying has been more elusive (Espelage & Swearer, 2003). Some research has examined racial and ethnic issues in bullying and the general consensus is that race and ethnicity are less of an issue compared with the racial and ethnic norms in a given school (Juvonen & Graham, 2001). Age is another issue that has been examined with respect to bullying and victimization, with the general consensus being that bullying behaviors increase over the elementary schools years, peak in middle school, and start to decline in high school (Nansel et al., 2001). Psychological factors, such as depression, anxiety, and anger, have all been studied in relation to bullying behavior and have been found to be related to bullying and/or victimization. There are no "classic" individual characteristics that can be identified in order to determine who will be likely to engage in bullying others or who will be likely to be victimized. Research certainly has explored the link between sex, age, race, and psychological variables; however, a "profile" does not exist.

Family Influences

With respect to the family context, research has been conducted on both children who chronically bully and those who are chronically victimized (Finnegan et al., 1998; Rodkin, 2004). Consistently, bullies, as a group, report that their parents are authoritarian, condone "fighting back," use physical punishment, lack warmth, and display indifference to their children (Baldry & Farrington, 2000; Loeber & Dishion, 1984; Olweus, 1995). McFadyen-Ketchum and colleagues (McFadyen-Ketchum et al., 1996) found that parents can also contribute to a *decrease* in children's aggression over time; aggressive children who experienced affectionate mother–child relationships showed a significant decrease in their aggressive–disruptive behaviors. Furthermore, these positive parental connections appeared to buffer the long-term negative consequences of aggression. Another area of investigation related to the potential influences of the family context includes studies on parental attachment and those focused on perceived social support among bullies and bully-victims. In a widely cited study, Troy and Sroufe (1987) found that children who had insecure, anxious-avoidant, or anxious-resistant attachments at the age of 18 months were more likely than children with secure attachments to become involved in bullying at the age of 4 and 5 years. In a recent study, middle school students classified as bullies and bully-victims indicated receiving substantially less social support from parents than those students who were in the uninvolved group (Demaray & Malecki, 2003). Accordingly, in a more recent study among 784 ethnically diverse youth a significant interaction between bully/victim groups and peer social support was found (Holt & Espelage, in press). Specifically, bullies, victims, and bully-victims who reported moderate peer social support also indicated the least anxiety/depression; however, parental support did not play a role. However, with few exceptions, most of the research on the family contextual influences has evaluated the perceptions of the children and adolescents. Future research needs to consider the family environment from the parents' perspective rather than focusing solely on the children's self-report.

Peer Influences

Dominance Theory

Early adolescence is also a time when there is an increase in the amount of bullying (Pellegrini, 2002b; Pellegrini & Long, 2002; Smith et al., 1999). A potential explanation for this increase is dominance theory. Dominance is viewed as a relationship factor in which individuals are arranged in a hierarchy in terms of their access to resources (Dunbar, 1988). Pellegrini (2002b) argues that the transition to middle school requires students to renegotiate their dominance relationships, and bullying is thought to be a deliberate strategy used to attain dominance in newly formed peer groups. In an empirical test of dominance theory of proactive aggression and bullying, Pellegrini and Long (2002) found that bullying was used more frequently by boys who targeted their aggression toward other boys during this transition. Certainly, this research supports the idea that males engage in more bullying than do girls during the transition to middle school, but it also highlights the importance of studying this increase as a result of the complex interaction among the need for dominance, changes in social surroundings and peer group structure, and the desire to interact with the opposite sex. Extending this research to include a direct assessment of social networks, Mouttapa et al. (2004) argued that social dominance was at work in their sample of Latino and Asian sixth graders ($n = 1,368$). Friends' participation in aggressive behaviors was found to be positively associated with being a bully or an aggressive victim, and an interesting finding was that female bullies received fewer friendship nominations, but had the highest proportion of reciprocated friendships.

Attraction Theory

Attraction theory posits that young adolescents in their need to establish separation from their parents become attracted to other youth who possess characteristics that reflect independence (e.g., delinquency, aggression, disobedience) and are less attracted to individuals who possess characteristics more descriptive of childhood (e.g., compliance, obedience) (Bukowski et al., 2000; Moffitt, 1993). These authors argue that early adolescents manage the transition from primary to secondary schools through their attractions to peers who are aggressive. In their study of 217 boys and girls during this transition, Bukowski and colleagues found that girls' and boys' attraction to aggressive peers increased upon the entry to middle school. This increase was larger for girls, which is consistent with Pellegrini and Bartini's finding that at the end of middle school girls nominated "dominant boys" as dates to a hypothetical party (Pellegrini & Bartini, 2001). This theory, along with the homophily hypothesis and dominance theory, demonstrates the complex nature of bullying during early adolescence and underscores the need to move beyond descriptive studies of aggression among boys and girls.

School Influences

School influences on bullying behaviors cannot be understated. As many as 70% of middle school youth reported some type of involvement in bullying behaviors (Swearer & Cary, 2003). Students involved in bullying reported more negative views of their school environment (Nansel et al., 2001) and positive school climate is vital to reducing bullying behaviors (Orpinas & Horne, 2006). Essentially, the overall health of the adults in the school is related to the overall health of the students. Are the teachers happy? Do the teachers work hard? Do the teachers and administrators have a healthy relationship? Is there open communication between school personnel and parents? Do teachers and students have healthy relationships? Are the students happy to be in school? A positive school environment is created by the people who exist in that building and surrounding community. Finding ways to create healthy school environments is foundational for ameliorating bullying behaviors.

Classroom practices and teachers' attitudes are also salient components of school climate that contribute to bullying prevalence. Aggression varies from classroom to classroom, and in some instances aggression is supported (Rodkin & Hodges, 2003). Bullying tends to be less prevalent in classrooms in which most children are included in activities (Newman et al., 2001), teachers display warmth and responsiveness to children (Olweus & Limber, 1999), teachers respond quickly and effectively to bullying incidents (Olweus, 1993), and parents are aware of their children's peers relationships (Roberts & Coursol, 1996). Furthermore, Hoover and Hazler (1994) note that when school personnel tolerate, ignore, or dismiss bullying behaviors they are conveying implicit messages about values that victimized students internalize. Conversely, if school staff members have attitudes not supportive of bullying behavior, and these are translated into voicing their opinions and/or actively intervening in bullying episodes, the school culture as a whole becomes less tolerant of bullying.

Using Knowledge to Inform Prevention Strategies

Need for Teacher Training

Very little research has been conducted on teacher's attitudes toward bullying. What is known from the extant literature is that teachers might foster bullying by failing to either promote respectful interactions among students or speak out against teasing and other behaviors consistent with bullying. More specifically, extant studies have documented that teachers (1) tend to report lower prevalence rates of bullying than do students (e.g., Stockdale et al., 2002), (2) do not always correctly identify bullies (e.g., Leff et al., 1999), and (3) typically do not feel confident in their abilities to deal with bullying (e.g., Boulton, 1997). Teachers are not only unaware of the extent to which bullying occurs in their schools, but appear to be unwilling to intervene should they recognize instances of bullying. Therefore, interventions should include an assessment of teachers' attitudes toward bullying and how they relate toward students. Education about bullying for teachers is also necessary. In fact, this training should extend to preservice teachers, lunchroom supervisors, and school bus drivers (Boulton, 1997).

Home–School Collaboration

Extending teacher training in order to embrace a prevention focus can be accomplished via home–school collaboration. Home–school collaboration refers to a dynamic process whereby parents and educators work together to improve the social and educational experiences of all students (Cowan et al., 2004). This type of collaboration demands mutual respect and a true appreciation for developing partnerships in order to facilitate healthy student functioning. Thus, parents are involved in their children's school by volunteering in schools, attending parent-teaching conferences, being active members of the school Parent Teacher Organization (PTO), and positively reinforcing education and school activities. Educators are involved in their students' family's lives by communicating openly with parents, creating opportunities for parents to get involved in school activities, and accepting family members as educational partners.

School–Community Collaboration

Further extending a true preventative approach to the problem of bullying includes the notion of school–community partnerships, whereby families, schools, and community agencies work in tandem to create a positive social climate that pervades a broader community (Sheridan et al., 2002). Inherent in the process of school–community collaboration is a genuine respect for diversity, a commitment to positive, healthy relationships, and a collaborative relationship that is mutually beneficial. When schools, families, and community agencies work together to improve the lives of youth, a positive social climate can be developed.

Counseling Services

Victims, bullies, and bully-victims often report adverse psychological effects and poor school adjustment as a result of their involvement in bullying, which warrant individual counseling services (Juvoven et al., 2000; Nansel et al., 2003).

For example, targets of bullying reveal more loneliness, greater school avoidance, more suicidal ideation, and less self-esteem than do their nonbullied peers (Hawker & Boulton, 2000; Kochenderfer & Ladd, 1996; Olweus, 1992; Rigby, 2001). Depression also has been found to be a common mental health symptom experienced by male and female victims of bullying (Kaltiala-Heino et al., 2001; Neary & Joseph, 1994). These effects are not necessarily transitory in nature. As discussed by Olweus (1995), results from his longitudinal work indicate that at age 23, individuals who had been chronically victimized in their youth had lower self-esteem and were more depressed than nonvictimized members of their cohort.

Whereas victims tend to report more internalizing behaviors, bullies are more likely than their peers to engage in externalizing behaviors, to experience conduct problems, and to be delinquent (Haynie et al., 2001; Nansel et al., 2001). Furthermore, long-term outcomes for bullies can be serious; compared to their peers, bullies are more likely to be convicted of crimes in adulthood (Olweus, 1993). One study conducted in the USA revealed that youth identified as bullies in school had a 1 in 4 chance of having a criminal record by age 30 (Eron et al., 1987). These data suggest that these bullies would benefit from individual interventions, such as the Bullying Prevention Program developed by Dr. Susan Swearer at University of Nebraska-Lincoln (UNL) (described earlier).

Finally, considerable research has documented that the most at-risk group of youth is bully-victims and therefore another group to be considered for referral to individual counseling. For instance, bully-victims demonstrate more externalizing behaviors, are more hyperactive, and have a greater probability of being referred for psychiatric consultation than their peers (Kumpulainen et al., 1998; Nansel et al., 2001, 2003).

Although there exists a plethora of research documenting the link between peer harassment and negative outcomes, recent research suggests that there is in fact heterogeneity in victims' adjustment to harassment (Salmivalli et al., 1996; Skinner & Kochenderfer-Ladd, 2000; Smith et al., 2001). Specifically, some victims, despite being exposed to chronic peer harassment, find ways to overcome long-term harmful consequences. Therefore, researchers have shifted their focus to delineating the factors that might buffer the negative effects of peer harassment. One such area of interest is the role of victim attributions on adjustment outcomes. Attributions, or how people tend to explain the causes of events or behaviors, have gained attention in the peer harassment literature particularly because of their implications for intervention strategies (Graham & Juvonen, 2001). In a recent study of 661 middle school students (grades five to eight), bullying victimization was associated with higher levels of characterological self-blame and characterological self-blame was found to be a strong predictor of depressed affect, after controlling for general levels of depression and anxiety (Kingsbury & Espelage, in press). Victims and bully-victims reported higher self-blaming attributions and greater depressed affect than did uninvolved students, bullies, and aggressive bullies. Furthermore, victims and bully-victims were more likely to cope by keeping to themselves compared to other groups. These findings have implications for intervention programs, namely, that for them to be most beneficial, one must recognize the complex interplay among individuals' appraisals and coping strategies to better understand heterogeneity across victim subtypes. Counselors should collaborate with school administrations to develop such programs guided by theory integrating complex relations among multiple factors.

In sum, students involved in bullying in any capacity appear to suffer negative effects, and these outcomes might be heightened over the transition from elementary to middle school when all students are experiencing a time of change and stress.

How to Implement Prevention Strategies?

The most effective prevention and intervention programming will exist when a coordinated effort exists between primary, secondary, and tertiary strategies. As previously mentioned, Positive Behavior Supports (PBS; Sprague & Golly, 2004; Sprague & Walker, 2005) is an example of coordinating these strategies. Clearly, coordinating school, family, and community prevention and intervention efforts is essential in reducing aggressive and bullying behaviors in students (Sprague & Walker, 2005). However, despite the fact that there are more than 300 violence prevention programs (Howard et al., 1999), there is little guidance for school personnel and parents on how to implement these programs.

Successful implementation of any prevention or intervention strategy depends in large part on the people involved. Any program will fail if the adults in the system are not supportive. If the adults in the school are enthusiastic, positive, and emotionally healthy and have a unified focus on doing what is in the best interests of students, then the school climate will be a healthy and positive environment. This environment in itself will help create a prevention-oriented atmosphere and will help prevent problems before they start. At the primary prevention level, strategies that help promote a positive school climate, positive relationships in the school, and positive home–school relationships are vital.

Teachers in the school must be supported in their classroom management strategies and classroom-based interventions. Secondary prevention strategies are more likely to be successful when teachers are supported in their work and they are able to identify the students who are struggling. When schools adhere to a unified referral system for at-risk students, they decrease the likelihood that a student might fall through the cracks or does not get additional help (i.e., social skills training). Positive relationships between teachers, administrators, and school support staff (i.e., school social workers, school psychologists) are critical.

Schools must support their counseling departments, as these personnel are trained in working with difficult students. At the tertiary level, there are many interventions that can be utilized in working with students who are involved in bullying behaviors. These interventions typically occur at the individual level, such as individual therapy. However, small group work, such as support groups, and family therapy may also be effective. It is incumbent upon counseling departments to have a solid referral system for teachers and parents and to develop strong links to providers in the community. Primary, secondary, and tertiary prevention and intervention efforts that are coordinated, positive, supportive, and data-based are vital for the reduction of bullying behaviors in our schools.

References

Baldry, A. C. & Farrington, D. P. (2000). Bullies and delinquents: Personal characteristics and parental styles. *Journal of Community and Applied Social Psychology*, 10, 17–31.

Bandura, A. (1986). *Social Foundations of Thought and Action: A Social Cognitive Theory*. Englewood Cliffs, NJ: Prentice Hall.

Boulton, M. J. (1997). Teachers' views on bullying: Definitions, attitudes, and ability to cope. *British Journal of Educational Psychology*, 67, 223–233.

Bronfenbrenner, U. (1979). *The Ecology of Human Development: Experiments by Nature and Design*. Cambridge, MA: Harvard University Press.

Bukowski, W. M., Sippola, L. K., & Newcomb, A. F. (2000). Variations in patterns of attraction to same- and other-sex peers during early adolescence. *Developmental Psychology*, 36, 147–154.

Casella, R. (2003). Zero tolerance policy in schools: Rationale, consequences, and alternatives. *Teachers College Record*, 105, 872–892.

Cowan, R. J., Swearer, S. M., & Sheridan, S. M. (2004). Home-School collaboration. In C. Spielberger (Ed.), *Encyclopedia of Applied Psychology* (pp. 201–208). San Diego, CA: Elsevier, Inc.

Craig, W. M. (1998). The relationship among bullying, victimization, depression, anxiety, and aggression in elementary school children. *Personality and Individual Differences*, 24, 123–130.

Craig, W. M. & Pepler, D. J. (1997). Observations of bullying and victimization in the school yard. *Canadian Journal of School Psychology*, 13(2), 41–59.

Crick, N. R. & Dodge, K. A. (1994). A review and reformulation of social information-processing mechanisms in children's social adjustment. *Psychological Bulletin*, 115, 74–101.

Demaray, M. K. & Malecki, C. K. (2003). Perceptions of the frequency and importance of social support by students classified as victims, bullies, and bully/victims in an urban middle school. *School Psychology Review*, 32(3), 471–489.

Dishion, T. J., McCord, J., & Poulin, F. (1999). When interventions harm: Peer groups and problem behavior. *American Psychologist*, 54, 755–764.

Dodge, K. (1991). The structure of function of reaction and proactive aggression. In D. J. Pepler & K. H. Rubin (Eds.), *The Development and Treatment of Childhood Aggression* (pp. 201–215). Hillsdale, NJ: Lawrence Erlbaum Associates.

Dodge, K. A. & Coie, J. D. (1987). Social-information-processing factors in reactive and proactive aggression in children's peer groups. *Journal of Personality and Social Psychology*, 53, 1146–1158.

Doll, B. & Swearer, S. M. (2005). Cognitive behavior interventions for participants in bullying and coercion. In R. B. Mennuti, A. Freeman & R. Christner (Eds.), *Cognitive Behavioral Interventions in Educational Settings*. New York: Brunner-Routledge.

Dunbar, R. I. M. (1988). *Primate Social Systems*. Ithaca: Cornell University Press.

Eder, D. (1995). *School talk: Gender and adolescent cultures*. New Brunswick, N. J.: Rutgers University Press.

Edstrom, L. V., Hirschstein, M., Frey, K., Snell, J. L., & MacKenzie, E. P. (2004, May). Classroom Level Influences in School-Based Bullying Prevention: Key Program Components and

Implications for Instruction. Paper presented at the annual meeting of the Society for Prevention Research, Quebec City, Canada.

Eron, L. D., Huesmann, L. R., Dubow, E., Romanoff, R., & Yarnel, P. W. (1987). Aggression and its correlates over 22 years. In D. H. Crowell & I. M. Evans (Eds.), *Childhood Aggression and Violence: Sources of Influence, Prevention, and Control* (pp. 249–262). New York: Plenum Press.

Espelage, D. L. & Holt, M. K. (2001). Bullying and victimization during early adolescence: Peer influences and psychosocial correlates. *Journal of Emotional Abuse*, 2, 123–142.

Espelage, D. L. & Swearer, S. M. (2003). Research on bullying and victimization: What have we learned and where do we go from here? In S. M. Swearer & D. L. Espelage (Eds.), Bullying prevention and intervention: Integrating research and evaluation findings [Special issue]. *School Psychology Review*, 32(3), 365–383.

Espelage, D. L., Holt, M. K., & Henkel, R. R. (2003). Examination of peer-group contextual effects on aggression during early adolescence. *Child Development,* 74(1), 205–220.

Finnegan, R. A., Hodges, E. V. E., & Perry, D. G. (1998). Victimization by peers: Associations with children's reports of mother-child interaction. *Journal of Personality and Social Psychology*, 75(4), 1076–1086.

Fonagy, P., Twemlow, S. W., Vernberg, E., Sacco, F., & Little, T. D. (2005). Creating a peaceful school learning environment: The impact of an antibullying program on educational attainment in elementary schools. *Medical Science Monitor*, 11, 317–325.

Frey, K. S, Hirschstein, M. K, Snell, J. L., Edstrom, L., Van Schoiack, MacKenzie, E. P. & Broderick, C. J. (2005). Reducing playground bullying and supporting beliefs: an experimental trial of the *Steps to Respect* program. *Developmental Psychology*, 41, 479–491.

Garbarino, J. & deLara, E. (2002). *And Words Can Hurt Forever: How to Protect Adolescents from Bullying, Harassment, and Emotional Violence.* New York: Free Press.

Graham, S. & Juvonen, J. (2001). An attributional approach to peer victimization. In S. Graham & J. Juvonen (Eds.), *Peer Harassment in School: The Plight of the Vulnerable and Victimized* (pp. 49–72). New York: Guilford Press.

Gordon, A. (2001). School Exclusions in England: Children's Voices and Adult Solutions?. *Educational Studies,* 27(1), 69–85.

Hawker, D. S. J. & Boulton, M. J. (2000). Twenty years' research on peer victimization and psychosocial maladjustment: A meta-analytic review of cross-sectional studies. *Journal of Child Psychology and Psychiatry and Allied Disciplines*, 41, 441–455.

Haynie, D. L., Nansel, T., & Eitel, P. (2001). Bullies, victims, and bully/victims: Distinct groups of at-risk youth. *Journal of Early Adolescence*, 21, 29–49.

Hirschstein, M. & Frey, K. S. (2006). Promoting behavior and beliefs that reduce bullying: The *Steps to Respect* Program. In S. R. Jimerson & M. Furlong (Eds.). (2006). *Handbook of School Violence and School Safety: From Research to Practice* (pp. 309–323). Mahwah, NJ: Lawrence Erlbaum Associates.

Holt, M. K. & Espelage, D. L. (in press). Perceived social support among bullies, victims, and bully-victims. *Journal of Youth and Adolescence.*

Hoover, J. H. & Hazler, R. J. (1994). Bullies and victims. *Elementary School Guidance and Counseling*, 25, 212–220.

Howard, K. A., Flora, J., & Griffin, M. (1999). Violence-prevention programs in schools: State of the science and implications for future research. *Applied & Preventative Psychology*, 8, 197–215.

Juvonen, J. & Graham, S. (2001). *Peer Harassment in School: The Plight of the Vulnerable and Victimized.* New York: Guilford Press.

Juvoven, J., Nishina, A., & Graham, S. (2000). Self-views versus peer perceptions of victim status among early adolescents. In J. Juvonen & S. Graham (Eds.), *Peer Harassment in Schools: The Plight of the Vulnerable and Victimized* (pp. 105–124). New York: Guilford Press.

Kaltiala-Heino, R., Rimpela, M., Rantanen, P., & Rimpela, A. (2000). Bullying at school: An indicator of adolescents at risk for mental disorders. *Journal of Adolescence*, 23, 661–674.

Kaltiala-Heino, R., Rimpelae, M., & Rantanen, P. (2001). Bullying at school: An indicator for adolescents at risk for mental disorders. *Journal of Adolescence*, 23, 661–674.

Kingsbury, W. & Espelage, D.L. (in press). Self-blaming attributions as mediators between victimization and psychological outcomes during early adolescence. *European Journal of Educational Psychology*.

Kochenderfer, B. J. & Ladd, G. W. (1996). Peer victimization: Cause or consequence of school maladjustment? *Child Development*, 67, 1305–1317.

Kumpulainen, K., Rasanen, E., & Henttonen, I. (1998). Children involved in bullying: Psychological disturbance and the persistence of the involvement. *Child Abuse & Neglect,* 23, 1253–1262.

Kumpulainen, K., Räsänen, E., & Puura, K. (2001). Psychiatric disorders and the use of mental health services among children involved in bullying. *Aggressive Behavior*, 27, 102–110.

Leff, S. S., Kupersmidt, J. B., Patterson, C. J., & Power, T. J. (1999). Factors influencing teacher identification of peer bullies and victims. *School Psychology Review*, 28, 505–517.

Leslie, A. M. (1987). Pretense and representation: The origins of "theory of mind." *Psychological Review*, 94, 412–426.

Loeber, R., & Dishion, T. (1984). Boys who fight at home and school: Family conditions influencing cross-setting consistency. *Journal of Consulting & Clinical Psychology*, 52(5), 759–768.

McFadyen-Ketchum, S. A., Bates, J. E., Dodge, K. A., & Pettit, G. S. (1996). Patterns of change in early childhood aggressive-disruptive behavior: Gender differences in predictions from early coercive and affectionate mother-child interactions. *Child Development,* 67(5), 2417–2433.

Moffitt, T. E. (1993). Adolescent-limited and life-course-persistent anti-social behavior: A developmental taxonomy. *Psychological Review*, 100, 674–701.

Mouttapa, M., Valente, T., Gallaher, P., Rohrbach, L. A., & Unger, J. B. (2004). Social network predictors of bullying and victimization. *Source Adolescence*, 39(154), 315–335.

Nansel, T. R., Overpeck, M., Pilla, R. S., Ruan, W. J., Simons-Morton, B., & Scheidt, P. (2001). Bullying behaviors among US youth: Prevalence and association with psychosocial adjustment. *Journal of the American Medical Association*, 285, 2094–2100.

Nansel, T. R., Haynie, D. L., & Simons-Morton, B. G. (2003). The association of bullying and victimization with middle school adjustment. *Journal of Applied School Psychology*, 19(45–61).

Neary, A. & Joseph, S. (1994). Peer victimization and its relation to self-concept and depression among schoolgirls. *Personality and Individual Differences*, 16, 183–186.

Newman, D. A., Horne, A. M., & Bartolomucci, C. L. (2000). *Bully Busters: A Teacher's Manual for Helping Bullies, Victims, and Bystanders*. Champaign, IL: Research Press.

Newman, R. S., Murray, B., & Lussier, C. (2001). Confrontation with aggressive peers at school: Students' reluctance to seek help from the teacher. *Journal of Educational Psychology*, 93(2), 398–410.

Olweus, D. (1978). *Aggression in the Schools: Bullies and Whipping Boys*. Washington, DC: Hemisphere.

Olweus, D. (1991). Bully/victim problems among schoolchildren: Basic facts and effects of a school based intervention program. In D. Pepler & K. Rubin (Eds.), *The development and treatment of childhood aggression* (pp. 411–448). Hills-dale, NJ: Erlbaum.

Olweus, D. (1992). Bullying among schoolchildren: Intervention and prevention. In R. D. Peters, R. J. McMahon, & V. L. Quinse (Eds.), *Aggression and Violence Throughout the Life Span* (pp. 100–125). London: Sage Publications.

Olweus, D. (1993). *Bullying at School*. Oxford, UK: Blackwell Publishing.

Olweus, D. (1995). Bullying or peer abuse at school: Intervention and prevention. In G. Davies & S. Lloyd-Bostock (Eds.), *Psychology, Law, and Criminal Justice: International Developments in Research and Practice*. Oxford, England: Walter De Gruyter.

Olweus, D. (2001). Peer harassment: A critical analysis and some important issues. In S. Graham & J. Juvonen (Eds.), *Peer Harassment in School: The Plight of the Vulnerable and Victimized* (pp. 3–20). New York: Guilford Press.

Olweus, D. & Limber, S. (1999). *Blueprints for Violence Prevention: The Bullying Prevention Program*. Boulder, CO: Center for the Study and Prevention of Violence.

Orpinas, P. & Horne, A. M. (2006). *Bullying Prevention: Creating a Positive School Climate and Developing Social Competence*. Washington, DC: American Psychological Association.

Pellegrini, A. D. (2002a). Bullying, victimization, and sexual harassment during the transition to middle school. *Educational Psychologist*, 37, 151–163.

Pellegrini, A. D. (2002b). Affiliative and aggressive dimensions of dominance and possible functions during early adolescence. *Aggression & Violent Behavior*, 7(1), 21–31.

Pellegrini, A. D. & Bartini, M. (2001). Dominance in Early Adolescent Boys: Affiliative and Aggressive Dimensions and Possible Functions. *Merrill-Palmer Quarterly*, 47, 142–163.

Pellegrini, A. D. & Long, J. (2002). A longitudinal study of bullying, dominance, and victimization during the transition from primary to secondary school. *British Journal of Developmental Psychology*, 20, 259–280.

Reynolds, W. (2003). *Bully-Victimization Scales for Schools Bully-Victimization Scale (BVS), Bully-Victimization Distress Scale (BVDS), School Violence Anxiety Scale (SVAS)*. Harcourt Assessment, UK.

Rigby, K. (2001). Health consequences of bullying and its prevention in schools. In J. Juvonen & S. Graham (Eds.), *Peer Harassment in School: The Plight of the Vulnerable and Victimized* (pp. 310–331). New York: Guilford Press.

Roberts, W. B. & Coursol, D. H. (1996). Strategies for intervention with childhood and adolescent victims of bullying, teasing and intimidation in school settings. *Elementary School Guidance and Counseling*, 30(3), 204–212.

Rodkin, P. C. (2004). Peer ecologies of aggression and bullying. In D. L. Espelage & S. M. Swearer (Eds.), *Bullying in American Schools: A Social-Ecological Perspective on Prevention and Intervention* (pp. 87–106). Mahwah, NJ: Lawrence Erlbaum.

Rodkin, P. C. & Berger, C. (2005). Who bullies whom? Social status asymmetrics by victim gender. Unpublished Manuscript.

Rodkin, P. C. & Hodges, E. V. (2003). Bullies and victims in the peer ecology: Four questions for psychologists and school professionals. *School Psychology Review*, 32(3), 384–400.

Salmivalli, C., Karhunen, J., & Lagerspetz, K. M. J. (1996). How do the victims respond to bullying? *Aggressive Behavior*, 22, 99–109.

School-Wide PBS (n.d.). Retrieved May 15, 2006 from http://www.pbis.org/schoolwide.htm.

Sheridan, S. M., Napolitano, S. A., & Swearer, S. M. (2002). Best practices in school-community partnerships. In A. Thomas & J. Grimes (Eds.), *Best Practices in School Psychology IV* (pp. 321–336). Bethesda, MD: The National Association of School Psychologists.

Skinner, K. & Kochenderfer-Ladd, B. (2000, March). Coping strategies of victimized children. In A. Nishina & J. Juvonen (Chairs), *Harassment Across Diverse Contexts*. Symposium conducted at the biennial meetings of the Society for Research on Adolescence, Chicago.

Smith, P. K., Madsen, K. C., & Moody, J. C. (1999). What causes the age decline in reports of being bullied at school? Toward a developmental analysis of risks of being bullied. *Educational Research*, 41, 267–285.

Smith, P. K., Shu, S., & Madsen, K. (2001). Characteristics of victims of school bullying: Developmental changes in coping strategies and skills. In S. Graham & J. Juvonen (Eds.), *Peer Harassment in School: The Plight of the Vulnerable and Victimized* (pp. 332–352). New York: Guilford Press.

Sprague, J. R. & Golly, A. (2004). *Best Behavior: Building Positive Behavior Supports in Schools*. Longmont, CO: Sopris West.

Sprague, J. R. & Walker, H. M. (2005). *Safe and Healthy Schools: Practical Prevention Strategies*. NY: Guilford Press.

Stockdale, M. S., Hangaduambo, S., Duys, D., Larson, K., & Sarvela, P. D. (2002). Rural elementary students', parents', and teachers' perceptions of bullying. *American Journal of Health Behavior*, 26, 266–277.

Sutton, J., Smith, P. K., & Swettenham, J. (1999). Bullying and "theory of mind": A critique of the "social skills deficit" view of anti-social behaviour. *Social Development*, 8, 117–127.

Swearer, S. M. (2001). *The Bully Survey*. Unpublished manuscript. Lincoln: University of Nebraska.

Swearer, S. M. & Cary, P. T. (2003). Perceptions and attitudes toward bullying in middle school youth: A developmental examination across the bully/victim continuum. *Journal of Applied School Psychology*, 19, 63–79.

Swearer, S. M. & Doll, B. (2001). Bullying in schools: An ecological framework. *Journal of Emotional Abuse*, 2, 7–23.

Swearer, S. M. & Espelage, D. L. (2004). Introduction: A social-ecological framework of bullying among youth. In D. L. Espelage & S. M. Swearer (Eds.), *Bullying in American Schools: A Social-Ecological Perspective on Prevention and Intervention* (pp. 1–12). Mahwah, NJ: Lawrence Erlbaum.

Swearer, S. M. & Givens, J. E. (2006). Designing an Alternative to Suspension for Middle School Bullies. Paper presented at the annual convention of the National Association of School Psychologists, Anaheim, CA.

Swearer, S. M., Song, S. Y., Cary, P. T., Eagle, J. W., & Mickelson, W. T. (2001). Psychosocial correlates in bullying and victimization: The relationship between depression, anxiety, and bully/victim status. *Journal of Emotional Abuse*, 2, 95–121.

Troy, M. & Sroufe, L. A. (1987). Victimization among preschoolers: Role of attachment relationship history. *Journal of the American Academy of Child and Adolescent Psychiatry*, 26, 166–172.

Twemlow, S. W., Fonagy, P., & Sacco, F. C. (2001). An innovative psychodynamically influenced intervention to reduce school violence. *Journal of the American Academy of Child and Adolescent Psychiatry*, 40, 377–379.

Twemlow, S. W., Fonagy, P., & Sacco, F. C. (2005). A developmental approach to mentalizing communities: II. The Peaceful Schools experiment. Bulletin of the Menninger Clinic, 69, 282–304.

Chapter 18
School Shootings in Middle School, High School, and College: Clinical Management and School Interventions for High-Risk Students

Thomas W. Miller, William Weitzel, and Janet Lane

Introduction

School shootings have occurred at several levels of education including middle school as in Paducah, Kentucky, high school at Columbine and others, and at the college and university levels as with the University of Texas and Virginia Tech violence. School violence has gained considerable attention nationally. Examined in this chapter are theoretical considerations involving escape theory, the risk and protective factors for school violence, case analyses of case studies, and discussion of school shootings involving fatal injuries involving others. Identifying at-risk and high-risk students is essential as a part of prevention of school violence. Also examined are diagnostic issues in understanding children who are at risk for school violence and ways school violence may be managed in the schools and clinical management and school interventions aimed at the prevention of school violence. Offered are suggestions and recommendations including recommendations provided by the National School Safety Center (2006) for school personnel as are steps to be taken in creating a safe school environment. Our intent in the chapter is to provide information that may be useful for prevention to educational, medical, health care professionals, law enforcement personnel, and school boards who oversee administratively and who provide services to school-aged children.

Identifying At-Risk Students: Theory Applied to School Violence

Escape theory (Baumeister, 1990; Heatherton & Baumeister, 1991) postulates that peer victimization or bullying is driven by the desire to escape a state of painful self-awareness, characterized by inadequacy, negative affect, and low self-esteem. The emotions associated with this state of self-awareness are focused on the self-perceived failure to achieve acceptance among peers and are often based on rigid self-standards. According to the theory, certain individuals attempt to escape these negative self-perceptions and emotions by narrowing their consciousness to an immediate action, like bullying, which results in irrational cognitions that predominate over normal inhibitions against self-destructive behaviors. The psychological profile for bullies characterizes people who engage in escape behaviors. According to escape theory, the personality characteristics of bullies which predispose them to episodes of negative self-perceptions affect low self-esteem and high levels of self-awareness. These risk factors set the stage for frequent episodes of acting out against others in the form of bullying accompanied by irrational thoughts which, in turn, activate the desire to escape. Frequent repetitions of this cycle create high levels of residual negative affect and irrational thinking. Children and adolescents who engage in escape behaviors on a regular basis tend to display more negative affect, irrational thinking, negative self-awareness, unrealistically high self-standards, and low self-esteem. We predict that this profile will distinguish both binge eaters and those with suicidal thoughts from normalcy.

While there is a dearth of empirical research that has been done investigating escape theory and bullying behavior, there is reason to believe that escape theory has applicability to perpetrator motives in some school violence situations. Studies that have investigated aspects of escape theory have examined differing constellations of variables, with mixed findings (Beebe et al., 1995). While escape theory does not address how different "escape behaviors" emerge, it does aid in understanding risk factors that school personnel must be alert to in the school environment end that may result in violent behaviors.

The National School Safety Center offers the following checklist derived from tracking school-associated violent deaths in the United States. Follow this link to the School Associated Violent Deaths Report. After studying common characteristics of youngsters who have caused such deaths, the National School Safety Center has identified the following behaviors which could indicate a youth's potential for harming himself/herself or others.

_____ Has a history of tantrums and uncontrollable angry outbursts.
_____ Characteristically resorts to name calling, cursing, or abusive language.
_____ Habitually makes violent threats when angry.
_____ Has previously brought a weapon to school.
_____ Has a background of serious disciplinary problems at school and in the community.
_____ Has a background of drug, alcohol, or other substance abuse or dependency.
_____ Is on the fringe of his/her peer group with few or no close friends.
_____ Is preoccupied with weapons, explosives, or other incendiary devices.
_____ Has previously been truant, suspended, or expelled from school.
_____ Displays cruelty to animals.
_____ Has little or no supervision and support from parents or a caring adult.
_____ Has witnessed or been a victim of abuse or neglect in the home.
_____ Has been bullied and/or bullies or intimidates peers or younger children.
_____ Tends to blame others for difficulties and problems she/he causes herself/himself.
_____ Consistently prefers TV shows, movies, or music expressing violent themes and acts.

_____ Prefers reading materials dealing with violent themes, rituals, and abuse.

_____ Reflects anger, frustration, and the dark side of life in school essays or writing projects.

_____ Is involved with a gang or an antisocial group on the fringe of peer acceptance.

_____ Is often depressed and/or has significant mood swings.

_____ Has threatened or attempted suicide.

Developed by the National School Safety Center

Published with permission

Dr. Ronald D. Stephens, Executive Director

These characteristics should serve to alert school administrators, teachers, and support staff to address needs of troubled students through meetings with parents, provision of school counseling, guidance, and mentoring services, as well as referrals to appropriate community health/social services and law enforcement personnel. Further, such behavior should also provide an early warning signal that safe school plans and crisis prevention/intervention procedures must be in place to protect the health and safety of all school students and staff members so that schools remain safe havens for learning.

School administrators are advised to take the following steps in creating a safe learning environment:

- Develop a safety plan and implement the plan.
- Inspect the premises on a regular and predictable basis.
- Identify areas that individual schools are not controlling.
- Direct students to supervised areas when they arrive at school. Security personnel & school administrators.
- Identify and conduct routine inspections of secluded areas. Kentucky School Boards Association (KSBA) officials suggested searching school grounds for a heavy concentration of cigarette butts; that is likely to be where students are gathering unobserved.
- Inspect playgrounds regularly and on a daily basis.
- Monitor and inspect hallways and restrooms between classes.
- Document everything, from hallway inspections to follow-ups on sexual harassment complaints.
- Make decisions that relate to the health and benefit of students. Decisions that promote character development; helpful and assure the students, models, and boundary experience with home, school, and peers.

Risk Factors in the School Environment

Many of the risk factors that emerge in the school environment are symptomatic of other problems, such as learning disabilities, emotional problems, or a temporary difficulty in the family's situation (Parker et al., 1995; Dean & Range, 1996; West et al., 1993). In addition, more serious symptoms may be caused by major problems associated with family dysfunction, domestic violence, or substance abuse (Miller, 1998; Puka, 1994). Some of the following risk factors in the school environment are symptomatic of problems experienced outside of school. In school, children and adolescents may behave aggressively or violently toward other students and teachers in the classroom or on the playground. They may use money as a means of winning other students' approval and acceptance. They may disrupt the classroom by failing to attend to the tasks of the class, to stay in their seats, to respond appropriately to the teacher, and to participate in appropriate classroom behavior. These are students who may vandalize school property and classroom materials, make sexual gestures toward other students and teachers, or perform poorly in academic work, regularly scoring low on tests and consistently failing to complete classroom and homework assignments. Often these students spend free time with older students who behave aggressively in and out of the classroom and fail to show self-respect or respect for others. These patterns of behavior are often an indicator of low self-esteem and poor self-confidence levels in these children (Veltkamp & Miller, 1994).

Case Examples

Postincident committees and school districts in Mississippi, Kentucky, Arkansas, Oregon, Colorado, and Virginia have experienced a strikingly similar pattern of behavior among perpetrators, all in rural communities. Several of the critical factors realized in each instance are summarized in Table 18.1. While this does not suggest an all-inclusive summary, what does emerge are demographic, interpersonal, and family factors that demonstrate consistency across incidents.

Critical data have been collected on five of the eight cases and is summarized in a sequential fashion for the Kentucky, Arkansas, Oregon, Colorado, and Virginia events and the subsequent observations of teachers, parents, professionals, and peers are summarized. In addressing some of the clinical factors, Table 18.1 summarizes demographic factors, interpersonal factors, and violence and family factors across the five cases. The Kentucky case involves a 14-year-old who stole a .22 caliber pistol from a neighbor. He comes from a sound home with both parents in the home and an older sister who is bright and socially well accepted by peers. The Jonesboro, Arkansas, involved two adolescents aged 11 and 13. Again, three firearms were used and they were stolen from relatives. In this case, one set of parents was divorced, the other intact and at home. The Springfield, Oregon, case involved a 15-year-old who used a semiautomatic and two pistols, which were gifts from his father. He, like his counterpart in Kentucky, was described as a loner. Both parents are in the home, and like the Kentucky case, there is a bright older sister. The Colorado case involved two young men 17 and 18 years of age. Both from the parent homes and in one case a brother is a well-recognized athlete. Access to guns in this case involved gaining access through friends who purchased the weapons.

Table 18.1 Clinical factors in school violence

	CO	OR	KY	AR	VA
Demographic factors					
Rural setting	X	X	X	X	X
Age	17/18	15	14	11/13	
Sex	M	M	M	M	M
Interpersonal factors					
Felt humiliated	X	X	X	X	X
Teased/Bullied by peers	X	X	X	X	X
Involved in deviant or antisocial behavior	X	X	X	X	X
Need for power and control	X	X	X	X	X
Competition with siblings or peers	X	X	X	X	X
Advance signals to cause harm	X	X	X	X	X
Angry loner	X	X	X	X	X
Peers knew of premeditation		X	X	X	
Access to violence					
Ready availability of weapons	X	X	X	X	X
Exposure to violence in media	X	X	X	X	X
Influenced by music and movies	X	X	X	X	X
Video games/Doom, Quake	X	X	X	X	X
Boundary difficulties	X	X	X	X	X
Carried weapons	X	X	X	X	X
Motive of anger/hate	X	X	X	X	X
Identity diffusion	X	X	X	X	X
Family factors					
History of disruptive home life		X		X	X
Psychopathology present	X				X
Being treated with medication	X	X	X		X
Prevention intervention					
Conflict resolution skills lacking	X	X	X	X	X
Lacking empathy	X	X	X	X	X
Anger control and management skills lacking	X	X	X	X	X

In the Virginia Tech case, Cho Seung-Hui, a 23-year-old senior English major from Centreville, Virginia, and attending Virginia Tech, who had a history of mental illness acted out against others because of anger and hostility that may have been the product of bullying and humiliation.

He was taking medication to combat depression and his recent behavior was troubling, including setting a fire in a dormitory and stalking women on campus. His anger led to the wounding and killing of fellow students and teachers at Virginia Tech. Bullying again became a critical marker in mass school shootings in the United States (Figs. 18.1–18.5) (Espelage & Swearer, 2004; Boxer et al., 2005; Edwards et al., 2005).

Risk factors identifying critical issues that heighten the potential for adverse behavior in the group of young men that acted out with lethal consequences are identified. In addition to the riffle factor noted, the presence of a psychiatric disorder or symptoms consistent with a psychiatric disorder must be addressed. In addressing the psychiatric stability of each of the cases, there is reason to believe that there

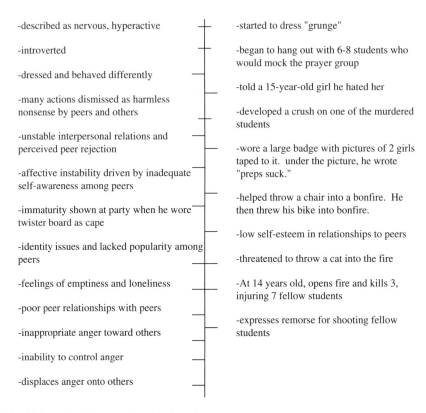

Fig. 18.1 Paducah, Kentucky, critical markers

are psychiatric markers in each instance. The Kentucky teen has been described as depressed, with erratic fears, but had not received psychiatric treatment. He pleaded guilty and mentally ill at the time of his arraignment. The Arkansas youth was described as an aggressive, impulsive, and bully-type of youngster, with his counterpart being described as tough and mean-spirited individual. The Springfield, Oregon, case has similarities to the Kentucky case in that this youngster was also described as depressed, was on Ritalin then Prozac. Most notable is the fact that this adolescent was described as a loner and was known to torture animals. In the Virginia Tech case, the perpetrator was described as having mental illness and was a person who showed symptoms from early childhood.

There are well-researched protective factors that may buffer against the likelihood of acting-out behavior as unstressed in Arkansas, Kentucky, Oregon, and Virginia. Figure 18.6 summarized some of the protective factors that may serve this benefit and reduce the chances of the level of activity and lethality in these situations.

Perpetrators with self-esteem problems, a reservoir of anger, or confusion brought on by a dysfunctional family system often disclose their pathology through their behavior. One of the adolescent perpetrators, in the weeks before he shot and

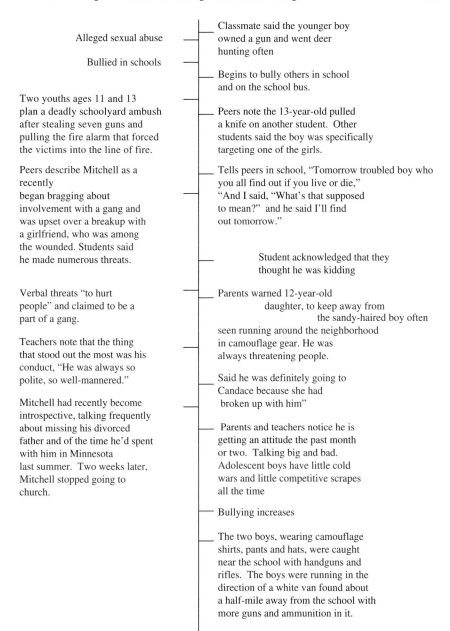

Alleged sexual abuse — Classmate said the younger boy owned a gun and went deer hunting often

Bullied in schools — Begins to bully others in school and on the school bus.

Two youths ages 11 and 13 plan a deadly schoolyard ambush after stealing seven guns and pulling the fire alarm that forced the victims into the line of fire. — Peers note the 13-year-old pulled a knife on another student. Other students said the boy was specifically targeting one of the girls.

Peers describe Mitchell as a recently began bragging about involvement with a gang and was upset over a breakup with a girlfriend, who was among the wounded. Students said he made numerous threats. — Tells peers in school, "Tomorrow you all find out if you live or die," "And I said, "What's that supposed to mean?" and he said I'll find out tomorrow."

troubled boy who

Student acknowledged that they thought he was kidding

Verbal threats "to hurt people" and claimed to be a part of a gang. — Parents warned 12-year-old daughter, to keep away from the sandy-haired boy often seen running around the neighborhood in camouflage gear. He was always threatening people.

Teachers note that the thing that stood out the most was his conduct, "He was always so polite, so well-mannered." — Said he was definitely going to Candace because she had broken up with him"

Mitchell had recently become introspective, talking frequently about missing his divorced father and of the time he'd spent with him in Minnesota last summer. Two weeks later, Mitchell stopped going to church. — Parents and teachers notice he is getting an attitude the past month or two. Talking big and bad. Adolescent boys have little cold wars and little competitive scrapes all the time

— Bullying increases

— The two boys, wearing camouflage shirts, pants and hats, were caught near the school with handguns and rifles. The boys were running in the direction of a white van found about a half-mile away from the school with more guns and ammunition in it.

Fig. 18.2 Jonesboro, Arkansas, critical markers

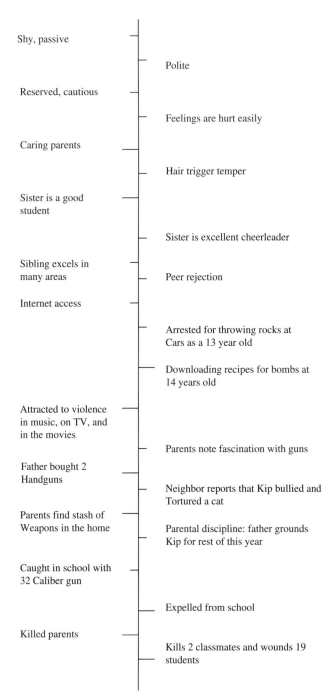

Fig. 18.3 Springfield, Oregon, critical markers

- Eric Harris (18)
- comes from a good family
- brother is a star athlete
- descriptive childhood moving often from the air force base to another
- took a prescribed antidepressant for depression
- Wanted to go into the military like his father but was rejected by the Marines.
- He liked violent video games and the German rock group Rammstein
- Viewed by peers as a manipulator
- Once threw a chunk of ice at a car, cracking its windshield. Website bad geysers of hate like the one saying he longed to "blow up and shoot everything he could kill."
- Described by friends as incredible
- Fact no remorse, no sense of shame
- Expressed belief that he didn't care if he lived or died in the shoot out and note "all I want to do is kill and injure as many of you (expletive) as I can."
- Favorite Music: Marilyn Manson
- Favorite Heroes: Hitler and Nietzsche
- Launched the Columbine massacre, murdering 13 and wounding 23 before killing themselves
- Dylan Klebold (17)
- good family background with intact two parent family
- described by others as shy and sad, a loner
- Teased by jocks, labeled "Trench Coat Mafia," and called "faggots" by peers at school
- Dylan becomes Eric's new best friend but had a hateful website.
- His website offered bomb-building instructions and boasted that he and a friend, cod-named "VoDka," had made four pipe bombs and detonated one ("Flipping thing was heart-pounding gut-wrenching brain-twitching ground-moving insanely cool!"
- Liked the music of Marilyn Manson; hero was Hitler; video games: Doom and Quake were his favorite
- Played fantasy baseball on the not having made the school computer team
- Girlfriend bought three of the guns used in the shooting

Fig. 18.4 Columbine critical markers

killed three classmates and injured five other students, revealed the behavior pattern that communicated his rage, his confusion, and his desire to strike out against others. These words and actions displayed elements of hostility and destructive behavior just a few weeks before his shooting rampage. The perpetrator told a fellow classmate in his school that he hated her and this was based on what he likely perceived as rejection on her part. She was a close friend of three of the eight victims whom the 14-year-old has been charged with shooting in the lobby of the local high school. On another occasion, the perpetrator was seen wearing a large button onto which he had pasted pictures of one of his victims and her twin sister. Under their pictures, he had written the words: "Preps suck." This victim now lies partially paralyzed by one of the bullets fired in the shooting spree. In another instance, the perpetrator helped throw a chair into a bonfire attended by a number of Heath students, most of whom, like him, were members of the school band. After the chair went into the fire, he threw his bike in and talked about throwing a cat into the fire. Hostility directed toward animals is a serious predicator of hostility directed toward humans. Another instance is the perpetrator had previously shown hostility toward another member of a school group, who was wounded in the shooting. Two

-Cho Seung-Hui, a 23-year-old senior English major at Virginia Tech

-born into poverty with two parents working a great deal of time.

-Little time for him during developmental years His father, Seung-Tae Cho worked in oil fields and on construction sites in Saudi Arabia away from home.

-In an arranged marriage, he wed Kim Hwang-Im, the daughter of a farming family that had fled North Korea during the Korean War.

-Their son was well behaved as a child and responsive to strict parental control

-his pronounced bashfulness deeply worried his parents. Relatives thought he might be a mute.or mentally ill.

-The kid didn't say much and didn't mix with other children,"

-In 1984, relatives who had moved to the United States invited the family to join them.

-In 1992, arrived in Detroit and then moved on to Centreville, Va., home to a bustling Korean community on the fringe of Washington.

-They found jobs in the dry-cleaning business-

-family was uncommonly private They shunned the more prominent Korean-language Christian churches, and prayed at a small church outside of town.

-High school did not help Seung-Hui Cho surmount his miseries. He went to Westfield High School, one of the largest

- He was unresponsive in class, and unwilling to speak.

-Classmates recall some teasing and bullying over his taciturn nature.

-The few times he was required to speak for a class assignment, students mocked his poor English and deep-throated voice.

-Neighbors saw him shooting baskets by himself.

-Cho's older sister, Sun-Kyung Cho, went to Princeton University and was scholarly

-Cho developed draft scripts for two plays for a writing class that contain "really twisted, macabre violence," according to a student who was in class with him

-His writing was "very graphic" and "extremely disturbing. The plays had really twisted, macabre violence that used weapons

-before Cho got to class that day, we students were talking to each other with serious worry about whether he could be a school shooter.

-Cho was extremely quiet, and efforts by other students to draw him out were rebuffed.

-Cho took his own life as police closed in on him, Thirty other bodies were found in Norris Hall along with Cho

-Federal agents describe Cho as having many of the same characteristics of a criminal behavioral profile called the "Collector of Injustice," or someone who considers any misfortune against him the fault or responsibility of others

-Eventually, the person's compilation of wrongs becomes overloaded, and he lashes out violently to right them and get even with those who he believes have caused him misfortune and ridicule

-Cho Seung-Hui, a 23-year-old senior English major from Centreville, Virginia, Virginia Tech

-a note has been found indicating Cho showed anger against "rich kids."

-Cho had a history of mental illness

-Cho left a note in his dorm in which he railed against "rich kids," "debauchery" and "deceitful charlatans" on the Virginia Tech campus

-Cho may have been taking medication to combat depression and that his recent behavior was troubling, including setting a fire in a dorm and stalking women.

Fig. 18.5 Virginia tech critical markers

students told others that he had developed a crush on one of his victims, who died in the shooting. Peers revealed that it was no secret among students that he had a romantic interest in one of the victims. Peers said students in her circle of friends knew the perpetrator had a crush on one of his victims, but that she might not have known about it. Students thought he had asked the girl out once or twice, but she did not accept his invitation. A fellow sophomore and band member was the girl to whom the perpetrator said "I hate you" repeatedly during the prior 6 months to the shooting. The adolescent perpetrator in recent months had seemed attracted to a

In Four Cases of School Violence

	Risk Factors	Protective Factors
Peer Group	Emotional Problems	Respect Authority
	Inability to delay gratification	Responsible
	Aggressiveness	Independent thinking
	Sensation seeking	Communication skills
School	No home support	Caring
	Low achievement expectations	Social skills
	Family dysfunction	Cooperative learning
	Lack of school commitment	Teacher/child relationship
Family	Distress/low stability	Positive child/parent relationship
	Marital/family conflict	Support and affection
		Parental abuse/neglect
		High expectations regarding behavior
	Lack of discipline	Discipline and rule enforcement
Community	Concentrated poverty	Trustworthy role models
	Schools w/ high failure/dropout rates	Adults helping with students
		Firearms and crime
		Responsibility & relationship
	Lack of positive role model	Respect

Fig. 18.6 Risk and protective factors

group of older students who dressed "grunge." He would wear oversized, "greasy" pants, tie-dyed T-shirts, and attention getting symbols. Fellow students reported that the perpetrator often stood with some of his friends on the fringes of the student group that gathered every morning before school in a ring and hold hands. The perpetrator would often mock the group and bully group members.

Case Study
Bill your case information here.

Diagnostic Issues

Clinical indicators (American Psychiatric Association, 1994) of at-risk and high-risk students, which is important to school personnel related to psychopathology, include several diagnostic factors including, but not limited to, the following: Is there a pervasive pattern of disregard for and violation of the rights of others occurring as indicated by three (or more) of the following: (1) failure to conform to social norms with respect to lawful behaviors as indicated by repeatedly performing acts that are grounds for arrest or reprimand; (2) deceitfulness, as indicated by repeated lying, use of aliases, or conning others for personal profit or pleasure; (3) impulsivity or failure to plan ahead; (4) irritability and aggressiveness, as indicated by repeated physical fights or assaults including bullying; (5) reckless disregard for safety of self or others; and (6) consistent irresponsibility, as indicated by repeated failure to sustain consistent work behavior or honor financial obligations.

Is there a pervasive pattern of instability in interpersonal relationships, self-image, and affect, and marked impulsivity beginning by early adulthood and present in a variety of contexts, as indicated by five (or more) of the following: (1) frantic efforts to avoid real or imagined abandonment; (2) a pattern of unstable and intense interpersonal relationships characterized by alternating between extremes of idealization and devaluation; (3) identity disturbance: markedly and persistently unstable self-image or sense of self; (4) impulsivity that is potentially self-damaging; (5) recurrent behavior, gestures, or threats of harm to self or others; (6) affective instability due to a marked reactivity of mood; (7) chronic feelings of emptiness; (8) inappropriate, intense anger or difficulty controlling anger; and (9) transient, stress-related paranoid ideation or severe dissociative symptoms.

Clinical Management and School Intervention

Educators and clinicians can be very helpful in consulting with school administrators and teachers and can play an effective role in limiting and mitigating the influence of problematic behavior, including violence. The effectiveness of such efforts depends on the level of communication among school personnel and the speed of their response: school personnel must be in constant communication with one another, each employee must have a clearly designated response role, and employees must respond rapidly to any threat of violence. The National School Safety Center (1999) suggests the following actions to limit violence in the schools: acknowledge the student's problem immediately and seek help from local health or mental health care professionals, police, and community resources, educate all school personnel about risk factors for both individuals and groups, establish an informed communication network with students, institute a strict visitor/trespassers policy in the schools, monitor and control points of access to the school, work closely with local police, and establish procedures to share information with them and consider the use of cameras to monitor potential sites for socially deviant behavior.

Observing and confronting agitated and troubled students send an important indicator that should be addressed. There are several markers to consider when encountering these students. Observe thinking and behavior change; a troubled child's behavior is reflective of a sharp shift in thinking. Individuals who are troubled may show signs of anxiety and depression, irritability, and acting out. Monitor these individuals. Be truthful to these children and be realistic. They need to know that they can manage with help. Send simple and direct communication that identifies the problems and the expected behavior. Troubled individuals need to know that they can count on the adults in their lives to listen to them, support them, and care for them. School is a home away from home, a place for students to share their lives with others. When students are troubled, they need to share their thoughts and feelings with an adult. Students need to know that school has expectations and requirements that require discipline and will be a stable and supportive refuge. When talking to students, move to their level of understanding and use good eye contact. Use open-ended questions to solicit their thoughts and feelings. Enhance your own knowledge of individuals at risk through training opportunities and refer to Fig. 18.2 for risk and protective factors. Know your own assumptions and beliefs about what is troubling the individual. Address "character development" in your class, which emphasizes respect of self, respect for others, and responsibilities we have to one another when there are threats of harm to self or others. Recognize the "teachable moment." The teachable moment occurs when an opportunity to teach students about respect and responsibility arises through events happening around them. Create that moment by using opportunities in the curriculum. Model your own thoughts and feelings to offer students an appropriate way of dealing with life's stressful events. Observe clinical warning signs indicating the need for professional help and advise appropriate authorities immediately.

Clinical warning signs may include the following:

1. An extended period of anxiety and/or depression in which the child loses interest in daily activities and events and seems inwardly preoccupied.
2. Inability to sleep, loss of appetite, prolonged fear of being alone, has few peer or adult contact.
3. Immature behavior for an extended period may be an indication of regressive behavior as a way of coping.
4. Suicidal or homicidal ideation or intent.
5. Withdrawal from friends and shifting to other troubled peers.
6. Lower school performance and/or refusal to attend school.

A child or adolescent psychiatrist, clinical or school psychologist, school counselor, clinical social worker, nurse practitioner, or qualified member of the health care community can help the student and assist persons associated with the individual through the process or referral. Many individuals express anxiety and depression by acting out. This behavior usually varies depending on the person's age and developmental level. The person may become unusually loud and noisy, have temper outbursts, start fights, defy authority, or simply rebel against everything. Drawing again on escape theory, escape in fantasy or reality may show itself in getting poor grades, assuming a general "I don't care about anything" attitude, or even running away from home or school to seek support for this anxiety and depression.

Clinical Issues and Implications

Some students who are at high risk for acting-out behaviors fail to successfully negotiate adolescence, because the behaviors that predispose them to negative experiences are a function of failure to bond with home and family, school and teachers, and peers. Egocentrism is crucial to the adolescent. Elkind (2004) defines egocentrism as the stage which adolescents differentiate between the thoughts of others and their own, but they do not differentiate between the objects of their thoughts and the objects of the thoughts of others. They think all others are personally concerned with them. Since adolescents feel peers are as concerned and admiring of him as he is, he constructs, reacts, and plays to an imaginary audience, constantly on stage, and may wear outlandish clothing, sass adults, or engage in other risk-taking behavior to please this perceived audience.

However, other adolescents have their own imaginary audiences they are performing for and are not that concerned with other peers. This explains the power of the peer group over the individual during early or middle adolescence, and illustrates how easily the adolescent can misinterpret others' perceptions. Most of the cases saw themselves as an outcast with peers, a failure, lost all self-worth, self-love, and self-esteem. Although most were not a known troublemaker, they did exhibit a number of behaviors that got them the attention and, in some cases, the acceptance that they so desperately wanted from others, which to them, as Elkind points out in his theory, is quite real (Miller, 1996).

Deemed totally driven by a perceived lack of and need for acceptance, the perpetrator repeatedly told students something big would happen on a specific day at school for attention, but never intended to do anything. He had hoped if he showed the guns, he would have friends and be liked, but they kept ignoring him, he said. He strove for approval in his family continuously acting out the role of the good son. He printed information off the Internet to gain favor with friends. He and his friends regularly tried to disrupt the prayer group. They often talked about taking over the school with firearms, as a prank to get attention from peers. These issues of vulnerability and resilience have stimulated an interest in the identification of protective factors in the lives of adolescents—factors that, if present, diminish the likelihood of negative social outcomes that result in the violence we have witnessed in this decade.

Of the constellation of forces that influence adolescent risk behavior, the most fundamental are the social contexts in which adolescents are embedded, in the family, their school, and their peers. Adolescents' connection to these contexts shapes their risk behaviors and necessitates further study. Other researchers (Zager & Arbit, 1998) report that adolescents may know and experience more violence than parents are aware. Although most young people reported never having been the victim of violent behavior, 24.1% indicated they had been a victim of violent acts. Additionally, 12.4% of students indicated that they had carried a weapon during the previous 30 days.

Taken within the *family context*, demographic factors and family variables explained relatively little of the variability in violence perpetration, 7% and 5% among younger and older students, respectively. Items associated with higher levels of violence for all students included household access to guns and a recent history of family suicide attempts or completions. Factors associated with somewhat lower levels of interpersonal violence included parental and family connectedness. In addition, higher parental expectations for school achievement were weakly associated with lower levels of violence among older adolescents. Of interest is the *school context*. School context accounted for 6–7% of the variability in violence among students. Specifically, higher levels of school bonding were correlated with somewhat lower levels of violence.

Finally, individual characteristics accounted for 44% of the variability in violent behavior among 7th and 8th graders and 50% of the variability among 9th through 12th graders. Among both younger and older adolescents, involvement in violence was associated with having been a victim or witness to violence, frequency of carrying a weapon, involvement in deviant or antisocial behaviors, and involvement in selling marijuana or other drugs within the past year. Among younger students, interpersonal violence was associated with lower grade point average and higher perceived risk of failure in peer, parent, and teacher relationships (Centers for Disease Control 2003).

Recently, there has been interest in whether high or low self-esteem underlies violent behavior. New research suggests that the most dangerous people are those who have a strong desire to regard themselves as superior beings. They conducted two studies in which they explored the connection between narcissism, negative interpersonal feedback, and aggression in 540 students. Narcissists were found to be emotionally invested in establishing their superiority, yet while they care passionately about being superior to others, they were not convinced that they have achieved this superiority. While high self-esteem entails thinking well of oneself, narcissism involves passionately wanting to think well of oneself. In both studies, narcissism and self-esteem were measured, and subjects were given an opportunity to act aggressively toward a neutral third party, toward someone who had insulted them, or toward someone who had praised them. Results found that the most aggressive respondents in both studies were narcissists who were attacking someone who had given them a bad evaluation. Narcissists were exceptionally aggressive toward anyone who attacked or offended them, yet when they received praise, their level of aggression was not out of the ordinary. In both studies, self-esteem was not related to aggression, suggesting that the relationship between self-esteem and aggressive behavior is small at best. In light of the recent school shootings, the authors of the study note that many schools are attempting to increase their students' self-esteem, which will probably have no effects on violent behavior. But excessive self-love, or narcissism, could actually increase violence in schools (McEvoy & Welker, 2000).

Researchers (Miller, 1996; Taub, 2002) assert that people with high self-esteem are a heterogeneous group that may be more different than alike since high self-esteem can be an accurate recognition of one's positive traits, or it may be a highly doubtful sense of personal superiority that is not reality-based. While some individuals with high self-esteem are largely unaffected by feedback, others may require frequent confirmation and validation of their favorable self-image by others. The researchers suggest that aggression by narcissists is an interpersonally meaningful and specific response to an ego threat. Narcissists mainly want to punish or defeat someone who has threatened their highly favorable views of themselves. Critical to our knowledge of acts of violence in the schools is the realization that there is a contagious effect in society that provides the vulnerable perpetrator a model of aggression sometimes seen in the angry loner.

Clinician researchers Zager and Arbit (1998) suggest that the following factors predict with high accuracy teens who are likely to commit crimes similar to those in Paducah, Jonesboro, Colorado, and Springfield. A child's odds of committing such crimes are doubled when the child comes from criminally violent families, has a history of being abused, belongs to a gang, and uses alcohol and drugs. The authors further contend that the odds are tripled when along with these factors, the child uses weapons, has arrest records, has a neurological disorder, is truant, and has other school-related problems.

The cultural influences give clues to the possible motives and the resulting use of violence in the course of the patterns of behavior exhibited by each. All were loners, did not mix into the mainstream of the peer group, some had strong emotions for a girl that had resulted in perceived rejection. Peers teased most if not all and with the exception of the Arkansas youth who was seen as a perpetrator who used bully tactics, all were assessed after the fact as victims of bullying. The Kentucky youth was called gay, and the Colorado youth were both teased by athletes, labeled "faggots," and called "the trench coat Mafia." The motive for a response is certainly possible in these clinical indicators. The cultural influence for each comes consistently from the contemporary portrayal of violence in music and motion picture. It was the Basketball Diaries and video games such as Doom and Quake in the Kentucky case, the music of Tupac Shakur along with the video game mortal combat in the Arkansas case. In both the Oregon and the Colorado cases the music of Marilynn Manson and Nirvana. And with the Colorado case, video games like Quake and Doom have been documented. The influence of Hitler is also noted in the Colorado case although it is not clear the extent to which this influenced their thinking and behavior.

Recommendations

Violence in the schools is sometimes random but often premeditated by the perpetrator. The following recommendations should be considered (National School Safety Center, 2006). Train teachers and school officials on recognizing signs and symptoms, better control exposure of youth to violence in the media, voluntary self-control, character education, and anger management skills training. Become aware of the identity issues in a child's life. Rejection, anger, and poor conflict resolution skills are found in most perpetrators. Provide education and training for all teachers, students, and parents. It appears from such behavior that males because of "inadequacy to feelings" find that power and control can be achieved primarily through violence. Anonymous tip lines should be considered in the schools. Stricter gun control is needed and access for children and adolescents should be monitored.

Understanding the spectrum of psychopathology offers clues to potential reasons for the aggressive nature of these young perpetrators toward their peers. Further research needs to address the role of narcissism and other personality disorders in addressing the etiology and subsequent acts of violence we have observed in children and adolescents who have come to employ lethal methods as they displace their anger, hatred, frustration, and despair on peers, parents, and other victims of school violence.

What Have We Learned from a Forensic Perspective?

The news came suddenly. The now familiar sickening and frightening report was made on the evening of April 16, 2007. A student had shot and killed fellow students and teachers of the campus community at Virginia Tech University. Once again, a local community and a nation were plunged into self-recrimination and self-examination with an aching desire to "Fix what needs to be fixed."

Events such as these caused one to reflect again, on one's involvement as a forensic examiner. As our society attempts to deal with these episodes of chaos after the fact, our own efforts have been plagued with glitches. It reminded me of my experience with a senior faculty member at University Kentucky Medical Center, during years past. Psychiatric house staff regularly had the opportunity to present the more difficult psychiatric cases from the hospital ward to this expert for his thoughts about evaluation and treatment. The recurring script was that as the house staff member would complete his/her case presentation, the consultant would respond, "Yes, but what is the question?"

The most obvious questions that needed to be answered after the Paducah, Kentucky, shootings, which involved the deaths of three classmates and the shooting and injuring of five additional classmates, were the following:

1. Does the defendant meet the Kentucky Revised Statutes (KRS) standards for competency to stand trial?
2. If competent to stand trial, does he lack substantial capacity to appreciate the wrongfulness of his act, and does his conduct conform to the standards of the law?

Two teams of professional experts were assembled for the purposes of determining the status of this defendant. Those on the side represented by the Commonwealth's Attorney Office included Elissa Benedect, M.D., Child and Adolescent Psychiatrist—University of Michigan; William D. Weitzel, M.D., General Psychiatry—University of Kentucky (coauthor of this chapter); and Charles C. Clark, Ph.D., an academic neurophychologist at the University of Michigan. This team of professionals, who evaluated the defendant with the intent of presenting a report to the Commonwealth's Attorney, posed the relevant questions earlier. The Defense employed two clinicians: Diane Schetky, M.D., Child and Adolescent Psychiatrist—University of Vermont at School of Medicine, Maine Medical Center, and Dewy Cornell, M.D., Academic neuropsychologist—University of Virginia Medical School. Dr. Schetky concluded for the defense that although the defendant had evidence of a dysthymia, traits of schizotypal personality disorder with borderline and paranoid features, he did not lack responsibility for his acts during the event of December 1, 1997.

Axis I:	No diagnoses
Axis II:	No diagnoses
Axis III:	General medical conditions: None
Axis IV:	Schizotypal personality problems
	Criminal prosecution and separation from family routine
Axis V:	Global Assessment of Functioning: "78"

The diagnoses rendered by the Commonwealth Attorney's team (which incorporates the DSM-IV1 terminology) included the following:

These conclusions were delivered in the format recommended by the *Diagnostic and Statistical Manual* (American Psychiatric Association, 1994) published periodically by the American Psychiatric Association. It is the official tone and provides the official vocabulary to be used by mental health clinicians worldwide. The defense team did not appear to adhere closely to this orientation, and so their data were more varying in quality, as they reached their opinions. These findings by these two independent and adversarial employed teams of professionals are remarkably similar, and yet both teams violated the DSM-IV admonition, which stresses that it is inappropriate to describe an individual as having a personality disorder until that individual has reached the chronological age of at least 18. Further, it is the professional opinion of this author that this "Over reaching," by both teams, highlights the restricted usefulness of DSM-IV in our attempts to explain anything more than narrowly drafted questions, for example, with respect to competency and criminal responsibility. But, then again these questions were the ones that were proposed, among many others that could be proposed, as we attempt to understand these awful events.

In this case the original examiners were interested in finding differences on how the defendant told his story about his different experiences and feelings. During that fall and early winter of 1997, these questions and reviews were in depth, repetitive, and tended to be factual-oriented. Therefore, the information sometimes came across as colorless. The defense psychiatrist advocated publicly that the defendant had many of the features of a schizo-typical personality disorder, and in addition suffers from a depression. This would first appear in his first year of junior high school. Then it would appear in the fall of 1997, just prior to the killings. She further implied that this was due to his rejection, and the teasing in school.

During the course of interviewing the defendant for the State Attorney General, at the Lexington Detention Center, this coauthor was asked about the early reports that there had been a conspiracy of classmates, who had agreed to participate in this shooting and chaos. The defendant admitted that he had told that story to the deputy sheriff who was transporting him that evening, but then he recanted and said that was not true. That information chilled me to the core. The defendant was then asked why he would lie about such a sensitive issue. His response was that he had lied about the conspiracy because the deputy sheriff wanted such a story, "so I gave it to him." When later confronted with the same question, by the defense attorney, the defendant reported that he did not want anyone else involved, because he would lose his status, that is, if other people brought shot guns and shot them during the event, he would no longer be able to consider himself as the "Alpha dog."

The reports of these sterile and antiseptic-like evaluations, involving the facts and some of the feelings, did not meet the needs of the many people around the country, who felt that the descriptions offered by DSM-IV were incomplete and incompletely unacceptable. Why should the evaluations about criminal responsibility and competence be restricted to those with the qualifications of psychologist and psychiatrist? The field of "mental health" includes many other practitioners of various disciplines, who have something of value to offer, in terms of a more complete explanation.

There was also the issue of "duality of roles." It became known during the early months of this case that one of the expert witnesses for the prosecution and one for the defense were beginning the preparation of a coauthored text on how to do forensic evaluations with child murders. Once the decision was made, that the defendant would plead guilty and accept the 25 year of incarceration without the opportunity of parole, most of the concerns about these collaborations ceased.

One of the fears expressed was that these two expert witnesses might participate in this trial with an almost academic perspective rather than "real life." Any alternative perspective would be to approach this event with a new question of "what happened." Kathleen S. Newman may have done just that, with her book entitled *Rampage, Social Rules of School Shootings* (Newman, 2000). In her book she lists five criteria which she says even one would make it less likely that the shooter would act on his feelings. Presence of all five makes it very likely that there would be an incidence. So although this approach is not good at forecasting, it is a good present state measure of the degree of disharmony that a student is feeling. The criteria include the following:

1. The shooter perceives himself as extremely marginal in the social world that means something to him.
2. School shooters must suffer from psychiatric/psychological problems that magnify the impact of other marginality.
3. Cultural roll scripts shaped the design of the rampage.
4. School shooters often fall under the radar because they tend not to exhibit the extreme types of behavior that the schools officials tend to associate with potential violent or troubled kids.
5. Access to guns.

The sociological approach of this author seems to allow for more speculation and more probing questions. As she deals with the issue of "what went wrong in the group that morning, which lead to this expression of behavior?" In these sensational cases, with so many players involved and so many agendas, both financial and academic issues emerge. This makes the search for a clear, well-defined, explanation and reconstruction of the event unlikely to happen. If those of us, who are consumers of this kind of information in our society, would acknowledge the restrictions and the limitations that our current investigative approach presents, then the disappointment would be less. The need to continue the quest for information about chaos involved in school shootings needs to be pursued with a broader inclusion of other specialized disciplines, not just that of a psychiatrist or neuropsychologist. A spectrum of specialists in cultural anthropology and criminal sociology should be considered for such evaluations.

Lessons Learned on Clinical Management and School Intervention

The need for students to have access to mental health, immediately, is being recognized by schools and juvenile justice systems. For a lot of these families, access to mental health is problematic. The barriers presented to families are issues such as lack of income, lack of health insurance, no or limited transportation, and very limited knowledge on how to access facilities. In addition, for a majority of these families, the fear of having their children taken out of their custody, or the fear of being labeled as "a bad parent," also presents itself as a barrier for families to seek mental health. Moreover, the family dysfunction is a "way of life" and the adults within the family system appear to not know any other way to live.

When students arrive at school, they bring with them issues that are also occurring within their family. Some students witness drug use and abuse, drug dealing, domestic violence, and drive by shootings. Others witness emotional abuse between parents as well as severe depression or other mental health concerns among family members. It has become apparent that mental health and schools need to work together to ensure that at-risk students have a better chance in succeeding in school and life. One way is to have the mental health community work in the school system on a daily basis. In other words, have mental health where there is easy and fast access for students and their family. In Lexington, Kentucky, one elementary school has recognized this need and through a grant now has a therapist and case manager on site throughout the school year. Key players meet weekly to discuss students who were referred by their teacher. Referrals range from academic problems to truancy to behavioral problems. If it is determined that mental health intervention is appropriate, then steps are taken to get permission for treatment. Once permission is obtained, then these students are able to participate in individual and group therapy all while staying at school. In addition, the case manager is able to provide services that will "wrap around" the family. Services can range from financial help to providing more intensive family interventions.

Once a student's behavior becomes problematic, whether it is from aggression or truancy, most parents feel that the school does not "like" their child, and they (the parent) avoid communicating with school personnel. A key component for mental health is to open up the lines of communication between the parent and the school. Getting parents to volunteer at the school is one such way. Children appear to respond more positively when their parent is involved with the school.

Summary and Conclusions

Examined herein are clinical issues and case analyses of five school violence situations in the United States involving lethal peer victimization by the perpetrator(s). Escape theory suggests that peer victimization is driven by the desire to escape a state of painful self-awareness characterized by inadequacy, negative affect, and low self-esteem. Reviewed have been several diagnostic indicators of at-risk children as well as diagnostic issues that should be considered in their diagnosis and treatment. Suggestions and recommendations are offered that may benefit physicians, child psychiatric professionals, health care staff, teachers, counselors, school administrators, attorneys, and educational personnel in the recognition, prevention, and interventions with children who are at risk to act out against their peers, parents, and significant others in the school environment.

Acknowledgment The authors acknowledge the assistance of James Clark, Ph.D., Lane J. Veltkamp, M.S.W., A.C.S.W., B.C.D., Brenda Frommer, Tag Heister, M.L.S., Deborah Kessler, M.L.S., Katrina Scott, M.L.S., and Jill Livingston, M.L.S.; Library Services are acknowledged for their support and assistance in the completion of this manuscript.

References

American Psychiatric Association. (1994). *Diagnostic and Statistical Manual of Mental Disorders*, 4th edition. Washington, D.C.: American Psychiatric Association.

Baumeister, R. F. (1990). Suicide as escape from self. *Psychological Review*, 97, 90–113.

Beebe, D. W., Holmeck, G. N., Albright, J. S., Noga, K., & DeCastro, B. (1995). Identification of "binge-prone" women: An experimentally and psychometrically validated cluster analysis in a college population. *Addictive Behaviors*, 20, 451–462.

Boxer, P., Goldstein, S., Musher-Eizenman, Gubow, E. F., & Heretick, D. (2005). Developmental issues in school based aggression prevention. *The Journal of Primary Prevention*, 26(5), 383–400.

Centers for Disease Control. Web-based Injury Statistics Query and Reporting System (WISQARS [Online]. (2003). National Center for Injury Prevention and Control, Centers for Disease Control and Prevention (producer). Retrieved February 17, 2003, from http://www.cdc.gov/ncipc/wisquars

Dean, P. J. & Range, L. M. (1996). The escape theory of suicide and perfectionism in college students. *Death Studies*, 20, 415–424.

Edwards, D., Hunt, M., Meyers, J., Grogg, K., & Jarrett, O. (2005). Acceptability and student outcomes of a violence prevention curriculum. *The Journal of Primary Prevention*, 26(5), 401–418.

Elkind, D. 2004. The problem with constructivism. The Educational Forum 68(4), 306–312.

Espelage, D. L. & Swearer, S. M. (Eds.). (2004). *Bullying in American Schools: A Social-Ecological Perspective on Prevention and Intervention*. Mahwah, NJ: Lawrence Erlbaum Associates Incorporated.

Heatherton, T. F. & Baumeister, R. F. (1991). Binge eating as escape from self-awareness. *Psychological Bulletin*, 110, 86–108.

McEvoy, A. & Welker, R. (2000). Antisocial behavior, academic failure, and school climate: A critical review. *Journal of Emotional and Behavioral Disorders*, 8, 130–141.

Miller, T. W. (1996). *Theory and Assessment of Stressful Life Events.* Madison, Connecticut: International Universities Press Incorporated.

Miller, T. W. (1998). *Children of Trauma.* Madison, Connecticut: International Universities Press Incorporated.

National School Safety Center. (2006). *Guidelines for a Safe School Environment.* Washington D.C.: Task Force on School Violence (Website: www.nsscl.org).

Newman, K. S. (2000) Rampage, Social Rules of School Shootings. New York: Basic Books Publishers Inc,

Puka, B. (Ed.). (1994). *Fundamental Research on Moral Development.* New York: Garland. Publishers.

Parker, G., Hadzi-Pavolvic, D., Greenwald, & Weissman. (1995). Low parental care as a risk factor to lifetime depression in a community sample. *Journal of Affective Disorders*, 33, 173–180.

Taub, J. (2002). Evaluation of the second step violence prevention program at a rural elementary school. *School Psychology Review*, 31, 186–201.

Veltkamp, L. J. & Miller, T. W. (1994). *Clinical Handbook of Child Abuse and Neglect.* Madison, Connecticut: International Universities Press, Inc.

West, M. L., Keller, A. E. R., Links, P., & Patrick, J. (1993). Borderline personality and attachment disorders. *Archives of General Psychiatry*, 53, 502–505.

Zager, R. & Arbit, J. (1998). School violence in rural areas. *American Psychological Association Monitor*, vol 29(8). Washington, D.C.: American Psychological Association, pp 35–41.

Chapter 19
Character Education as a Prevention Strategy for School-Related Violence

Thomas W. Miller, Robert F. Kraus, and Lane J. Veltkamp

Introduction

Character education has been a valued partner in prevention-based strategies. Prevention education is seen as a key component in addressing school violence. Three hundred and three fourth-grade students in 9 of the 11 elementary schools in a predominantly rural community were provided a specialized program of character education as a prevention tool to reduce the potential for deviant behavior. Students in three schools were in the no treatment control condition. Students in the remaining six schools received a school-based and curriculum-driven character education program. These six schools were divided into two conditions. Two of the schools were in the curriculum-only condition while in four of the schools students were randomly selected to receive a protocol-driven summer academic (6 weeks) and experiential education/program. Those not selected were an embedded control group. The remaining one-third of the fourth-grade class in these four schools constitutes a comparison group. Primary prevention involves the provision of education and training along with efforts to promote school bonding. There are several approaches to addressing school-related violence.

Prevention education through character education is considered a critical component in a healthy school environment (Beane, 2001; U.S. Department of Education, 2002; DeVoe et al., 2002; Edwards & Mullis, 2003). There has been for some time support for character education in local and state governments, state departments of education, and educational organizations. Successful programs include the process of building community consensus and commitment helping different religions and cultures realize common values. Several state and federal court decisions refer to the obligation educators have to teach the values upon which democracy and social order depend.

The term character refers to those aspects of personality that are learned through experience, through training, or through a socialization process (The Josephson Institute of Ethics, 2007). Character is not everything one learns, but refers primarily to things a person learns about how he or she should conduct himself or herself or behave in social or interpersonal situations. Part of this shaping of our behavior is based on the need to be seen in a positive way, as moral or virtuous (i.e., as having a good reputation), but another part relates to how people want to see and feel about them. Character has as a primary characteristic, noted by virtually all theorists, consistency in behavior across time. Character is enduring, not transient like an interest, emotion, or attitude. Character is critical to moral and ethical development.

In considering the structure of character development, Benninga and Wynne (1997) documented the record-breaking rates of distress afflicting young Americans and form an essential backdrop for character development. The annual rates of death among youth (15- to 19-year-old) white males by homicide and suicide are at their highest points since national record keeping began. The rates of out-of-wedlock births among youth (15- to 19-year-old) white females are also at or near their highest points since national record keeping began. Benninga and Wynne (1997) argue that character educators want children and adolescents to learn to feel a sense of belonging to and responsibility for others. They believe that instability and individual feelings of anxiety and dissatisfaction sometimes result in depression, suicidal ideation, and other forms of disorder. Educators believe that children need age-appropriate responsibilities, in order to feel socially integrated and respected. They believe that adults with authority should feel comfortable disciplining youngsters who fail to carry out those significant duties. Benninga and Wynne (1997) argue that the responsibility of adults is to critically examine children's and adolescent's social environments and to design and manage them to those environments that guide school-aged children to maturity and morally responsible adults.

Educators, parents, and health care professionals are often involved with the several classroom disruptions teachers face and most are the result of antisocial behaviors. Walker et al. (1996) argue that well-developed antisocial behavior patterns and high levels of aggression evidenced early in a child's life are among the best predictors of delinquent and violent behavior years later. Such behavior patterns negatively affect the child in the school environment and become elaborated and more destructive over time; they poison the school environment and lower the quality of life for students and staff alike (Hawkins & Catalalano, 1992; Frey et al., 2000; McMahon et al., 2000). Clayton et al. (1996) provided a model intervention that offers educators a better understanding of the risk and protective factors associated with today's youth and provides a model for prevention intervention strategies that offer critical learning components to students, parents, teachers, and the necessary school bonding experience.

Purpose of the Study

This study was designed to evaluate the effectiveness of a universal, protocol-driven, school-based character education and problem behavior prevention program; a selective, comprehensive, protocol-driven, school-based summer program designed to reduce risk factors and strengthen protective factors related to school violence and bullying behaviors among youth; and a selective, protocol-driven family program for parents/guardians of at-risk fourth- and fifth-grade students. A component of the student–teacher bonding was targeted by matching incoming students with their new teachers during a summer camp program.

Methodology

Design and Sample

Informed parental consent was obtained on all fourth-grade students in 9 of the 11 elementary schools in a predominantly rural southeastern county (predominantly rural, highest percentage of African American population). Students in three schools were in the no treatment control condition. Students in the remaining six schools received a school-based curriculum-driven character education program. Students in two of these six schools not only received the curriculum, but one-third (chosen on the basis of poor academic achievement and externalizing behaviors [youth self-report and teacher appraisals]) also received a 6-week, protocol-driven, summer academic (4 weeks) and experiential education program for 2 weeks. In the final two schools, all fourth-grade students received the curriculum, one-third (chosen on the basis of poor academic achievement and externalizing behaviors) received the 6-week intervention, and the parents of these students received an eight-session version of the *Duke Family Coping Power* program. The summer camp intervention was delivered by the teachers with these students who they were scheduled to have in the fifth grade.

Gearing Up to Success (GUTS) (Hansen, 1997) program employed the combined experimental curriculum and the summer camp experience wherein high-risk students were able to utilize skills learned through the character education program involving both experiential and didactic components. Teacher and counselors utilized the involvement of the GUTS program with their fourth and fifth grades to assess the effectiveness of the prevention intervention on academic performance and social competence.

Results and Discussion

Based on the results obtained, the predictor variable of academic achievement for children aged 9–11 years yielded a χ^2 of 8.21 ($p = .76$) with 12 degrees of freedom. A key dimension of the targeted predictor variable, Academic Achievement, was school bonding. Here it is shown that the summer program participants had stronger gains in bonding to school personnel and school activities then did those students who did not receive the intervention. There were no significant differences between the participants in summer camp whose parents received the family program and those who just received the summer program. However, this result is not surprising given that the family program was targeted more toward the direct effect of strengthening interactions among family members rather than strengthening the academic performance of students. Noteworthy is the statistically significant differences noted between treatment groups as summarized in Table 19.1 which favor the effectiveness of school bonding when children were exposed to the curriculum, parent involvement, and teacher–student bonding through the camp experience prior to entering sixth grade as realized through higher math scores.

It is clear that no single component of the program stands alone as strong but when combined, the results suggested that school bonding was increased. The curriculum on character education was offered during the school year, the family intervention involved training in parenting skills, and the camp experience involved school bonding through teacher–student interaction in a social and educational setting. A one-way analysis of variance (ANOVA) which addresses the factors by each condition yields a significant result ($F = 3.056$, df = 167, $p < .30$), suggesting that of the conditions considered, the summer camp experience makes the greatest difference in these students participating in this study.

A dose–response relationship was observed among the intervention conditions for social competence. Here students who received the most comprehensive intervention (summer program, curriculum, and the family component) had the highest increases in social competence, followed by those who received both the curriculum and the summer program. The lowest increase in social competence was observed among those who received only the curriculum program.

The findings for parental investment show that the family program was effective at increasing the amount of parent and child interactions. These data demonstrate that students in the other two intervention conditions had fewer interactions with parents over the study period. From a developmental perspective, one would expect to find a decreasing amount of parental investment over time. When the child begins to assert independence and develop peer networks, they are drawn away

Table 19.1 Analysis of variance (ANOVA) summary table for change in mathematics ability by experimental condition

Source	df	SS	MS	F
Between subjects	211	4809.76		
Condit (A1)	3	509.38	169.796	08.20**
Sex (A2)	1	32.99	32.997	01.59
Race (A3)	1	0.71	0.710	00.03
Residual between	206	4266.68	20.712	
Within subjects	212	1280.53		
Time (B)	1	248.00	248.000	50.62***
A1 × B interaction	3	20.64	6.880	1.40
A2 × B interaction	1	02.46	2.469	0.50
A3 × B interaction	1	0.13	0.138	0.03
Residual within	206	1009.30	4.899	
Total	423	6090.29		

Note: $N = 216$.
*$p < .05$, **$p < .01$, ***$p < .001$.

from family activities and more toward those activities with peers. Therefore, the family component was efficacious at slowing the natural progression of detachment that occurs during adolescence from home and family members.

Transitions for At-Risk Behavior Children

Educators and clinicians must be aware of the developmental transitions that school-aged children face. The subjects in this study were best characterized developmentally as being in middle childhood (ages 9–11). Because of this, the majority are involved in at least two school-related transitions thought to influence both predictor variables and high-risk outcome variables. Other transitions they could be facing include parental conflict, parents' separation or divorce, and foster placement among others. The first of these transitions is puberty. Specific school-related transitions involve at least two findings from the study that are especially relevant: (a) puberty is a more continuous process for females than for males, for whom it is like a switch, and (b) there are substantial differences in onset of puberty. A limitation of this study involves the fact that we did not include an assessment that directly measures puberty through, for example, the Tanner Staging or other such measures of pubescence. The second transition overlaps with puberty but is more directly measured in this study. This transition is the migration from elementary school to middle school. Subjects in our study will be undergoing a major change in status, from the oldest to the youngest in the school. They will be moving from relatively smaller to relatively larger and more heterogeneous middle schools, so size of the population will be involved. Finally, they are moving from a more structured class schedule to one in which there are a number of changes in classrooms and teachers.

A prominent feature of the transition from elementary to middle school is crucial in the developmental progression of risk taking as exemplified by abusing substances and sexual risk taking, in that it is one of the key life course transitions that occurs during the life cycle. As academic climates change, the student is confronted with the potential of new friendship networks, increasing academic demands, and unfamiliar teachers. Among the events that occur during adolescent development, changes in school foster a loosening of social bonds that tie students to home, school, and family. The use of booster sessions aimed at this population might buffer the effects of this transition by inoculating against high-risk behavior, which may include risk taking involving illegal substances and sexual risk-taking behaviors.

Transforming Research into Practice

From the results obtained in this study, a practice guideline is presented to assist educators and prevention-oriented clinicians and practitioners in addressing a standardized model for addressing prevention strategies related to school-based violence and promoting healthy school bonding through a three-pronged approach involving curriculum, parent–child relations, and teacher–student bonding. Clinical algorithms and care pathways delineate specific steps and timelines in which interventions should occur. They further address the decision-making process, the clinical services offered, and the potential interactions among multidisciplinary health care professionals and providers for specific needs of patients referred. Clinical information systems capable of supporting the functional requirements of comprehensive critical pathway also provide direction to the development and implementation of algorithms appropriate for change (Miller, 1999). The clinical algorithm for school-related violence is summarized in Fig. 19.1. Sometimes the client will present with symptoms or complaints not of the abuse but of some other related symptom. The clinical algorithm provides the clinician, by moving through the history and systems review, the identification of symptoms and the diagnostic criteria for acute and/or chronic trauma. It also considers symptoms, specific treatment and supportive care, and how the clinicians can reassess and monitor the school-based violence and respond to it.

A clinical care pathway delineates the specific timelines in which assessment and treatment or interventions must occur. Note with specificity the importance of the legal and ethical responsibilities within the abuse spectrum. Specific emphasis here is on reporting and responding to the child or children who are both victims and perpetrators in the abuse. Reporting and follow-up with the appropriately designated state agency is critical. In addition, specific information related to office management for clients who present with problems associated with school-related violence are summarized in Fig. 19.2, the care pathway or guideline provided. These become the critical ingredients to be considered in a care pathway that would provide standardized care and treatment for the victim of school violence and abuse.

Children in the school setting who are victimized through bullying or other traumatic experiences including sexual abuse may well experience a more complex picture of psychopathology (Miller, 1998). They may well be victims of a disorder of extreme stress which must capture the manifestations of repeated and prolonged abuse and its resultant impact on personality development that is not usually seen in situations of more acute stressful nature. Clinicians have come to the realization that the significance of prolonged and repeated trauma as seen through school-based violence warrant careful consideration in providing an intervention.

Risk and Protective Factors in School Violence

Educators' recognition of risk and protective factors is crucial. Risk and protective factors can be identified in four domains: the peer group, the school environment, the home and family, and the community. Summarized in Table 19.1 are several of the critical risk and protective factors for each of these domains. Educators and clinicians may find these identified factors helpful in assessing the child and domains in which the child is experiencing exploitation and abuse (Table 19.2).

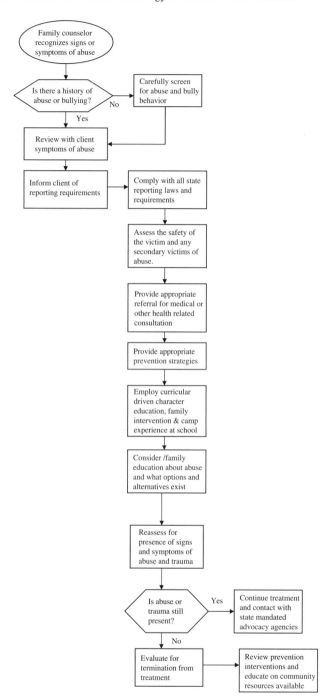

Fig. 19.1 Model algorithm for school-based violence

ACTIVITY	VISIT 1	VISIT 2-5	VISIT 6	VISIT 8
ASSESSMENT	Abuse Screening		PRN Assessment	Depression Screening
INTERVENTION	Abide by reporting requirements for abuse in your jurisdiction	Abuse focused Mental Health Counseling Brief Therapy		Considered for Individual Counseling; Family Counseling; Couples Therapy Cultural Specific Holistic Care
CONSULTS/ ASSESSMENTS CONSIDERED	Internist Psychologist Psychiatrist Mental Health Counselor OB/GYN Pediatrician	Follow-up with consultant	Integrate counsel and recommendations	
CLIENT/ FAMILY EDUCATION				Encourage client and family education, review "cycle-violence", theory and encourage victim-initiated interventions and control

Fig. 19.2 Model care pathway for school violence

Processing the Trauma of Abuse

Abuse can take several forms as has been realized in the chapters in this volume. Past discussion of child sexual abuse has focused on adult perpetrators and child victims. However, there is an increased incidence of peer sexual abuse in the school setting among both males and females. Among some of the more severe forms is early child sexual abuse among preschool and grade school peers. This has reached increased prominence because of the exposure to pornographic material and access children have had to Internet pornographic windows.

The trauma of physical and/or psychological abuse for the victim is often a difficult experience to understand and accommodate. The Trauma Accommodation Syndrome (Miller & Veltkamp, 1996) is based on DSM IV criteria (American Psychiatric Association, 1994) and outlines how trauma such as abuse is processed

Table 19.2 Risk and protective factors related to school violence

Risk factors	Protective factors
Peer group	
Emotional problems	Respect authority
Inability to delay gratification	Responsible
Aggressiveness	Independent thinking
Sensation seeking	Communication skills
School	
Failed home support	Caring
Low achievement expectations	Social skills
Family dysfunction	Cooperative learning
Lack of school commitment	Teacher–child relationship
Family	
Distress/low stability	Positive child/parent
Marital/family conflict	Support and affection
Parental abuse/neglect	High expectations regarding behavior
Lack of discipline	Discipline and rule
	Enforcement
Community	
Concentrated poverty	Trustworthy role models
Schools with high failure/dropout rates	Adults helping with responsibility and relationship
Lack of positive role model	Respect

by the victim. There is usually extreme difficulty in discussing any aspect of the victimization. The victim confronted with such abuse often passes through a series of stages in dealing with this trauma. The initial stage is one of *victimization*, which is recognized as the stressor and is usually realized as an acute physical and/or psychological trauma. The person's response is usually one of feeling overwhelmed and intimidated, and the locus of control for the victim is more of an external nature. It is not uncommon for the victim to think of the stressful experience and to focus on the intimidating act, as well as the physical pain associated with the abuse. Figure 19.3 summarizes the stages or phases the victim often experiences along with clinical indicators present during each stage.

This *acute stage* of trauma involving feelings of helplessness and fear is followed by a stage involving more cognitive disorganization and confusion. This stage is marked by a vagueness in understanding both the concept of abuse and the expectations associated with the demands of the perpetrator. The third stage may involve denial and a conscious inhibition wherein an effort is made on the part of the victim to actively inhibit thoughts and feelings related to the abuse. This can involve revisiting the cognitive disorganization phase and the earlier memories, with flashbacks to the acute physical and psychological trauma. This stage can also realize avoidance involving unconscious denial, wherein the victim is not aware of his effort to avoid the psychological trauma associated with the abuse. The victim, therefore, unconsciously denies or minimizes the abuse and/or any efforts to respond to the abusing experiencing. This results in stagnation, feelings of entrapment, and often results in the victim accommodating the pain of the abuse.

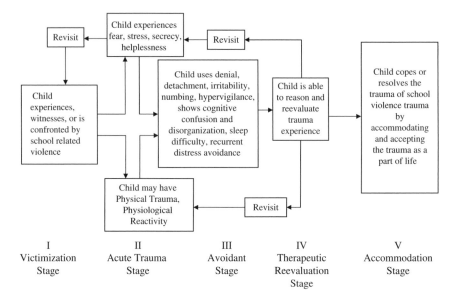

Fig. 19.3 Trauma accommodation syndrome related to school-based violence (Miller & Veltkamp, 1996)

This *avoidant stage* may be followed by a stage of *therapeutic reevaluation*, where a "significant other" usually supports the reasoning through a reevaluation of this psychological and physical trauma associated with the abuse. In this stage, the victim may begin to disclose specific content relevant to the abuse. The phase of therapeutic reevaluation and reasoning is significant in that it indicates that conscious support has been realized by the victim in passing from the avoidant phase to the issues, activities, and trauma of the abusing experience(s).

The final stage is one of accommodation that involves coping and/or resolution, wherein the victim has been able to deal with the issues of the abuse and comes to a better understanding of the significance of the abuse and the perpetrator. The victim is viewed at this stage as (1) being more open to talking about the incident, (2) being able to express thoughts and feelings more readily, and (3) being committed to both assessment and therapy where the victim may discharge some of the aggressive feelings toward the perpetrator. It is clearly at this stage that the victim has realized an alliance with the counselor, significant others, and/or other professionals in (1) exploring the original abusive experience, (2) dealing with both the physical and psychological stressors involved, (3) attending to the repressed material and the process of either conscious inhibition or unconscious denial utilized during the avoidant stage, (4) focusing on self-understanding and psychological and emotional support of others in comprehending the rationale for the abusing experiences, and (5) exploring appropriate psychosocial lifestyles to determine the degree of therapeutic intervention yet required.

Future Directions and Implications for Violence Prevention

This study investigated fourth-grade students in 9 of the 11 schools in a rural community. The results confirmed that the summer program participants had significant gains in school achievement, greater social competency as reported by self and teachers, greater increases in reading achievement, and a positive effect on parental–child interaction. The specialized curriculum, family program, and the experiential summer camp component contributed to the school bonding experience.

There are several important substantive issues and research questions raised by these findings. Future research should address the effects of character education programs on the predictor variables from the fourth- and fifth-grade interventions evident as youth make the transition to the sixth grade and the middle school culture. Other questions of interest include the following: What are the effects of the new boosters on the predictor variables? Will the sixth-grade interventions have an additive effect on the predictor variables and the outcome variables of interest? What is most clear is the realization that the students in the most comprehensive intervention curriculum, summer program, and family intervention had (1) the lowest increases in the number of friends who use drugs, (2) highest gains in resistance to peer pressure, (3) greatest increases in social competence, (4) the largest gains in reading achievement, and (5) largest increase in parental interaction of the students studied. This would suggest significant benefits may be realized from a standardized protocol-driven prevention intervention program incorporating character education in the curriculum, family skills intervention training, and the opportunity to practice and utilize these skills in an experimental environment.

Educators should take the following steps based on this study:

- Identify at-risk children and provide proven interventions that include a combination of curriculum, parent intervention, and experiential opportunities for students to utilize the skills they learn from these programs through a summer camp experience
- Offer primary, secondary, and tertiary prevention strategies for at-risk reduction in children and adolescents

Primary prevention strategies include the following:

- Programs that focus on family communication and effective parent–child interaction
- Programs that interrupt the at-risk behavior, bullying, and peer victimization
- Programs that increase understanding of enhancing protective factors in the home, school, and community
- Programs that maximize helping networks for at-risk children who have poor socialization and need peer social competency skills

Secondary prevention strategies include the following:

- Identify students and families at risk and provide referral to school and/or community services

- Monitor high-risk students through peer counseling programs
- Provide education and counseling strategies for students who need to develop social competency and self-regulation skills

Tertiary prevention strategies include the following:

- Reduce the incidence and prevalence of at-risk behaviors and promote protective factors
- Multiple strategies involving curriculum, active involvement of teacher, counselors, and parents facilitate school bonding

Educators need to

- Be aware of the risk and protective factors among peers, school, family, and community. These include the following: Peer group risk factors include emotional problems and an inability to delay gratification. Aggressive behavior and sensation seeking are major risk factors and lead to alcohol and substance abuse. Protective factors among peers often involve respect authority, responsible behavior, and effective independent thinking skills and good communication skills permit social competence and self-regulation.

School-based risk factors include no home support, low achievement expectations, family dysfunction, and lack of school commitment. Protective school factors include caring school personnel, social skills encouraged in the classroom, cooperative learning, and an effective teacher–child relationship. Risk factors in the family include distress/low stability, marital/family conflict, parental abuse/neglect, and lack of discipline. Protective family factors include a positive child–parent relationship, support and affection from family, high expectations regarding behavior and discipline, and rule enforcement in the home. Community risk factors often include concentrated poverty, schools with high failure/dropout rates, and firearms and crime. Often there is a lack of positive role models. Protective factors in the community include trustworthy role models, adults helping students, responsibility and relationship, and respect for both self and others.

There are several important substantive issues for the counselor and for future research. Among these is the question whether the effects on the four predictor variables, social competence, academic achievement, self-regulation, and parental attachment, from the fourth- and fifth-grade interventions are evident as youth make the transition to the sixth grade and the middle school culture. What are the effects of the new booster session on these predictor variables? Will the sixth-grade interventions have an additive effect on the predictor variables and the outcome variables of interest? What is clear from the present study is the realization that a protocol-driven, standardized program that involves curriculum in the schools, parental involvement, and opportunities as the summer camp experience sets tranquilly enhance the potential for improved self-regulation and social competence among at-risk children.

The National Institute of Mental Health (NIMH)-supported scientists are continuing to conduct research into the impact of prevention intervention and the role of character development and school bonding with children and adolescents confronted with violence in schools. Current protocols are examining prevention approaches that address the emotional, social, and academic effects of exposure to violence. In some of the children, the researchers will look at the role of stress hormones in a child or adolescent's response to traumatic experiences. Another study will deal specifically with the victims of school violence, attempting to determine what places children at risk for victimization at school and what factors protect them. It is particularly important to conduct research to discover which individual, family, school, and community interventions work best for children and adolescents exposed to specific forms of school violence, and to find out whether a well-intended but ill-designed intervention could set the youngsters back by keeping the trauma alive in their minds. Through research, NIMH hopes to gain knowledge to reduce the impact of school violence on children, adolescents, and their families.

Acknowledgments The authors acknowledge the guidance and support of our good colleagues at the Center for Prevention Research—Richard Clayton, Ph.D., Nancy Grant Harrington, Ph.D., William Turner, Ph.D., Donna Durbin, M.S., Thomas Holcomb, Ed.D., Janet Saier, M.S., Jill Livingstone, M.L.S., Tag Heister, M.L.S., Deborah Kessler, M.L.S., Amy Pierce, Katrina Scott, Library Services—and Cathy Martin, M.D., Department of Psychiatry, and Brenda Frommer for their contributions to the completion of this manuscript.

References

American Psychiatric Association (1994) *Diagnostic and Statistical Manual-Revised (DSM-IVR)*. Washington DC. American Psychiatric Association.

Beane, A. L. (2001). *The Bully Free Classroom*. Minneapolis, Minnesota: Free Press Publishing Incorporated.

Benninga & Wynne (1997). *Trends in Youth Character Development. The Construction of Children's Character*. (pp. 96–108) Chicago, Illinois: The National Society for the Study of Education.

Clayton, R. R., Nancy, G. H., William, T., Thomas, M., & Donna, D. (1996) Project REAP: Executive summary. Lexington, Kentucky: University of Kentucky, Center for Prevention Research. http://guide.helpingamericasyouth.gov/programdetail.cfm

DeVoe, J. F., Peter, K., Kaurfam, P., Ruddy, S. A., Miller, A. K., Planty, M., Synder, T. D., Duhart, D. T., & Rand, M. R. (2002). *Indicators of School Crime and Safety: 2002*. U.S. Department of Education and Justice. NCES 2003-009/NCJ 196753. Washington, DC.

Edwards, D. & Mullis, F. (2003). Classroom meeting: Encouraging a climate of cooperation. *Professional School Counseling*, 7, 20–28.

Frey, K., Hirschstein, M., & Guzzo, B. (2000). Preventing aggression by promoting social competence. *Journal of Emotional and Behavioral Disorders*, 8, 102–113.

Hansen, W. B. (1997). *All Stars Fourth and Fifth Grade Program*. Durham, North Carolina: Tanglewood Research Incorporated.

Hawkins, D. & Catalano, R. (1992). Communities that care. San Francisco: Jossey-Bass. Publishers.

The Josephson Institute of Ethics (2007). *Character counts*. Retrieved March 31, 2004, from http://www.rt66.com

McMahon, S., Washburn, J., Felix, E., Yakin, J., & Childrey, G. (2000). Violence prevention: Program effects on urban preschool and kindergarten children. *Applied and Preventive Psychology*, 9, 271–281.

Miller, T. W. (1998). *Children of Trauma*. Madison, Connecticut: International Universities Press Incorporated.

Miller, T. W. (1999). The Psychologist with 2020 Vision. *Consulting Psychology Journal*, 50(1), 25–35.

Miller, T. W. & Veltkamp, L. J. (1996). *Clinical Handbook of Child Abuse and Neglect*. Maadison, Connecticut: International Universities Press Incorporated.

U.S. Department of Education (2002). *Exemplary and Promising Safe, Disciplined, and Drug-Free Schools*. Portsmouth, North Hampshire: U.S. Department of Education.

Walker, H. M., Horner, R. H., Sugai, G., Bullis, M., Sprague, J. R., Bricker, D., & Kaufman, M. J. (1996). Integrated approaches to preventing antisocial behavior patterns among school-age children and youth. *Journal of Emotional and Behavioral Disorders*, 4, 194–209.

Chapter 20
The Bully Free Program: A Profile for Prevention in the School Setting

Allan Beane, Thomas W. Miller, and Rick Spurling

This chapter reviews the philosophy, targets, structure, and effective elements and components that should be present in any anti-bullying program. To provide a framework for discussion, the authors dissect and discuss the Bully Free Program (www.bullyfree.com), the most comprehensive anti-bullying program being adopted by schools and districts around the United States. It includes strategies (administrative and classroom based) and curriculum which address all of the elements and components that must be present. Some of its materials are available in eight languages and is being used around the world.

What Is Bullying?

In the school environment, bullying is considered to be the repeated exposure, over time, to negative actions from one or more other students. Activities generally include physical, verbal, or indirect actions that are intended to inflict injury or discomfort upon another student (Beane, 1997). Bullying prevention programs are generally built on a series of steps that include the establishment of a bullying prevention committee within the school and a series of programs that target bullying behavior. These include the use of students surveys to determine if there is a bullying problem; involving teachers and parents in planning, discussions, and action plans; establishing classroom rules against bullying behaviors; and creating a long-term anti-bullying plan to raise school and community awareness of the problem.

Bullying behavior is any form of hurtful behavior by one child toward another, which is disruptive to the emotional well-being of the victim. Olweus (1995) suggests there are three main features present when bullying occurs: (1) deliberate aggression, (2) an asymmetric power relationship, and (3) the aggression results in pain and distress. Barone (1997) surveyed 847 eighth-graders in upstate New York. He found that 58.8% of the students surveyed had been victims of bullies. Barone's study also reinforced the notion that school personnel are mostly unaware of bullying events. He surveyed 110 of the students' counselors, teachers, and administrators. They said they thought that 16% of their students had been victims of bullies.

T. W. Miller (ed.), *School Violence and Primary Prevention.*
© Springer 2008

Olweus argues that bullying is the repeated intimidation of a victim perpetrated by a more powerful person or group in order to cause physical, emotional, and/or emotional hurt. Bullying can take many forms including physical, emotional, and/or verbal abuse. It may involve one child bullying another, a group of children against a single child, or one group against another. Bullying involves an imbalance of power. It involves differing emotional tones; the victim is upset and the bully is cool and in control. The victim is blamed for what has happened. Bullying is also characterized by a lack of concern on the part of the bully for the feelings and concerns of the victim.

Incidence and Prevalence

Peer victimization has been studied more extensively in other countries than in the United States. However, there has been an intense increase in research over the last few years. In the United States, surveys have turned up a wide range of results, with anywhere from 10 to 75% (Hoover et al., 1992) of children saying they have been bullied recently in school. There is also evidence that 14% of both boys and girls suffer severe trauma from peer victimization (Oliver et al., 1994). In the United States, bullying starts as early as age three, peaks in middle school, and then decreases in high school.

The research on bullying shows a wide range in prevalence (Miller & Beane, 1999). Much of this variability is due to differences in how bullying is defined and how the data are collected. For example, some researches (Olweus, 1989) in Scandinavia have used a definition that requires bullying to be repeated, thus excluding the single episode, regardless of its severity.

Olweus (1995) at the University of Bergen found that 11% of primary school children experienced significant bullying. By secondary school age, the number of victims had been reduced by half. The number of children identified as bullies stayed fairly constant at around 7% at both primary and secondary school age. An overall figure of 15% of Scandinavian children is involved in bullying as victims or bullies. In Great Britain, Kidscape (Elliot, 1989) has attempted to study the prevalence of bullying; held in 1989 and 1990, over 12,000 letters and 4,000 telephone calls were received from parents, children, and teachers about the problems of bullying. Oliver et al. (1994) surveyed 207 small-town middle and high school students. Of the students surveyed, 88% reported observing bullying during their school careers. Of these students, 90% believe it to be a significant problems for the victim. Seventy-three percent of boys were reported as victims, far more often than were girls (27%). Most (60%) of the students reported that victims were bullied primarily by boys; 32% reported being bullied by both girls and boys, while 8% were bullied by girls only. It is also interesting to note that 69% of the students observing victimization believed that school professionals handled the situation poorly. *Childline*, a professional nonprofit organization in the United Kingdom, provides public education and services to the general public. *Childline* has an Internet

Web site. *Childline* set up a special bully line for 3 months in 1990. According to Hereward Harrison, *Childline's* Director of Counseling, they answered 5,200 calls and counseled ~2,000 distressed children and teenagers. In 1984, *Kidscape* conducted a 2-year study with 4,000 children. Sixty-eight percent had been bullied at least twice or had experienced at least one particularly bad incident. Eight percent of the students felt it had affected their lives to the point that they attempted suicide, ran away, refused to go to school, or became chronically ill. Most of the incidents occurred while traveling to or from school or while in school. The bullying usually took place when there was no adult present.

Several studies that have focused on bullying in schools suggest that the problem tends to be ignored by teachers and school administrators. Teachers' estimates of the incidence of bullying behavior among school children suggest that they greatly underestimate the amount of bullying that goes on in their schools (O'Moore & Hillery, 1989). For example, teachers identified only 17 (22.1%) of 77 self-confessed pure bullies and 38 (25.2%) of the 151 victims. Thus, only 24% of the total numbers of bullies were identified by their teachers. Perhaps this unawareness is due to the covert nature of bullying and the often subtle manner bullies use to intimidate their victims. Further, pupils may be reluctant to inform teachers about bullying incidents they have witnessed. They are often afraid that adults will only make the situation worse. Unfortunately, many teachers and principals are unsympathetic to pupils who tell on others. Rather than seeking solutions within their schools, some principals even suggest that victimized children be transferred to a different school.

The Victimizer

Studies have found that children who bully can be high-spirited, active, energetic children. They may be easily bored or envious and/or insecure (Miller, 1997). They may be jealous of another's academic or sporting success, or of a sibling/ new baby. They may have a learning disability, which makes them angry and frustrated; this may have the opposite effect and make them a target for bullies. They may be angry or down-trodden from abuse they themselves have suffered (Olweus, 1995).

In a 20-year study, Olweus identified the significance of the child rearing practices of the bully's family (Olweus, 1995). Patterns of perpetration may emerge from the following profiles.

The Neglected Child

If the child is neglected, picked on, or punished excessively at home, he or she may develop a very negative self-image. The child may become frustrated, anxious, and insecure. The child may then start to bully others in order to gain respect and prove that he or she is worthy of notice.

The Aggressive Family

The family of the bully may be aggressive or quick-tempered with lots of loud arguments and shouting. As this is the child's first behavior model, he or she will tend to reproduce this type of aggressive behavior when he or she is with other children.

"Anything Goes" Family

The child may be given a great deal of license at home and so have trouble recognizing what is appropriate with other people. He or she may react badly to discipline. He or she may be spoiled and used to being the center of attention at home.

Types of Bullies

Olweus (1995) identified three main types of bullies. The first is the *Aggressive Bully*. The majority of bullies fall in this category. They exhibit poor impulse control, a positive view of violence, the desire to dominate, and insensitivity to the feelings of others. The second category is the *Anxious Bully*. About 20% of bullies seem to have anxiety-related problems. This tends to be the most disturbed group, exhibiting low self-esteem, insecurity, friendliness, and emotional instability. The third category is the *Passive Bully*. Child perpetrators become involved in bullying as they become followers of a bully. The motivation for this is to protect themselves and to have the status of belonging to the dominant group. These bullies are easily dominated, passive, and easily led. They may not be particularly aggressive, may empathize with others, and may feel guilty after bullying.

The Victim

Children can become victims of bullying for a variety of reasons, but the most prominent cause is that the bully builds his or her self-esteem by hurting others (Olweus, 1994; Miller, 1997). Bullying is rarely caused by the victim. Victim profiles often include children who are gentle, physically weaker than bullies, and appear to lack confidence. They are often intelligent, lacking in social skills, and disruptive. They often cannot understand why they have been singled out. According to Byrne (1994), the shy, sensitive personality type is often at risk of being bullied. Such individuals tend to take everything to heart and personalize all negative comments. They look and act like easy targets. Bullies will carry on singling out victims until they find enough victims to satisfy their need to dominate and control others. However, the research of Olweus (1994) also suggests that physical attributes that are considered different/deviant may contribute more to short-term and direct bullying (e.g., hitting, shoving). Even though these characteristics may not initiate direct bullying, bullies often focus on them to maximize their mistreatment. However, bullying occurs because the bully wants to have power and control over the victims, not because the individuals look different (Beane et al., 1999).

Besag (1989) found that victims tend to fall into the category of passive "watchers" who remain on the sidelines of the playground, whereas bullies tend to be the "doers," confident and fully involved in a variety of activities. Finally, Olweus (1989) has found that some common targets of bullying include, but are not limited to, race, language, culture, sex, and religion.

Bullying results in immediate consequences for both the victim and the bully (Olweus, 1989; Beane, 1997). The consequences to the victim may include the following:

- Loss of confidence
- Lowered self-esteem
- Withdrawal from social experience
- Difficulty concentrating
- Academic work slides
- Truancy tendencies
- Development of school phobic responses
- Suicidal ideation

The bullies may

- Learn that using aggression/violence is a successful strategy for getting what they want;
- Realize that they can get away with violent and cruel behavior, eroding school discipline;
- Become divisive as a dominant group coalesces;
- Become more disruptive, perhaps eventually testing school administration and teachers to see how far they can be pushed.

Elliot and Kilpatrick (1994) surveyed young offenders in Britain. Seventy-nine young offenders ranging from age 16 to 21 in two institutions revealed their experiences of school bullying. They were asked whether bullying happened often in their school, whether they were involved in bullying, and what they thought schools should do to tackle bullying effectively. The majority of the young offenders (62%) had themselves been bullies at school. Twenty-three percent were involved as bystanders or witnesses who egged the bullies on, and 15% had been the victims of bullying. Of these victims, 7% subsequently became bullies, 5% committed crimes under the influence of bullies, and 3% remained victims.

O'Moore and Hillery (1989) studied Irish populations of young offenders. The study indicated that factors that contribute to bullying include (1) feelings of inadequacy, such as were expressed in relation to academic and school status, and

(2) popularity among peers. The authors suggest that as these factors remain, compensatory behavior will remain. There is a strong body of evidence which indicates that self-esteem is the single most influential factor in determining behavior (Burns, 1982). However, it may be wrong to assume that all bullies have poor self-esteem. According to Marano (1995), bullies may feel good about themselves because they are not aware of how little they are liked.

The development and implementation of an effective anti-bullying program requires several key components including a clearly defined definition, a strong program philosophy, appropriate program targets, critical elements, a systematic implementation plan, and evaluation process to assess the effectiveness of the program. Just such a model has been used and implemented with the Bully Free Program (Beane, 1997).

Acceptable Definition and Program Philosophy

An effective anti-bullying program will have an acceptable definition of bullying that is internationally accepted. It should view bullying as a form of overt and aggressive behavior that is intentional, hurtful (physical and/or psychological), and persistent (repeated). Bullied students are teased, harassed, and assaulted (verbally and/or physically) by one or more peers and often socially rejected by their peers. There is a real or perceived imbalance of strength (power).

An effective anti-bullying program will also have a program philosophy that reflects the research regarding effective program approaches and components. For example, the philosophy of the Bully Free Program states that anti-bullying programs should include not only policies and procedures but also prevention and intervention strategies (administrative and teacher-centered) and curriculum. The program should be implemented system/district-wide and school-wide. It should be comprehensive and seek to promote a sense of belonging and acceptance in all students as well as promote the Golden Rule—treat others the way you want to be treated. The program should also prevent students from becoming victims and bullies, help victims, help bullies change, empower bystanders, and educate all stakeholders (school personnel, parents, community representatives, etc.).

Appropriate Program Targets

Any effective anti-bullying program should have a broad-base of impact. It should impact the entire school and the community. Bullying is not just a school problem, it is also a school system and community problem (Beane, 1997). For example, the Bully Free Program targets students in preschool, elementary school, middle school or junior high school, and high school. Some of the strategies are designed specifically for potential victims, victims, bullies, followers, bystanders, parents, school personnel, and community representatives. System-wide, school-wide, classroom, and individual components interrelate throughout the program in order to enhance the impact.

Major Elements of Effective Anti-Bullying Programs

An effective anti-bullying program will address all the critical elements that contribute to the problem as well as prevent the problem. For example, the Bully Free Program has the following critical elements:

- Addresses all forms of bullying (e.g., physical, verbal, social, and relational).
- Utilizes comprehensive research-based strategies and curriculum developmentally tailored to be age appropriate and build on what is learned each year.
- Recognizes and allows for the creativity of school personnel and the use of other prevention and intervention strategies and curriculum.
- Includes practical teacher-generated lessons and activities that promote acceptance and a sense of belonging, that empower bystanders, and that address all forms of bullying behavior (physical, verbal, social/relational, cyberbullying, etc.).
- Includes a focus on all aspects of bullying.
- Addresses anger management, conflict resolution, peer mediation, friendship, information for victims, potential victims, bullies, empowerment of bystanders, parent education, community involvement, etc.
- Empowers school personnel, parents, volunteers, community representatives, and students.
- Focuses on process (as opposed to conducting only special events).
- Provides flexibility in delivering the curriculum through classroom meetings, lesson plans, and/or a curriculum schedules, yet ensure systematic and consistent implementation—offering options for incorporating the content into the curriculum.
- Includes an ongoing effort to promote the Golden Rule—treat others the way you want to be treated.
- Uses a whole school system and school-wide approach.
- Includes systematic implementation of prevention and intervention strategies (administrative, teacher-centered, student-centered, and parent-centered) coupled with curriculum.
- Includes procedures for investigating rumors and reports and responding to bullying.
- Utilizes a curriculum and strategies must be age appropriate and address the uniqueness of students, teacher preferences, parent–teacher relationships, school culture, and climate as well as community needs.
- Seeks to help all stakeholders (school personnel, students, parents, community representatives, etc.) understand the nature of bullying.
- Endorses the fact that bullying is a heart problem and recognizes that it is the little things done every day that make a difference in attitudes, thinking, and behavior.

- Includes a structure that is flexible enough to allow for the creativity of school personnel and the discovery of new effective strategies, activities, and resources.
- Promotes a sense of belonging and acceptance in students.
- Views student, parent, and community involvement as critical elements.
- Harnesses the energy and commitment of students.
- Empowers bystanders.
- Encourages adults to model the Golden Rule—to treat others the way they want to be treated.
- Requires adults to example their beliefs about bullying and seeks to dispel myths about bullying.
- Identifies high-risk areas and includes supervision strategies and supportive supervisory strategies (e.g., adding structure to unstructured activities) that should be used.
- Recognizes boys and girls bully and is sensitive to the differences in their behavior.
- Recognizes that bullies and victims come from all walks of life.
- Seeks to create a "telling environment"—all adults must be "safe places" to tell about bullying.
- Does not minimize any form of bullying behavior and does not classify such behaviors as mild, moderate, and severe—its impact varies too much from one child to another.
- Endorses findings that peer mediation and conflict resolution are usually not effective with bullies, but should be included for other students.
- Includes a program evaluation and assess plan to determine effectiveness and to make improvements.

Major Components of The Bully Free Program

The Bully Free Program (Beane, 1996) includes the following major components that should be present in any anti-bullying program:

- Coordinating committees(s) called the Bully Free Program Support Team(s)/Committee(s)
- Mission statement, goals, slogan/motto, and logo are established by the Bully Free Program Team
- Ongoing effort to promote acceptance and a sense of belonging in all students by promoting the Golden Rule—treat others the way you want to be treated
- Anti-bullying policies, procedures, and rules are developed
- *Response Plans* are developed to allow for immediate, consistent intervention by all adults
- Appropriate progressive negative/reductive consequences and positive consequences as well as nonpunitive/nonblaming approaches

- Comprehensive bank of research-based and proven prevention and intervention strategies are provided that are
  - System-centered (district-wide and school-wide)
  - Child-centered (victim, potential victims, bully, followers, bystanders)
  - Peer-centered (empowerment of bystanders)
  - Family-centered
  - Personnel-centered
  - Community-centered

- Bully Free training and program implementation training for all school personnel
- Bully Free awareness presentation for parents
- Bully Free awareness assembly for students
- Program "kick-off" assembly for students
- Program "kick-off" meeting for parents, school personnel, and community representatives
- Serious talks/interviews with victims, bullies, followers, and bystanders
- Curriculum delivery choices: Classroom Meetings Schedule, or Curriculum Schedule, or Lesson Plans
- Bulletin Boards, Posters, and Banners Schedule
- Adult involvement which models the Golden Rule—treat others the way you want to be treated
- Strategies for a *Student Involvement and Empowerment Plan*
- Strategies for a *Parent Involvement and Education Plan*
- Strategies for a *Community Involvement and Education Plan*
- Strategies for identifying high-risk areas
- Strategies for a *Supervision Plan*—developed to supervise high-risk areas—supervision strategies and supportive supervisory strategies (e.g., adding structure) included
- Training for supervisors of high-risk areas
- Strategies for the creation of a "telling environment"
- Strategies for identifying victims, potential victims, bullies, and followers
- *Intervention Plans* for potential victims, victims, and bullies
- Strategies for ongoing communication with stakeholders for maintaining momentum
- Strategies for communicating leadership's commitment
- Strategies for creating a "telling environment"—school personnel and parents must become "safe places" to tell
- Ongoing review and monitoring of program implementation and effectiveness
- Staff Focus Meetings, Student Focus Meetings, and Parent Focus Meetings
- Strategies and tools for evaluating the program (anonymous questionnaire)
- Baseline measurements of the nature and extent of bullying in the setting (e.g., anonymous self-report surveys and/or student focus groups) and follow-up assessments to determine the effectiveness of the interventions—based on reliable survey instruments and other assessment strategies.

Systematic Implementation

The mark of an effective anti-bullying program is systematic implementation that recommends district-wide programming and strategies. Bullying usually starts around age three and continues through high school. If district-wide implementation is not possible, it should be school-wide in as many schools as possible. The program should also be comprehensive and multifaceted in that it permeates policies, procedures, activities, events, instructional activities, operating procedures, codes of conduct, discipline procedures, and other areas.

The following steps to implementing the Bully Free Program are provided to illustrate a systematic approach. Some steps can be completed simultaneously through subcommittees and the rest of the steps can be taken, as the team deems appropriate. These steps may be customized to meet the needs of the school system or school(s). However, it is very important not to let planning delay helping students.

Step 1: Establish and train system-wide and/or school-wide Bully Free Program Support Team/Committee(s) as well as develop the Program Timeline/Calendar.

Step 2: Provide the Bully Free Awareness Training for school personnel and volunteers.

Step 3: Provide the Bully Free Awareness Assembly for all students.

Step 4: Provide the Bully Free Awareness Session for all parents and the community.

Step 5: Develop the Program Evaluation Plan and determine the status of bullying in the school(s)—collect baseline data.

Step 6: Develop the Bully Free Program mission statement, goals, slogan/motto, and logo.

Step 7: Develop and implement the Bully Free Program Administrative Strategies Plan.

Step 8: Identify high-risk locations and high-risk times as well as develop and implement a Bully Free Supervision Plan.

Step 9: Establish the Bully Free policies, rules, discipline rubrics, behavioral expectations in high-risk areas, and response plan(s).

Step 10: Train school personnel, volunteers, and other key individuals to adhere to policies, procedures, discipline rubrics, and response plan(s).

Step 11: Conduct a program kick-off meeting with faculty, staff, volunteers, community representatives, parents, and an assembly program for students to introduce the Bully Free Program and the new policies.

Step 12: Develop and implement the Bully Free Classroom Meeting Schedules, Curriculum Schedules, or Lesson Plans, and a Bulletin Boards, Posters, and Banners Schedule as well as provide training for school personnel related to these.

Step 13: Develop and implement a Student Involvement and Empowerment Plan to create a caring and action-oriented community of bystanders.

Step 14:   Develop and implement a Parent and Community Involvement and Education Plan.

Step 15:   Check the implementation of program plans and strategies.

Step 16:   Readminister survey instrument(s), analyze pre- and postdata, and make improvements.

Step 17:   Celebrate success and maintain momentum.

Evidence of Program Effectiveness

When adopting an anti-bullying program, there should be evidence of its effectiveness. As mentioned earlier, the Bully Free Program is research based and integrates the latest research with proven prevention and intervention strategies. The following is an example report addressing the effectiveness of the Bully Free Program (Table 20.1):

Table 20.1   Results on the effectiveness of the bully free program

Attendance improved...
- Baseline (2001–2002)—90.8%
- After 175 days of program implementation (2002–2003)—97.8%
- After 175 more days (2003–2004)—95.7%

Students who feel bullies exist at the school...
- Baseline (2001–2002)—74.6% of students
- After 175 days of program implementation (2002–2003)—38.9% of students
- After 175 more days (2003–2004)—49.7% of students

Students who have been bullied at school...
- Baseline (2001–2002)—44.8% of students
- After 175 days of program implementation (2002–2003)—20.2% of students
- After 175 more days (2003–2004)—24.6% of students

Students who believe they have avenues to report bullying at school...
- Baseline (2001–2002)—24.6% of students
- After 175 days of program implementation (2002–2003)—78.6% of students
- After 175 more days (2003–2004)—86.7% of students

End of grade (EOG) test scores
- Baseline (2001–2002)—74.3%
- After 175 days of program implementation (2002–2003)—84.3%
- After 175 more days (2003–2004)—87.6%

Number of aggressive occurrences...
- Baseline (2001–2002)—36 aggressive occurrences
- After 175 days of program implementation (2002–2003)—7 aggressive occurrences
- After 175 more days (2003–2004)—5 aggressive occurrences

Suspensions as a result of aggressive behavior...
- Baseline (2001–2002)—19 suspensions
- After 175 days of program implementation (2002–2003)—3 suspensions
- After 175 more days (2003–2004)—6 suspensions

In 2004, Dr. Rick Spurling, as his dissertation, tested the effectiveness of the Bully Free Program in five western North Carolina Middle schools (grades 5–8). A total of 54 participants were involved in this study with in-depth interviews that lasted from 30 min to 1.5 h. Fourteen administrator, 22 teachers, and 18 parents were interviewed using a qualitative design (action-research design) guided by the following inquiries. The following summary of his findings reflects the variety of areas that can be impacted by an effective anti-bullying program (Table 20.2). The research questions were as follows:

- What are the views of administrators, teachers, and parents concerning the current implementation of a Bully Free Program?
- What factors, as perceived by the participants, play a role in a well-organized Bully Free Program?
- What aspects are perceived as barriers to an effective Bully Free Program?
- What changes have occurred with attendance, aggressive/violent occurrences, and perceptions toward school safety by administrators, teachers, and parents since the implementation of the Bully Free Program?
- What ideas can administrators, teachers, and parents contribute to enhance the effectiveness of a Bully Free Program?

Table 20.2 Effectiveness of the bully free program[a]: major impact findings (from action research) in five middle schools

The Bully Free Program, in each of the five schools
- improved the dynamics of interpersonal relationships that exists in the school community (student/student, student/teacher, teacher/teacher, parent/teacher, parent/parent, and school/community).
- improved lines of communication between all stakeholders.
- significantly decreased incidences of aggressive and violent behavior.
- improved school attendance.
- improved state test scores.
- created trust among personnel working on the program.
- created trust in the program's philosophy.
- increased interactions between teachers and students during nonclass times.
- increased awareness of the need for and importance of adults modeling positive interactions as well as made adults more conscious of their behavior.
- increased students' understanding of their role in preventing and stopping bullying.
- increased personnel's comfort level and confidence in their ability to deal with bullying.
- dramatically decreased fighting among boys
- changed how discipline was administered.
- increased a sense of security.
- increased attendance and involvement of students at after-school events.
- resulted in a dramatic decrease in vandalism.

[a] Spurling, R. (2006). The Bully-Free School Zone Character Education Program: A Study of the Impact on Five Western North Carolina Middle Schools.

Lessons Learned and Recommendations for Effective Anti-Bullying Programs

Bullying occurs in every school and it takes the cooperation of school personnel, parents, students, and community representatives to adequately attack the problem. The anti-bullying program can be a once-a-month effort. Preventing and stopping bullying has to become a high-priority of the school and it has to become a way of living from preschool through high school. The program should not only teach students prosocial behaviors and promote the Golden Rule, but there also have to be consequences for bullying behaviors. These consequences need to be progressive, in that they progressively become more negative in the mind of the students. Since some students provoke students to the point of being mistreated, it is important that schools not only realize their responsibility in helping some victims change but also apply consequences to students who mistreat the provocative victim. The Golden Rule does not say, treat others the way you want to be treated if they do not irritate you, or if you like them. Too often, schools blame only the victim.

It is also important for adults to model the Golden Rule—treat others the way you want to be treated. They need to demonstrate that it is more than a belief, it is a conviction. It is a belief that controls their attitudes, thoughts, and behaviors. Unfortunately, some adults bully children and bully each other. They are poor role-models and do not model sensitivity, kindness, and empathy.

Another critical element is training. All school personnel need to be given training to help them understand the nature of bullying and rationale preventing and stopping it, to implement prevention and intervention strategies, to provide quality supervision (especially in high-risk areas) and to add structure to unstructured times, to implement the anti-bullying curriculum, to respond to bullying when it is observed, and to adhere to anti-bullying policies and procedures (including discipline rubrics). It is also important that students have a campaign against bullying and they are trained to be empowered to stop bullying. Their parents also need to be educated about the problem and involved in the campaign. There is a tremendous need for parent education.

Summary and Conclusions

The Bully Free Program is the most comprehensive anti-bullying program and its impact on schools has been far reaching. The initial research on its effectives has been encouraging. The program continues to be improved and expanded. More research is being conducted to determine its effectiveness.

Fortunately, more and more anti-bullying materials and resources are being developed and published by an array of companies. However, one of the greatest needs is low-cost technology-based solutions for reporting bullying, for monitoring and supervising high-risk areas, and for providing instruction. There is also a need for research and program development at the preschool level, especially in the area of discipline. Many children come from aggressive and/or permissive home environments. To compound the problem of poor structure and discipline in the home is the fact that many preschool programs do not have strong discipline plans. In fact, some of them are permissive and do not adequately correct bullying behavior. They are not even allowed to use timeout. Another area that needs to be developed is the prevention of bullying in high schools. Research needs to be conducted to determine effective prevention and intervention strategies for high school students, the attitudes of high school teachers regarding their role in preventing and intervening, and effective strategies for integrating the high school curriculum.

There is also a tremendous need for programs that prevent and stop bullying on buses and to prevent bullying while children walk to and from school. These continue to be problem areas that need attention. Solutions are waiting to be discovered and they eventually will be.

References

Barone, F. J. (1997, September). Bullying in School: It Doesn't Have to Happen. Phi Delta Kappan: 80–82. EA 533 807.

Beane, A. (1996). Steps to Implementing the Bully Free Program. Bully Free Systems, LLC: Murray, KY.

Beane, A. (1997). The trauma of peer victimization. In T. W. Miller (Ed.), *Children of Trauma*. Madison, CT: International University Press, Inc.

Beane, A. L., Jacobs, M., & Miller, T. (1999). Promoting acceptance to prevent discipline problems. ERIC (ED 420 723)—Clearinghouse on Assessment and Evaluation.

Besag, V. E. (1989). *Bullies and Victims in Schools*. London: Open University Press, Publishers.

Burns, R. B. (1982). *Self-Concept Development and Education*. London: Holt, Rinehart, and Winston.

Byrne, B. (1994). *Bullying: A Community Approach*. Mount Merrion, Blackrock, Co. Duglin: The Columbia Press.

Elliot, M. (1989). The Kidscape Kit. Kidscape, World Trade Center. Europe House, London E1 9AA.

Elliot, M. & Kilpatrick, J. (1994). *How to stop a bullying: A Kidscape training guide*. London: Kidscape, Inc.

Hoover, J.H., Oliver, R.L., & Hazler, R. J. (1992). Bullyng: Perceptions of adolescent victims in the midwestern U.S.A. School Psychology International, 13, 5–16.

Marano, H. E. (1995, September/October). Big. Bad. Bully. *Psychology Today*, 28(5), 50–82.

Miller, T. W. (1997). *Children of Trauma: Stressful Life Events and Their Effects on Children and Adolescents*. Madison, CT: International Universities Press, Inc.

Miller, T. & Beane, A. L. (1999). Clinical impact on child victims of bullying in the schools. *Directions*, 9, 121–129.

Oliver, R., Hoover, J. H., & Hazler, R. (1994, March/April). The perceived roles of bullying in small-town midwestern schools. *Journal of Counseling & Development*, 416–419.

Olweus, D. (1989). Bully/victim problems among school children: basic facts and effects of a school based intervention program. In K. Rubin & D. Pepler (Eds.), *The Development and Treatment of Childhood Aggression*. Hillsdale, NJ: Erlbaum Publishers.

Olweus, D. (1994). Bullying at school: Basic facts and effects of a school-based intervention program. Journal of Child Psychiatry 35(7): 1171–1190.

Olweus, D. (1995). *Bullying at school: What we know and what we can do*. Cambridge, MA: Blackwell Publishers.

O'Moore, A. M. & Hillery, B. (1989) Bullying in Dublin Schools. *The Irish Journal of Psychology*, 10(3), 426–441.

Roland, E. (1989). Bullying: The Scandinavian research tradition. In D. P. Tatum & D. A. Lane (Eds.), *Bullying in Schools*. London, England: Trentham Book Publishers Incorporated.

Spurling, R. (2006). *The Bully-Free School Zone Character Education Program: A Study of the Impact on Five Western North Carolina Middle Schools*. Department of Educational Leadership and Policy Analysis. East Tennessee University, Johnson City, TN.

Chapter 21
A Series of Culturally Relevant Models to Prevent School-Age Youth Violence: A 4-Year (2001–2005) Family and Community Violence Prevention Study

Laxley W. Rodney, Rameshwar P. Srivastava, and Dana L. Johnson

Overview The Family and Community Violence Prevention (FCVP) Program, a 12-year federally funded initiative, was established in 1994 to address the escalation of youth violence among ethnic minorities. The program was implemented through a cooperative agreement between Central State University, Wilberforce, Ohio, and the Office of Minority Health, U.S. Department of Health and Human Services and adapted the public health model which views violence as a public health disease. Through this cooperative agreement, a total of 45 Family Life Centers were organized in 23 states, the District of Columbia, Puerto Rico, and the U.S. Virgin Islands to serve youth who were considered to be at risk for violence and other abusive behaviors.

An article titled "The Impact of Culturally Relevant Violence Prevention Models on School-Age Youth" published in the September 2005 issue of the *Journal of Primary Prevention* featured a 3-year study, 1999–2002, on the effectiveness of the six-component curriculum of the FCVP Program in reducing violence among participants. Subsequent to the that study, the authors expanded their research and completed a new 4-year evaluation study of 3,094 at-risk minority youth who participated in the program during academic years 2001–2005.

This chapter revisits the 1999–2002 study published in the 2005 article in the *Journal of Primary Prevention* and uses it as the focal point for the background of the new 4-year study (2001–2005) with 2001–2002 being the only overlapping year. New data sets are analyzed and presented to see if they are consistent with 1999–2002 results as well as to report on new trends.

Statistically, significant results from this new 4-year study confirm and validate the earlier findings that showed the FCVP curriculum to be effective in improving participants' academic performance in the areas of spelling and arithmetic as measured by standard scores on the Wide Range Achievement Test. The youth's academic performance, particularly those with high arithmetic scores, was negatively correlated with involvement in violence and other risky behaviors (as measured by standard scores on the Violence Risk Assessment Inventory). A negative association was also found between participants' level of bonding to school (as measured by standard scores on the School Bonding

T. W. Miller (ed.), *School Violence and Primary Prevention.*
© Springer 2008

Index-Revised) and their involvement in violence and risky behaviors. A very strong positively correlated relationship between participants' exposure and subsequent involvement in violence was also found. Adolescent girls showed a high tendency to be involved in violence and other abusive behaviors and there were differential effect of the FCVP curriculum among the four ethnic and culturally distinct groups, namely, African American, Hispanics, Native American, and Native Hawaiian.

The authors' conclusion and discussion points include strong academic performance being a protective factor against school-age violence, exposure to violence is a risk factor for later involvement in violence, more research is recommended to clarify the observed increase in the number of older girls getting involved in aggressive and risky behaviors. Are they simply getting bad or are they simply displaying symptoms of abuse by their boyfriends and other male associates? Although ethnic and cultural groups such as those being served by the FCVP Program may be experiencing similar risk factors, prevention programs should be designed to reflect differences norms.

The Family and Community Violence Prevention Program: A Series of Culturally Relevant Models to Prevent School-Age Youth Violence

Youth violence remains a major public health problem in the USA. The homicide rate for children younger than 15 is 16 times the combined rates of 25 other industrialized countries (Junger-Tas et al., 1994; Maguire & Pastore, 1999). According to Trump (2002), some 5,506 young people between the ages 15 and 24 were victims of homicide during 1998. For youth aged 10–14, homicide is the third leading cause of death and for youth aged 15–19 is the second leading cause of death. One in every eight people murdered in 2000 was younger than 18 years old (Satcher, 2001; Stinson, 2002).

Ethnic minorities are disproportionately victimized and are more likely to become perpetrators of violent acts themselves. Young Black boys and girls are 11 and 4 times, respectively, more likely to be killed than White youth. Blacks, Pacific Islanders, and American Indians are more likely than Whites to be victimized with the use of a firearm. American Indians aged 12 and older were victims of violent crime at about twice the rate of Blacks, Whites, or Asians. During 1998, American Indians experienced 110 violent victimizations per 1,000 compared to 43 victimizations per 1,000 for Blacks, 38 per 1,000 for Whites, and 22 per 1,000 for Asians (Bureau of Justice Statistics, 2001; Rennison, 2001). Review of the literature by Edwards et al. (2005) shows that in 2000, homicide was the number one cause of death among African American youth (aged 15–24) and the second leading cause of death for Latino youth.

High Profile School Shootings Versus Low Profile, Nonfatal In-School and Out-of-School Violent Acts

Over the past decade, homicides associated with high profile school shootings (such as those at Jonesboro, Arkansas, 1997; West Paducah, Kentucky, 1997; Columbine, Colorado, 1999; and Red Lake, Minnesota, 2005) have received extensive media coverage and tend to be the points of reference for the general public whenever a discussion on school violence is initiated. These high profile shootings, like the one at Columbine High School in Littleton, Colorado, were responsible for the adoption of "threat assessment protocols" to address school-based attacks by the National Threat Assessment Center, an entity within the Department of Education. The authors reported on an extensive examination of 37 incidents of targeted school shootings and school attacks that occurred between 1974 and June 2000. The study involved extensive review of police records, school records, court documents, and other source materials, and included interviews with 10 school shooters.

The focus of the study was on developing information about the school shooters' pre-attack behaviors and communications. The goal was to identify information about a school shooting that may be identifiable or noticeable before the shooting occurs. This was to help inform efforts to prevent school-based attacks. The study found that school shootings are rarely impulsive acts. Rather, they are typically thought out and planned in advance. In addition, prior to most shootings, other children knew the shooting was to occur—but did not alert an adult. Very few of the attackers ever directed threats to their targets before the attack. The study findings also revealed that there is no "profile" of a school shooter; instead, the students who carried out the attacks differed from one another in numerous ways. However, almost every attacker had engaged in behavior before the shooting that seriously concerned at least one adult. The findings from the study suggest that some school attacks may be preventable, and that students can play an important role in prevention efforts. Using the study findings, the Secret Service and Department of Education modified the Secret Service threat assessment approach for use in schools to give them and law enforcement professionals tools for investigating threats in schools, managing situations of concern, and creating safe school climates (Vosselkuil et al., 2002).

Although serious and dramatic in nature and scope, the above high profile shootings described previously accounted for a relatively small number of homicides over a 9-year period. On the other hand, nonfatal in-school and out-of-school violent acts or violence associated with school-age children continue to receive relatively little media exposure. However, these violent acts remain a major concern to educators and parents. In the year 2000 alone, students between the ages of 12 and 18 were victims of ~700,000 violent crimes (Edwards et al., 2005). A large number of these crimes included rape, sexual assault, robbery, and aggravated assault. Overall, students were victims of about 1.9 million crimes while they were in school in 2000, and about 2.0 million away from school (National Center for Education Statistics, 2002).

Factors Associated with School Violence: How They May Be Reduced and Prevented

Researchers have identified five interdependent categories of adolescent risk factors which are likely to negatively impact youth behavior. These factors are associated with the individual, community, family, peers, and school (Stinson, 2002; Rodney et al., 1999a; Garbarino, 1999; Hawkins, 1995; Howell, 1995; Satcher, 2001). Although all categories are important for understanding the context of a given act of youth violence, only those that are associated with schools are discussed in this chapter.

Rodney et al. (1999b), in their review of the literature for a study on variables contributing to retention, found that school-related variables contributed more to delinquent behavior than did the effect of either family or friends. Academic failure was found to be one of the largest and most consistent predictors of delinquency and other abusive behaviors. This prediction was further found to be very profound among African American males, as illustrated in the testimony of citizens testifying before an Ohio public hearing in the early1990s. These citizens suggested "the failure of African American males in the education system is a major contributor to their involvement in the criminal justice system..." (Rodney et al., 1999b). These results are in keeping with earlier work by Siegel and Senna (1988) who found delinquents to be more academically deficient and thus more likely to leave school and become involved in antisocial behavior than nondelinquents. Also, Pianta et al. (1995) found that youth who perform poorly on measures of underlying ability tend to do poorly in school and are more likely to be retained. In more recent studies, other researchers also found poor academic performance to be directly linked to delinquent behaviors. Those who perform poorly are among the most likely to violate the law (Kaufman et al., 2000). It is common to find that school failure is a stronger predictor of delinquency than such personal variables as economic class membership, racial or ethnic background, or peer-group relations (National Center for Educational Statistics, 2002).

Over the years, many school- and community-based programs have been implemented to boost students' academic performance and other social skills in an effort to delay or prevent involvement in delinquent behaviors. In their review of the literature for their article in the *Journal of Primary Prevention*, Rodney et al. (2005a) cited research findings which showed: the integration of extracurricular activities such as those sponsored by schools and community organizations to be safeguards against risk-taking behaviors; youth participating in after-school activities tend to also have better grades and less-deviant behavior participation in extracurricular activities can sometimes facilitate bonding the school and may also enhance family bonding. Another effective strategy to help prevent and reduce violence associated with school-age youth seems to be one which incorporates extracurricular activities and other interventions that are culturally relevant.

A promising national program that has adapted a comprehensive approach to youth violence by incorporating academic enhancement, extracurricular activities, and other social and personal development skills in culturally relevant settings is the FCVP Program.

The FCVP Program

At the time of the writing of this chapter (December 2007), the FCVP Program was one of the nation's largest and most culturally diverse violence prevention initiatives. In the early 1990s, a group of 16 presidents of Historically Black Colleges and Universities (HBCUs) decided to address the escalating and devastating waves of violence across the USA, particularly among African American males. The psyche of young people in communities of color in those days was aptly captured in a quote from Louis Stokes, retired Congressman (D-Ohio11) who noted that "… young people who live in crime-ridden environments are beginning to accept violence as a way of life. Instead of planning their futures, they are planning their funerals… because they anticipated their death before reaching the age of 20." The congressman went on to express his disgust with the state of affairs when he noted that "It is a sad day in America when its children are preoccupied by the possibility of premature death due to violence…" (2008, p xx) (Rodney & Rodney, 1995 p 30).

According to Rodney (2008), it was within this background that the presidents of the following 16 HBCUs signed a memorandum of understanding in 1992 to establish The Consortium on Research and Practicum on Minority Males which later became known as The Minority Male (Min-Male) Consortium.

1. Central State University, Wilberforce, Ohio
2. Chicago State University, Chicago, Illinois
3. Clark Atlanta University, Atlanta, Georgia
4. Knoxville College, Knoxville, Tennessee
5. LeMoyne College, Memphis, Tennessee
6. Lincoln University, Lincoln, Pennsylvania
7. Morgan State University, Baltimore, Maryland
8. Morehouse College, Atlanta, Georgia
9. North Carolina A&T University, Greensboro, North Carolina
10. Philander Smith College, Little Rock, Arkansas
11. Talladega College, Talladega, Alabama
12. Texas Southern University, Houston, Texas
13. Tougaloo College, Tougaloo, Mississippi
14. University of the District of Columbia, Washington, DC
15. Wilberforce University, Wilberforce, Ohio
16. Xavier University, New Orleans, Louisiana

With the initial funding of $4,335,000 from the Office of Minority Health in the Department of Health and Human Services, the Min-Male Consortium, under the leadership of a management team located at Central State University, in Wilberforce, Ohio, lunched a 3-year cooperative agreement (1994–1997) known as "A Series of

Models to Prevent Minority Male Violence" (U.S. Department of Health and Human Services Notice of Award # D67MP94001-01, 1994). After establishing Family Life Centers (FLCs) on or near the campuses of the 16 participating colleges and universities to provide violence prevention services to at-risk minority youth, The Min-Male project was redesigned in 1997 by the Office of Minority Health to bring about a more structured approach to evaluation and its four-component curriculum—academic development, personal development, career development, and cultural enrichment. The newly redesigned program was renamed the FCVP Program.

By the summer of 2006, the FCVP Program had evolved into one of America's most comprehensive and dynamic initiatives designed to combat youth violence from minority and traditionally marginalized populations. From an almost 100% African American cohort, consisting overwhelmingly of adolescent boys in 1994, the FCVP Program evolved into a truly culturally and ethnically diverse initiative serving both under 12 and 12 and older male and female youth in equal proportions. Rodney and Johnson (2006) report that between the 1999–2000 and the 2003–2004 program years, the percentage of African Americans dropped from 81 to 54 while that of Native American increased from 3 to 14. Over the same period, the percentage of Hispanic/Latinos increased from 8 to 21 while Mixed (Multiracial) increased from 2 to 6.

The program's longevity spanned 12 years, and during that time period received ~$70 million in federal support. Forty-five colleges and universities located in 23 states, the District of Columbia, Puerto Rico, and the U.S. Virgin Islands participated and provided prevention services to more than 13,000 community youth and 3,200 college students. Six National Conferences on Family and Community Violence Prevention were held since the inception of the FCVP Program and its predecessor, the Min-Male Consortium. These conferences convened in Atlanta, Georgia (October 1996); Baltimore, Maryland (November, 1997); New Orleans, Louisiana (October, 1998); Houston, Texas (October, 1999); Los Angeles, California (April, 2001); and Honolulu, Hawaii (April, 2005). Scholarly papers, monographs, and reports have been published from these conferences as well as from evaluation and research studies (Rodney & Johnson, 2006).

According to the FCVP Web page at www.fcvp.org, in July 2006, the following 19 colleges and universities were actively participating in its national initiatives:

1. Albany State University, Albany, Georgia
2. California State University, Fullerton, California
3. Chicago State University, Chicago, Illinois
4. Howard University, Washington, DC
5. Lady of the Lake University, San Antonio, Texas
6. LeMoyne-Owen College, Memphis, Tennessee
7. Lincoln University, Jefferson City, Missouri
8. Little Priest Tribal College, Winnebago, Nebraska
9. New Mexico State University, Las Cruces, New Mexico
10. Pontifical Catholic College, Ponce, Puerto Rico

11. Sinte Gleska University, Rosebud, South Dakota
12. South Carolina State University, Orangeburg, South Carolina
13. Southern University-Baton Rouge, Baton Rouge, Louisiana
14. Texas A&M University-Corpus Christi, Corpus Christi, Texas
15. Tougaloo College, Tougaloo, Mississippi
16. University of Hawaii-Hilo, Hilo, Hawaii
17. University of North Carolina-Pembroke, Pembroke, North Carolina
18. University of the Virgin Islands, St. Thomas, U.S. Virgin Islands
19. Xavier University, New Orleans, Louisiana.

Over the years, individuals and groups associated with the FCVP Program have reported, through workshops, national conferences, monographs, and articles in referred journals, that its initiatives are effective in preventing and reducing participants' involvement in violence and other risky behaviors. The following is a summary of a recent article titled "The Impact of Culturally Relevant Violence Prevention Models on School-Age Youth" written by the authors of this chapter and published in the *Journal of Primary Prevention*, (Rodney et al., 2005a, pp. 439–454).

Highlights from the FCVP 3-Year (1999–2002) Study

The purpose of the 3-year study was to determine the effectiveness of the FCVP curriculum in reducing violence among youth participants. Comprehensive evaluation data were gathered at the time of pretest from 2,548 at-risk youth and from 2,315 of them at the time of the posttest. Boys comprised 59% or 1,357 and girls 41% or 958 of those who completed the posttest. In terms of ethnicity, the percentages were 72 for African American, 10.3 for Hispanics, and a combined percentage of 15 for Native American and Native Hawaiian. Most of the participants (61.5%) were 12 years and older, with under 12 comprising 38.5%. The authors believe that this representation of the different ethnic groups provided an accurate picture of the at-risk youth within the communities being served by the FCVP Program.

Eight common cross-site instruments were used to collect pre- and posttest data from participant and comparison groups in each of the three years. However, only the Wide Range Achievement Test, Third Edition (WRAT 3), a nationally normed, three-part instrument, the School Bonding Index-Revised (SBI-R), and the Violence Risk Assessment Inventory (VRAI), both of which were developed and pilot tested by the FCVP Program during the 1997–1998 academic year, were used to collect data for the study reported in the 2005 article in the *Journal of Primary Prevention*. Copies of the SBI-R and the VRAI are presented in Appendices 1 and 2 rein under the section dealing with the 2001–2005 4-year study.

In terms of the research question, "What were the effects of the overall FCVP curriculum on youth's involvement in violence and other abusive behaviors, compared to those who did not participate in the program?" the combined 3-year results showed that the FCVP intervention was more effective for youth under 12 years old, who showed greater reduction in delinquency than their older cohorts. The mean standard score on the violence risk (VR) subscale of the VRAI—items 1–20—showed a significant reduction [$t(2088) = 2.998, p < .01$] between pre- and posttest. While the results for the under age 12 participant and comparison groups showed a significant reduction in the VR standard scores, the reduction for the participant group had a higher level of significance [$t(2088) = 2.998, p < .01$] than the comparison group [$t(129) = 1.953, p = .05$], effect size, $d = .10$.

On the basis of the above results, the authors feel very strongly that violence initiatives, especially those which focused on enhancing basic academic skills, are critically important in the early years of the at-risk youth.

For the question, "What were the relationships between youth's academic performance and their involvement in violence and other risky behaviors?" the results showed that youth's academic performance (spelling and arithmetic) and their involvement in violence was negatively correlated, as measured by the Pearson's correlation for WRAT 3 and VRAI standard scores. During the last 2 years, the arithmetic and VRAI correlation was statistically significant ($r = -.149, p < .01$ in 2000–2001 and $r = -.164, p < .01$ in 2001–2002). During 2001–2002, the correlation between the spelling and VRAI was statistically significant ($r = -.115, p < .01$).

An interesting finding was that youth who scored high on the arithmetic section of the WRAT 3 showed lower involvement in violence and other abusive behaviors at the posttest. More research is being recommended to determine why this is the case because further elucidations could help educators and prevention professionals to design more meaningful activities that would stimulate youth to use higher level cognitive skills such as those required in logical reasoning in arithmetic and other mathematical problems. Although only spelling and arithmetic concepts were tested under the 3-year academic component of the FCVP Program, it seems logical that if youths achieved academic competence in other subject areas, their involvement in violent behaviors should be reduced.

In terms of the question, "What were the relationships between youth's level of bonding to school and their involvement in violence and other abusive behaviors?" the standard scores on three of the subscales of the SBI—school experience, school involvement, and school pride—had negative correlations with the standard T scores on the VRAI over the 3-year period. Standard scores on the school delinquency subscale showed a positive correlation with standard scores on the VRAI (r in the range 0.224–0.272, $p < .01$). These correlations were statistically significant in all three years.

The above results showed that youth were less likely to be involved in violence and other abusive behaviors if they feel bonded to their school. This implies that educators should endeavor to create and nurture a positive school environment for children. This idea is congruent with previously published research that shows a safe, secure, and positive environment in which youth can interact helps to shelter them from negative influences and prepares them to make good decisions regarding their academic and personal well-being (Walker, 1995). The difference between those schools that experience low levels of violent behaviors and those with high levels is the presence of a positive social climate that fosters nurturing and feelings of inclusiveness. The structures that attempt to teach and reinforce basic prosocial behaviors and develop caring relationships between youth and staff will reduce the likelihood of antisocial behavior (Walker, 1995; Walker et al., 1995; Kadel & Follman, 1993).

To obtain the answer for the question, "What was the relationship between youth's exposure to violence and their involvement in violence?" a detailed analysis of 2000–2001 data showed a positive correlation between the responses of participating youth on two items of the VRAI: Item 3 ("In the past three months, someone in my family has gotten in a physical fight") and Item 16 ("In the past three months, I have physically fought someone I knew"). Pretest results for these items showed almost an identical percentage of youth who responded in the affirmative, 38.3% for Item 3 and 41.7% for Item 16. On the posttest, responses for the same two items were 26.6% and 26.4%, respectively.

The above result shows that exposure to violence is a risk factor. The authors feel that this vicious cycle of violence must be broken because children model the behaviors of significant adults in the lives (parents, teachers, coaches, etc.). Thus, it is not surprising that the youth in this study became involved in violence after they were exposed to it. The authors feel that elements of the social learning theory ("…most human behaviors are learned observationally through modeling others…"), originally postulated by Bandura, can be used as a theoretical framework for understanding these correlation results. The results can be interpreted within the context of Goldstein's (1991) familial modeling theory which claims that the physically abused child who becomes an adult often batters his or her own child because the abused person acquires his or her behavior from observing the abuse used by parents. It is within this framework that the investigators recommend that prevention programs include opportunities for positive role modeling.

In terms of the question, "What types of changes in youth behavior were observed at 2001–2002 posttesting according to age, gender, and ethnicity?" detailed analysis of 2001–2002 data indicated that the under age 12 group, particularly the boys, was more likely to show a statistically significant reduction in deviant behavior than the older youth after being exposed to the FCVP curriculum. On 17 of the 20 items on the VR subscale, girls aged 12 and older showed increased involvement in violent and other abusive behaviors. A statistically significant increase was observed for three items: Item 8 ("Been away from home without permission"), $t(462) = 2.007$, $p < .05$; Item 12 ("Used a weapon like a knife, gun, stick in a fight"), $t(357) = -2.724$, $p < .01$; and Item 17 ("Been mad enough to fight") $t(470) = -3.045$, $p < .01$.

As alarming as these results may appear to be, they are consistent with emerging national trends that show that the gap between boys and girls is narrowing with respect to involvement in violence. Between 1983 and 1993, the ratio of boys to girls committing violent acts was 7.4:1 and 7:1, respectively; however, by 1998, the ratio narrowed to 3:1 (Satcher, 2001). This trend presents a serious challenge to educators, prevention practitioners, and researchers. More research is recommended to determine factors contributing to this trend and to develop more gender-appropriate prevention strategies.

Based on changes in the 2001–2002 mean pre-and posttest VRAI raw scores, there were differences in the behavior patterns among the ethnic groups. African American youth showed decreased involvement in violence and other abusive behaviors as shown on 12 of the 20 items on the VR subscale. This ethnic group showed statistically significant reduction, $t(928) = 2.062$, $p < .05$, on Item 16 ("Someone in my family has gotten in a physical fight"). On the contrary, Hispanics showed an increased involvement in violence and other abusive behaviors on 18 of the 20 items of the VR subscale, with the increase being statistically significant, $t(123) = -1.993$, $p < .05$, on Item 2 ("Fought with a group against another group"), $t(112) = -2.04$, $p < .05$, on Item 4 ("Physically fought someone I did not know"), $t(80) = -2.679$, $p < .01$, on Item 11 ("Damaged or destroyed school, private property"), and $t(124) = -3.135$, $p < .01$, on Item 20 ("Been so angry I acted without thinking of the consequences"). Native Americans also showed increased involvement in violence and abusive behaviors between pre- and posttest on every item except Item 8 ("Being away from home without permission"), which remained unchanged. On Item 14 ("Held a real gun in my hands"), the increased involvement was statistically significant, $t(167) = -2.049$, $p < .05$. Native Hawaiians showed high involvement with drug and alcohol-related items both at pretest and posttests, such as Item 6 ("Been with someone smoking pot, weed, bliss"), Item 7 ("Been offered drugs or alcohol"), Item 9 ("Drank alcohol or been drunk"), and Item 10 ("Argued with my parent(s) or guardian(s))," but there was no significant increase or decrease among Hawaiians. In contrast to their high involvement with drugs and alcohol, Native Hawaiians had a very low level of involvement with weapons such as guns and knives.

These results suggest that while minority groups may have common risk factors for violence and other abusive behaviors, prevention programs must be designed to reflect the unique culturally appropriate norms of each group.

Overall, results from the 1999–2002 study suggest that the FCVP presents a useful model for approaching violence within the context of a broad social setting requiring collaboration between schools, community agencies, families, and grassroots organizations (Rodney et al., 2005a).

A Series of Culturally Relevant Models to Prevent School-Age Youth Violence: A 4-Year (2001–2005) Follow-Up FCVP Study

Subsequent to the above 1999–2002 study, the authors expanded their research and completed a new 4-year follow-up study of 3,094 youth who participated in the program during academic years 2001–2005. Data sets were analyzed to fulfill the purpose of the study which was to determine if they were consistent with the 1999–2002 results and report on new trends that might have emerged over the period.

Specifically, the study set out to provide answers to the following questions:

1. What were the effects of the overall FCVP curriculum on youth's involvement in violence and other abusive behaviors, compared to those who did not participate in the program during the period 2001–2005?
2. What were the relationships between (a) youth's academic performance and their involvement in violence and other risky behaviors; (b) youth's level of bonding to school and their involvement in violence and other abusive behaviors?
3. What was the relationship between youth's exposure to violence and their involvement in violence?

A total of 3,228 elementary, middle, and high school youth were recruited and pre-tested by 21 FLCs located in 16 states, the District of Columbia, Puerto Rico, and the U.S. Virgin Islands. The list of the 21 FLCs follows:

1. Albany State University, Albany, Georgia
2. California State University, Fullerton, California
3. Chicago State University, Chicago, Illinois
4. Fort Peck Community College, Poplar, Montana
5. Florida A&M University, Tallahassee, Florida
6. Howard University, Washington, DC
7. Lady of the Lake University, San Antonio, Texas
8. LeMoyne-Owen College, Memphis, Tennessee
9. Lincoln University, Jefferson City, Missouri
10. Little Priest Tribal College, Winnebago, Nebraska
11. New Mexico State University, Las Cruces, New Mexico
12. Pontifical Catholic College, Ponce, Puerto Rico
13. South Carolina State University, Orangeburg, South Carolina
14. Southern University-Baton Rouge, Baton Rouge, Louisiana
15. Stillman College, Tuscaloosa, Alabama
16. Texas A&M University-Corpus Christi, Corpus Christi, Texas
17. Tougaloo College, Tougaloo, Mississippi
18. University of Hawaii-Hilo, Hilo, Hawaii
19. University of North Carolina-Pembroke, Pembroke, North Carolina
20. University of the Virgin Islands, St. Thomas, U.S. Virgin Islands
21. Xavier University, New Orleans, Louisiana.

The ethnic composition of the participants consists of four minority groups: African Americans (57.2%), Hispanics (16.3%), Native Americans (13.6%), and Native Hawaiians and multiracial (8.6%). To facilitate their developmental ages, youth whose median age was 12 were placed into two groups—under age 12 and age 12 and over, where they received the appropriate FCVP curriculum offerings. The average numbers for participant and comparison youth at each FLC were 40 and 31, respectively. Of the participating institutions, nine had comparison youth who were matched with participants based on associated risk factors and demographic characteristics.

All youth were deemed to be at risk for violence and other abusive behaviors and were from low- to moderate-income families. They were referred to the FLCs by local school officials based on FCVP accepted risk factors associated with the individual, community, family, peers, and school. The level of risks associated with each factor was left to the discretion of the local center.

Instruments

Eight common cross-site instruments were used to collect data to evaluate the effectiveness of the prevention strategies: The VRAI, SBI-R, WRAT 3, Rosenberg Self-Esteem Scale, Family Environmental Scale, Hansen Life Skills Battery, Ethnic Identity Scale, and Career Maturity Index. Descriptions of all eight instruments can be found in the FCVP Evaluation Newsletter # 6 (Rodney et al., 2005b) and is available at www.fcvp.org. For 2001–2005, data were collected through the use of only three of these instruments, namely, WRAT 3, SBI-R, and the VRAI. The reliability coefficients (Chronbach's alpha) computed over the 4 years from FCVP participants' scores for these three instruments are presented in Table 21.1. Examination of Table 21.1 shows that the reliability coefficients for all the three instruments are fairly high. The 4-year mean Chronbach's alpha values for WRAT 3 spelling and arithmetic were 0.77 and 0.72, respectively, while those for the SBI-R and the VRAI were 0.83 and 0.89, respectively.

The WRAT 3, which is a nationally normed test, is a three-part instrument for individuals aged 5 and older and is intended to measure spelling, arithmetic, and reading ability (Wilkinson, 1993). During the first 2 years of the study, only the spelling and arithmetic tests were administered to participant and comparison groups. Reading was added during the academic year 2003–2004.

The SBI-R, which is presented in Appendix 1, is a 24-item instrument developed and pilot tested by the FCVP Program during the 1997–1998 academic year (Srivastava & Rodney, 2003). It is designed to assess youth's level of attachment

Table 21.1 Reliability coefficient (Alpha) of three family and community violence prevention (FCVP) common cross-site instruments

	Program years			
	2001–2002	2002–2003	2003–2004	2004–2005
Wide Range Achievement Test, Third Edition (WRAT 3) spelling	0.76	0.78	0.78	0.77
	(N = 1,476)	(N = 1,491)	(N = 1,463)	(N = 1,501)
WRAT 3 arithmetic	0.67	0.73	0.73	0.77
	(N = 1,484)	(N = 1,550)	(N = 1,465)	(N = 1,567)
School Bonding Index	0.87	0.89	0.81	0.77
	(N = 1,289)	(N = 1,627)	(N = 1,588)	(N = 1,575)
Violence Risk Assessment	0.89	0.89	0.91	0.88
	(N = 1,497)	(N = 1,650)	(N = 1,588)	(N = 1,578)

to and comfort with school. The 24 items are divided into four subscales: school experience, school involvement, school delinquency, and school pride. Like the WRAT 3, the SBI-R produced consistently high reliability coefficient values over the 4-year period.

The VRAI, which is presented in Appendix 2, was used to measure the impact of the overall FCVP curriculum on youth's involvement in violence and other abusive behaviors. The 23-item VRAI has two subscales. The VR subscale covers items 1–20 and assesses behaviors and thoughts over the past 3 months. The high risk (HR) subscale assesses more dangerous activities over a 6-month period and is made up of items 21–23 (Srivastava & Rodney, 2003).

The VRAI was developed and pilot tested by the FCVP Program during the 1997–1998 academic year. It has since been administered to over 7,000 ethnic minority youth who have participated in the FCVP Program. During its development, the VRAI was critically reviewed by a team of evaluators and directors from FLCs across the country for evidence of content validity. The items that were retained based on results from factor analysis were found to be representative of the various domains of violence and abusive behaviors. Consequently, items 1–20, which constitute the VR subscale, are representative of information covering weapon possession and usage, possession and use of drugs and alcohol, exposure to and involvement in violence, involvement in fighting, and destruction of property. Further work on evidence on concurrent validity for the VRAI is being conducted through correlation of its scores with those of a nationally recognized instrument that assesses youth's involvement in violence and other abusive behaviors (Srivastava & Rodney, 2003).

The FCVP Curriculum

During the 4-year study under review, FCVP prevention activities or interventions were offered through a six-component curriculum.

The academic development component was designed to improve academic performance through the enhancement of cognitive skills, study skills, and other techniques which lead to achievement of short-term and long-term educational goals.

The personal development component provided a series of activities to promote social, emotional, physical, and spiritual well-being for the individual as participants learned to resolve problems, constructively reduce interpersonal aggression, and develop the capacity to negotiate experiences vital to improving the quality of life.

Family bonding activities were geared toward improving family relationships, parenting skills, and coping techniques that lead to enhanced family stability and increased social support networks.

Cultural development activities were provided to promote an awareness of and appreciation for one's heritage, traditions, values, and norms as well as those of other diverse populations. Activities were also provided to expose individuals and group to the creative expression of various ethnic and cultural groups.

Recreational enhancement activities promoted recreation and leisure, healthy lifestyles, and interpersonal skills by exposing individuals and groups to various games and activities designed to promote critical thinking, teamwork, cooperation, relaxation, and good health.

Career development provided youth with skills necessary for job readiness, promoted skills, and knowledge through exploration in a specific field. Activities were provided to assist youth in identifying career options.

Evaluation and research protocols, including parental informed consent and confidentiality assurances, were approved by the Internal Review Board of the universities and colleges of each FLC before programming began. At the beginning of each program year, individual FLCs administered the common cross-site instruments to participant and comparison groups. After pretesting at the beginning of the academic year, youth participants at all of the FLCs were exposed to the FCVP six-component curriculum and then posttested between May and June with the eight common cross-site instruments used during the pretest.

Analysis of scores obtained from the WRAT 3, SBI-R, and VRAI were carried out using standardized scores instead of raw scores. According to the WRAT 3 manual, raw scores are converted to standard scores with a distribution mean of 100 and a standard deviation of 15 (Wilkinson, 1993). Drawing from the researchers' earlier work (Srivastava & Rodney, 2003), raw scores from the SBI-R were converted to standard scores whose distribution has a mean of 100 and a standard deviation of 15. This conversion made it easier to work with WRAT 3 and SBI-R scores for assessing youth academic performance in the FCVP Program.

The formula for converting SBI-R raw scores to SBI-R standard scores is as follows:

Standard score = 100 + [{(Raw score – FCVP wide mean)/ FCVP wide SD}× 15]

In terms of the VRAI, raw scores were converted to standard T scores ($M = 50$, $SD = 10$). The formula used for the conversion is as follows:

Standard score = 50 + [{(Raw score – FCVP wide mean)/ FCVP wide SD}×10]

Results

The results of this study are based on data gathered from matching pre- and posttest scores for youth participants over the 4-year period, 2001–2005. The total number of participants at the time of the pretest was 3,228, with boys comprising 1,780 (55%) and girls comprising 1,444 (45%). After posttesting, a total of 3,094 matched pre and posttest scores were obtained for 1,677 (54.4%) boys and 1,404 (45.6%) girls. Thirteen youth did not indicate their gender. Overall, the retention rate was 95.8% between the pre- and the posttest. Girls were retained at a rate of 3.0 percentage point higher than boys (97.2% vs. 94.2%). African Americans made up 57% of the participants; Hispanics 16.3%. The combined group of Native Americans, Native

Hawaiians, and multiracial constituted 22% of the sample. Forty-nine percent of the participants were under age 12, with the remaining (51%) over age 12 at the time of the posttest.

As measured by standard scores on the VRAI at the time of the posttest, results in Table 21.2 indicate that for academic years 2003–2004 and 2004–2005, youth who participated in the FCVP Program had less involvement in violence and other risky behaviors than comparison youth who were not exposed to the FCVP curriculum. For academic year 2004–2005, the difference between the posttest scores for youth 12 years and older was statistically significant ($p < .05$); the effect size index (d) was 0.2.

In terms of the research question, "What was the relationship between youth's academic performance (WRAT 3 standard scores for spelling and arithmetic) and their involvement in violence and other risky behaviors (VRAI standard scores)?" results showed a negative correlation between these variables. As shown in Table 21.3, the arithmetic and VRAI correlation was statistically significant for each of the 4 years of

Table 21.2 Violence risk assessment inventory (VRAI) violence risk standard scores by age group for 2003–2004 and 2004–2005

	Youth under age 12		Youth age 12 or older	
	2003–2004	2004–2005	2003–2004	2004–2005
Participating youth				
Sample size (n_1)	353	406	400	365
Standard deviation (s_1)	9.07	9.03	13.33	10.59
Posttest mean	48.696	48.614	55.197	52.587
Comparison youth				
Sample size (n_2)	315	329	353	303
Standard deviation (s_2)	8.85	8.94	12.09	12.57
Posttest mean	49.227	49.077	55.021	54.849
T-test of significance for equality of means	0.445	0.85	0.488	0.013[a]
Effect size (d)	0.06	0.05	−0.01	0.20

[a] The difference between participants and comparison youth posttest means is significant at the $p < .05$ level (two-tailed).

Table 21.3 Correlation analysis of wide range achievement test, third edition (WRAT 3), standard scores and violence risk assessment inventory (VRAI) standard scores

		VRAI T score			
		2001–2002	2002–2003	2003–2004	2004–2005
	N	687	795	747	756
WRAT 3 Spelling	Pearson correlation (r)	−.115**	−.017	−.069	−.076*
Standardized score	Sig. (two-tailed)	0.003	0.646	0.059	0.040
WRAT 3 Arithmetic	Pearson correlation (r)	−.164**	−.096**	−.153**	−.095**
Standardized score	Sig. (two-tailed)	0.000	0.008	0.000	0.009

**Correlation is significant at the $p < .01$ level (two-tailed).
*Correlation is significant at the $p < .05$ level (two-tailed).

the study ($r = -.164, p < .01$ in 2001–2002; $r = -.096, p < .01$ in 2002–2003; $r = -.153$, $p < .01$ in 2003–2004; and $r = -.095, p < .01$ in 2004–2005). The correlation between the spelling and VRAI was statistically significant for two of the four years ($r = -.115$, $p < .01$), in 2001–2002 and during 2004–2005 ($r = -.076, p < .05$).

For the research question, "What is the relationship between youth's level of bonding to school and their involvement in violence and other abusive behaviors?" the standard scores on three of the subscales of the SBI—school experience, school involvement, and school pride—had negative correlations with the standard T scores on the VRAI over the 4-year period. Standard scores on the school delinquency subscale showed a positive correlation with standard scores on the VRAI (r in the range 0.272–0.354, $p < .01$). These correlations were statistically significant in all four years as shown in Table 21.4.

In terms of the question, "What was the relationship between youth's exposure to violence and their involvement in violence?" the results from 2003–2004 as well as earlier years showed a positive correlation between the responses of participating youth on two items of the VRAI: Item 3 ("In the past three months, someone in my family has gotten in a physical fight") and Item 16 ("In the past three months, I have physically fought someone I knew"). Pretest results for these items showed almost an identical percentage of youth who responded in the affirmative, 39.5% for Item 3 and 37.6% for Item 16. On the posttest, responses for the same two items were 35.8% and 34.6%, respectively. Pearson correlation coefficient r for the pair of scores (exposure to violence and anger involvement) on the pretest was 0.355 and on the posttest was 0.361. The correlation was significant at the .01 level.

One of the intriguing findings from the earlier 1999–2002 FCVP study was that adolescent girls, particularly in the 2001–2002 academic year, reported surprisingly high involvement in violence and other abusive behaviors. The investigators reexamined the question of differential involvement in risky behaviors according to gender. The results in Table 21.5 indicate a continued tendency for older girls to

Table 21.4 Correlation analysis of scores on school bonding index with violence risk assessment inventory (VRAI) t score

		VRAI T score			
		2001–2002	2002–2003	2003–2004	2004–2005
	N	595	795	783	769
Standardized score School Experience	Pearson correlation (r) Sig. (two-tailed)	−.074 0.072	−.051 0.152	−.223** 0.000	−.167** 0.000
Standardized score School Involvement	Pearson correlation (r) Sig. (two-tailed)	−.098* 0.017	−.065 0.065	−.225** 0.000	−.215** 0.000
Standardized score School Delinquency	Pearson correlation (r) Sig. (two-tailed)	0.272** 0.000	0.284** 0.000	0.294** 0.000	0.354** 0.000
Standardized score School Pride	Pearson Correlation (r) Sig. (two-tailed)	−.050 0.220	−.149** 0.000	−.174** 0.000	−.207** 0.000

**Correlation is significant at the $p < .01$ level (two-tailed)
*Correlation is significant at the $p < .05$ level (two-tailed)

Table 21.5 Violence risk assessment inventory (VRAI) violence risk standard scores for "age 12 and older girls" for 2003–2004 and 2004–2005

	Girls age 12 or older	
	2003–2004	2004–2005
Pretest		
Sample size (n_1)	168	163
Standard deviation (s_1)	11.23	11.31
Mean	52.06	52.43
Posttest		
Sample size (n_2)	168	163
Standard deviation (s_2)	11.98	9.17
Mean	53.88	50.80
T-test of significance for equality of means	0.153	0.149
Effect size (d)	−0.16	0.16

have a fairly high involvement in violence and other risky behaviors as measured by standard scores on the VRAI over the 2003–2004 and 204–2005 academic years. Although the differences between pre- and posttest scores for the two years under review were not statistically significant ($p > .05$) and the effect size index (d) only 0.16, the mean standard pre- and posttest scores for both years were relatively high, that is, all scores were above the established FCVP mean of 50.

To get a better understanding of the increase in deviant behavior of adolescent girls in the 2001–2002 and 2003–2004 academic years, the researchers conducted group discussions with the staff of the participating FLCs during the 2003 and 2004 winter and spring national technical assistance workshops. The groups reported that school officials were referring more girls to local FLCs because of their disruptive behaviors in and outside of the classroom. It was also expressed that as girls reach puberty, some seem to feel that it is necessary to appear tough so that they will not be "picked on" by peers, abusive boyfriends, or adult family members. Some staffers expressed the view that girls at this age are simply modeling the behavior of disruptive boys who have been receiving much attention from teachers and other adults.

Discussion and Conclusion

Results of the 2001–2005 4-year FCVP study confirms and reinforced earlier findings. Overall, the FCVP six-component curriculum has been found to be effective in improving youth's academic performance as measured by standard scores on the spelling and arithmetic subtests of the WRAT 3. This is considered significant in light of literature cited earlier in this chapter that shows high academic performance to be a protective factor against school failure and delinquency.

Examination of results in Table 21.3 showed academic performance (spelling and arithmetic standard scores on WRAT 3) to be highly negatively correlated with youth's involvement in violence and other risky behaviors as measured by their standard scores on the VRAI. In other words, as youth's academic performance increases, their involvement in violence and other delinquent behaviors decreases. It is worth noting that the correlations between the WRAT 3 arithmetic scores and VRAI scores were statically significant ($p < .01$) for all four years. This suggests that arithmetic—a basic component of the discipline of mathematics which uses logical and higher order cognitive skills—could be a powerful protective factor for young children who are at risk for delinquent behaviors.

In an effort to clarify the negative association between high arithmetic scores and low level of involvement in risky behaviors, the researchers theorized that individuals who demonstrate competence in arithmetic are likely to have acquired the capability of logical and rational thinking. These individuals are therefore more likely to be able to transfer this competence of rationality and logical thinking to social interactions with others. As such, they are better able to foresee, through reasoning, the negative consequence of certain social actions, such as fighting, use of alcohol, and drugs and involvement in risky sexual activities. In other words, they are less likely to act impulsively than their peers who do not possess a similar level of competence of rationality and logic. To test this theory, the researchers examined the literature relating to research on the impact of certain cognitive and psychomotor activities, such as music and fine arts, on the stimulation of those sections of the brain associated with special memory, logic, and analytical capabilities. In the review of the literature for their article "Whole Brain Learning: The Fine Arts with Students at Risk," which was recently published in the *Journal of Reclaiming Children and Youth*, Respress and Lufti (2006) reported that the studies of Rausher and Shaw confirm an unmistakable causal link between music and spatial intelligence; Repress and Lufti provide additional literature reviews which show: spatial reasoning is involved with many things, such as solving mathematical problems and creative scientific processes, and the ability to plan almost anything; there is a central processing region of the brain—the right cerebellum; the left frontal cortex; and the "gate" between the two, the anterior cingulate. It appears that the fine arts stimulate the functioning of this region, which in turn develops capabilities in reading, math, and science.

Other literature deemed relevant to the theory of the acquisition of the capability of logical and rational thinking through activities such as mathematics which are believed to stimulate certain sections of the brain can be found in an unpublished 2006 research paper by Offman (2006) who cites several research studies relating to music and brain stimulation to make them more proficient in mathematics. In her literature review for her graduate proposal, Offman points out that music instruction can have a positive effect on other areas of learning, like mathematics and spatial temporal reasoning, which are crucial to learning proportional reasoning and geometry skills; she also who points out that many researchers agree that mathematics and music are very similar because both are concerned with linking abstractions together, along with making patterns of ideas. The work of Gardner was also cited by Offman to show that music and mathematics are among the seven forms of multiple intelligences that contribute to the development of a child. The seven multiple intelligences are as follows:

Linguistic Intelligence:	The capacity to use words effectively, orally or written.
Logical-Mathematical Intelligence:	The capacity to use numbers effectively and to reason well.
Spatial Intelligence:	The ability to perceive the visual-spatial world accurately and to perform transformations upon those perceptions.
Bodily-Kinesthetic Intelligence:	Expertise in using one's whole body to express ideas and feelings and facility in using one's hands to produce or transform things.
Musical Intelligence:	The capacity to perceive, discriminate, transform, and express musical forms.
Interpersonal Intelligence:	The ability to perceive and make distinctions in the moods, intentions, motivations, and feelings of other people.
Intrapersonal Intelligence:	Self-knowledge and the ability to act adaptively on the basis of that knowledge.

Gardner's model of multiple intelligences as summarized by Offman (2006) seem to add credence to the FCVP investigators' theory of acquisition of capability of logical and rational thinking by youth through activities such as mathematics and their ability to transfer these competencies to social interaction with peers. The youth in the FCVP study who displayed high arithmetic scores and low involvement in delinquent behaviors seem to possess at least four of Gardner's seven multiple intelligences, namely:

1. Logical-Mathematical Intelligence
2. Spatial Intelligence
3. Interpersonal Intelligence
4. Intrapersonal Intelligence

Much more research is recommended to test and validate the researchers' theory of acquisition of capability of logical and rational thinking by youth through activities such as mathematics and their ability to transfer these competencies to social interaction with others. In the meantime, the researchers are recommending that prevention programs for at-risk minority youth incorporate academic activities that require them to use higher order thinking skills rather than only exposing them to basic skills and remedial experiences. A combination of interesting activities including mathematical concepts and the fine arts (music, drama, and dance) that incorporate emerging technology might be a very effective prevention approach.

The results relating to the question dealing with the relationship between youth's exposure to violence and their subsequent involvement in violence confirm those of the earlier study. The positive correlation between the two variables once again indicates that exposure to violence and abusive behavior is a very powerful risk factor that needs to be curtailed. As in the previous study, positive role modeling by adults, such as parents, teachers, coaches, and mentors who are significant in the life of the youth, is highly recommended.

One of the intriguing findings from the earlier 1999–2002 study as well as from the 2001–2005 was that adolescent girls reported surprisingly high involvement in violence and other abusive behaviors. The researchers were initially shocked at these results but further exploration through focus group discussions with staff of the FLCs and review of the literature showed that the findings may not be isolated but may be part of a growing national trend. In a 2005 FCVP Evaluation Report, Rodney et al. (2005b) cited the work of Chester-Lind who reported that results of her research studies in the 1990s showed that girls were members of female gangs, carried guns, killed people, and practiced brutal initiation rituals. She cited literature that shows violent girls reported higher rates of victimization than their nonviolent counterparts; those who were violent reported greater fear of sexual assault, especially from their boyfriends; roughly one out of four violent girls have been sexually abused compared to nonviolent girls. The FCVP researchers now believe that girls' aggressive behavior can be viewed as symptoms of violence and other abuse that have been committed against them in the past. More research is recommended to gain a better insight into the growing national trend of female violence.

Acknowledgments The authors recognize and thank the Office of Minority Health in the U.S. Department of Health and Human Services for its generous support over the period 1994–2006 (Grant # D67MP001-12-0) through a cooperative agreement with Central State University in Wilberforce, Ohio. This cooperative agreement allowed Central State University, through the use of a management team, to coordinate the implementation of demonstration and evaluation of violence prevention projects at 45 colleges and universities located in 23 states, the District of Columbia, Puerto Rico, and the U.S. Virgin Islands. Special thanks are in order for the directors and staff of the FLCs at the various institutions and members of the FCVP Management Team at Central State University and members of the Advisory Board for their dedicated work that help to build a truly great national program with one of the largest databases in the USA on ethnic minority youth prevention programs.

Appendix 1

School Bonding Index-Revised (SBI-R)

Read the following statement ......Mark 1 for Strongly Disagree, 2 for Disagree, 3 for Agree, and 4 for Strongly Agree. Shade your response under the School Bonding Index Revised (SBI-R) on Page 3 of the answer sheet booklet.

1. I think my school is a good place to be.
2. I like most of the students in my school.
3. My classmates and I want the same things from school.
4. I feel at home in this school.

5. I have influence over what this school is like.
6. If there is a problem in this school, the principal, teachers, and students can get it solved.
7. It is very important to me to go to this school.
8. Students in this school get along well with others.

9. I want to stay in this school until I go to or through high school.
10. I care about what my classmates know about me.
11. I like to stand in front of the class and speak.
12. I like to help the teacher in class.

13. I like to talk to my teachers before or after class.
14. When I have a problem, I can talk to a teacher or a counselor at school.
15. I am involved in a lot of activities at school.
16. I don't care if people throw paper on the floor at school.

17. I use profanity at school.
18. There is nothing really wrong with breaking bottles outside of the school building.
19. I often disrupt class.
20. Every chance I get, I cut class.

21. It bothers me when students break the windows at my school.
22. It bothers me when students write on the walls or desks at my school.
23. I don't think it's right to throw food in the cafeteria at school.
24. It really bothers me when students talk back to teachers.

Note: There are four subscales: The School Experience subscale is made up of the first 9 items on the SBI-R. The School Involvement subscale is made up of items 10 through 15. The School Delinquency subscale is made up of items 16through 20. The School Pride subscale is made up of items 21 through 24.

Appendix 2

Violence Risk Assessment Inventory (VRAI)

Read the following statements and choose the answer that BEST fits you. Please shade the appropriate response in the answer sheet provided and do not leave any blank. Mark N for "No," 1 for "once," 2 for "twice," 3 for "three times," and 4+ for "four or more times." Shade your responses in the spaces provided under the Violence Risk Assessment Inventory Revised (VRAI-R) on Page 2 of the answer sheet.

In the past three months, I have
1. carrie.d a weapon in public such as in school or on the street.
2. fought with a group of my friends against another group of people.
3. physically fought someone I knew.
4. physically fought someone I did not know.

5. been with someone who was selling drugs.
6. been with someone smoking pot, weed, bliss, and marijuana.
7. been offered drugs or alcohol.
8. been away from home without permission.

9. drank alcohol or been drunk.
10. argued with my parent(s) or guardian(s).
11. damaged or destroyed school, private, or public property.
12. used a weapon like a knife, stick, bat, etc. in a fight.

13. taken something that did not belong to me without paying for it.
14. held a real gun in my hands.
15. been so mad that I thought I was going to lose control.
16. seen someone in my family has gotten in a physical fight.

17. been mad enough to fight.
18. seen at least one person close to me—like a family member, parent, guardian, teacher, or friend—settle an argument by fighting.
19. felt like there is no way out of a situation without using violence.
20. been so angry that I acted without thinking about what would happen.

In the past six months, I have
21. used a weapon like a knife, stick, or bat, etc. in a fight.
22. held a real gun in my hands without permission from my parents/guardians.
23. carried a weapon in a public place like to school or the store.

References

Bureau of Justice Statistics (2001). *Differences in rates of violent crime experienced by Whites and Blacks narrow*. Washington, DC: Bureau of Justice.

Edwards, D., Hunt, H. H., Myers, J., Grogg, K. R., & Myers, J. (2005). Acceptability and student outcomes of a violence prevention curriculum. *Journal of Primary Prevention*, 26, 401–418.

Elliott, D. S. & Huizinga, D. (1989). Improving self-report measures of delinquency. In M. Klein (Ed.), *Cross-national research in self-reported crime and delinquency* (pp. 155–186). Boston: Kluwer.

Garbarino, J. (1999). *Lost Boys: Why our sons turn violent and how we can save them*. Los Angeles: The Free Press.

Goldstein, A. (1991). *Delinquent Gangs*. Illinois: Research Press.

Hawkins, J. D. (1995). Controlling crime before it happens: Risk-focused prevention. *National Institute of Justice Journal, August* (Issue Number 229), 10–18.

Howell, J. C. (Ed.) (1995). *Guide for implementing the comprehensive strategy for serious, violent and chronic juvenile offenders* (NCJ No. 153681). Washington, DC: U.S. Government Printing Office.

Junger-Tas, J., Terlouw, G. J., & Klein, M. W. (1994). *Delinquent behavior among young people in the western world: First results of the international self-report delinquency study*. Amsterdam: Kugler.

Kadel, S. & Follman, J. (1993). Reducing school violence in Florida. *Hot topics, usable research*. [ED 355614]. Washington, DC: Southeastern Region Vision for Education.

Kaufman, P., Chen, X., Choy, S. P., Ruddy, S. A, Miller, A. K., & Fleury, K. K., et al. (2000). *Indicators of school crime and safety, 2000*. (NCES 2000–017/NCJ-184176). Washington, DC: US Department of Education.

Maguire, K. & Pastore, A. L. (1999). *Sourcebook of criminal justice statistics, 1998*. US Department of Justice, (NCJ 176356). Washington, DC: U.S. Government Printing Office.

National Center for Education Statistics (2002). *Indicators of school crime and safety: 2002* (NCES Electronic Catalog No. 2003009). Washington, DC: National Center for Education Statistics.

Offman, J. (2006). The Effect of Early Music Education on Mathematical Achievement. Unpublished Graduate Research Proposal, College of Education, Prairie View A&M University, Prairie View, Texas.

Pianta, R. C., Steinberg, M., & Rollins, K. (1995). The first two years of school: Teacher-child relationships and deflections in children's classroom adjustment. *Development and Psychopathology*, 7, 297–312.

Rennison, C. (2001). *Criminal victimization 2000: Changes 1993–2000* (NCJ-187007). Washington DC: US Department of Justice, Office of Justice Programs, Bureau of Justice Statistics.

Respress, T. & Lufti, C. (2006). Whole brain learning: The fine arts with students at risk. *Journal of Reclaiming Children and Youth*, 15, 24–31.

Rodney, L. W. (2008). The Historical Evolution of the Family and Community Violence Prevention (FCVP) Program. In Martha Heggins, Laxley Rodney and Cashmir Kowalski (Eds.), Diverse Approaches to *Family and Community Violence Prevention: A National Perspective, Monograph*

Rodney, L.W. & Johnson, D. L. (2006). A salute to reclaiming children and youth from the family and community violence prevention program. *Journal of Reclaiming Children and Youth, 15*, 2–4.

Rodney, L. W., Johnson, D. L., & Srivastava, R. P. (2005a). The impact of culturally relevant prevention models on school-age youth. *Journal of Primary Prevention*, 26, 439–454.

Rodney, L. W., Srivastava, R., & Johnson, D. (2005b). Bad Girls or Fighting Angels? Evaluation Report # 6. Family and Community Violence Prevention (FCVP), Wilberforce, Ohio.

Rodney, L. W. (1999). Collaboration diversity and self-help in violence prevention. In L. Rodney (Ed.), *Proceedings from fourth national conference on family and community violence prevention*. Wilberforce, OH: Family and Community Violence Prevention Program.

Rodney, H. E., Tachia, H. R., & Rodney, L. W. (1999a). The home environment and delinquency: A study of African American adolescents. *Families in Society*, 80(6), 551–559.

Rodney, L. W., Rodney, H. E., Crafter, B., & Mupier, R. M. (1999b). Variables contributing to grade retention among African American adolescent males. *Journal of Educational Research*, 92, 185–190.

Satcher, D. (2001). *Youth violence: A report of the surgeon general*. Rockville, MD: US Government Printing Office.

Siegel, L. J. & Senna, J. J. (1988). *Juvenile Delinquency: Theory, Practice, and Law* (3rd Ed.). West, NY: Wadsworth.

Srivastava, R. & Rodney, L. W. (2003). *FCVP Program Instrument Scoring Manual*. Retrieved December 2003, from http://www.fcvp.org/0306evaluationforms/03–04_Draft_Scoring_Manual.pdf.

Stinson, N. (2002). Cooperative agreement with Central State University for the family and community violence prevention program. *Federal Register*, 67, 10413–10417.

Trump, K. (2002). *School-Related Violent Deaths, Shootings, Bomb Incidence and Crisis*. Cleveland, OH: National School Safety and Security Services.

Vosselkuil, B., Fein, R., Reddy, M., Boren, R., & Modzeleski, W. (2002). *The Final. Report and Findings of the Safe School Initiative. Implication for Prevention of School attacks in the United States*. Published by the United states Secret Service and the United States Department of Education, Washington, DC Retrieved 6/30/06 from www.secretservice.gov/ntac/ssi final report-.pdf.

Walker, H. (1995). *School Violence Prevention*. Eugene, OR: ERIC Clearinghouse on Educational Management.

Walker, H., Colvin, G.,& Ramsey, E. (1995). *Antisocial Behavior in School Strategies and Best Practices*. Pacific Grove, CA: Brooks/Cole.

Wilkinson, G. S. (1993). *The Wide Range Achievement Test (WRAT 3): Administration manual*. Wilmington, DE: Wide Range.

Chapter 22
Prevention of School Violence: Directions, Summary, and Conclusions

J. Robert McLaughlin and Thomas W. Miller

This volume has addressed critically important issues in understanding and providing a prevention model for school-related violence. We have learned much, and more remains to be learned to address this most important community issue. A review of the chapters follows with some concluding thoughts, personal comments, and lessons that we have hopefully learned.

Theory, Assessment, and Forms of School Violence

The first section of this volume focuses on the theory, assessment, and various forms of school violence, and we start with an interesting discussion by Drs. Miller and Kraus as they provide a clear and cogent definition of school violence that clearly shows the complexity and extent of the problem. It includes physical aggression as well as psychological trauma, sexual abuse, and numerous other "boundary" violations. The scope presented is vast and the risk factors discussed—childhood substance use and delinquency, and poor peer relations among early adolescents (weak ties with "good" peers and strong ties with "bad" peers), and gang membership—make it apparent that the prevention of and responses to school violence will require a complex set of communication and intervention strategies.

Drs. Miller and Kraus further present clear information on prevention goals, levels of prevention, and program interventions that seem to hold promise for helping to eliminate school violence as a public health issue. They outline some of the more effective models that use social skills training, parent involvement and training, school bonding between teachers and students, mentoring as a key strategy, and counseling support for both victims and perpetrators of school violence (Miller, 1996). A compelling case is made that the solution to school violence lies in a comprehensive, multidisciplinary approach with extensive involvement and collaboration among school staff, health educators, police, mental health experts, and other concerned social agencies. The issues around school violence are complicated and yet Miller and Kraus lay the groundwork for a hopeful response based on the research that currently exists and that which is needed.

T. W. Miller (ed.), *School Violence and Primary Prevention.*   431
© Springer 2008

Chapter 3 by Dr. William French is also very comprehensive as he examines a framework for understanding the neurobiology of violence and victimization. French outlines numerous biological variables that interact with the environment, which, in turn, impact violence and aggressive responses in children and youth. The key according to his review and research is not to focus on nature versus nurture, but rather, to focus on how the two interact to impact various aggressive and violent responses in our youth.

This chapter further explores the impact of trauma, abuse, and neglect on the development of our children in relation to violence and victimization. Various domains of trauma are outlined and discussed as they relate to aggressive responses. The concepts of "hot" and "cold" aggression are presented and used to further our understanding of the various types of youth violence and aggression. French discusses a strong connection between victimization and violence, the psychopathic implications of violence which may be summarized as a lack of conscience and a lack of moral sense, and how the concepts of "hot" and "cold" aggression help us to further understand the connections. And finally, he offers an integrated model of neurobiology in terms of how the brain functions to help us understand victimization and violence at yet an even deeper level.

Chapter 4 provides a thorough overview of the potential effectiveness of well-designed and implemented "Threat Assessments" in our schools to help prevent school violence from occurring. Dr. Callahan views the Threat Assessment as part of a comprehensive plan where school safety strategies are used in conjunction with positive, proactive, learning strategies such as teaching social skills, developing connectedness, classroom and school management, resiliency development, clear crisis procedures, and training all in recognizing at-risk factors. While threat assessment is difficult because no single profile has emerged from the literature, it can be effective if used with well-defined interventions. Dr. Callahan advocates for a comprehensive approach to addressing school violence.

She advocates in this chapter for a school violence prevention approach that focuses on building climates and cultures that emphasize respect, safety, and emotional support. The threat assessment is one tool to help in this ongoing process. The protocol calls for assessing actions, communications, and circumstances around an individual of concern. Professor Callahan provides thorough threat assessment information via a referral form, worksheet, threat assessment concepts, risk for harm categories, an interview outline, and questions for mental health professionals to use during an interview. A summary table of early warning signs of potential at-risk students is provided as a practical tool for all school administrators and teachers to identify help that a student may need. She provides some very useful tools for the school practitioner.

In Chap. 5, Amy Nigoff presents a thorough discussion on a social information processing model that may contribute to violent responses by students in certain social situations. The model is based on the theory that how children process and interpret social situations will lead to either violent or nonviolent responses. More specifically, if children misinterpret certain cues or parts of the situation then violence is likely to occur. Nigoff suggests that if children can learn about the model and learn the skills needed to successfully use it, then violence can be reduced significantly.

The model presented combine both social and cognitive psychology. Nigoff explains the six-step process used in the model and discusses a variety of research that has been conducted around the use of it. She further explains the concepts of proactive and reactive aggression and how they relate to the model. And as an advantage, she explains how easy it is to teach the model to children as long as they are not cognitively impaired. Prevention of and treatment for violence in schools is discussed with a clear focus on how to use the model: train specific skills so that skill deficits are removed, assist with removing biases, deficiencies in thinking are limited, and mistakes in assessing social cues are eliminated. All of the latter can lead to violence per the social information model. A school-based example is provided.

In Chap. 6, Drs. Kyle and Thompson present a model based on moral development and personal power. They show how the greater the knowledge about the conditions that lead to school violence, the greater the chance of future prevention in the form of policies and interventions. Their argument and model revolve around specific premises: ethics are important, students are influenced by their relationships with peers, poor socialization impacts moral development, and schools frequently reward competition as opposed to cooperation. They further present an overview of mass shootings and information about the possible causes.

While Drs. Kyle and Thompson recognize that a clear profile of a mass shooter has not been developed, they recognize that one clear difference in those who tend to not engage in extreme violence is a strong sense of ethics or moral development. While social factors must also be addressed, a strong, effective ethical system will assist the individual in developing alternate responses to extreme violence. They review thoroughly how adolescents develop morally and discuss personal power as a key factor in that development. Bullying and the school environment are proposed as other key factors in developing an effective antiviolence model. They suggest that an effective intervention plan will center on the family, peer relationships, self-esteem, bullying, and the reduction of conflict and competition in our schools.

In Chap. 7, Drs. Card, Isaacs, and Hodges provide an in-depth overview and discussion on the personal and ecological risk factors for peer victimization. They identify a variety of personal and social variables that appear to put certain peers more at risk to be victims of peer aggression. They focus on a multi-level approach to help provide a comprehensive framework for better understanding the risk factors involved in being a victim. They further discuss the many implications of the research available in this area, and they focus on prevention and intervention strategies that may hold some promise even though much more research is needed in this area. The intervention potential centers on Bullying Programs and outlines the seminal work of Olweus, and some of the evaluations of the impact of those strategies. They conclude by offering some challenges for addressing peer victimization and some possible future research directions.

In Chap. 8, Dr. Sapp outlines an in-depth discussion on childhood sexual abuse. He covers the clinical measures of such abuse, its assessment, and the treatment needed for the victims. A broad, thorough definition of sexual abuse is provided and the possible link to adolescent aggression is discussed and recognized as an area that needs more focus and research. Various at-risk populations for such abuse and assault are explored, and a variety of indicators of abuse and assault are reviewed. He concludes this section with an in-depth discussion on how sexual abuse may be assessed effectively.

The next section of this chapter covers the medical and psychological consequences of sexual abuse and assault. They are vast and detrimental to both the individuals directly involved and the communities where the abuse occurs. Sapp further discusses possible prevention strategies, interventions, and the great need for education in this area. The key to prevention seems to be education about sexual abuse and the early detection of it, a proper diagnosis, and management of abuse cases. While the ultimate goal is prevention, it is clear that quality care for all of the victims must be provided.

Chapter 9 presents an overview of the impact that trauma may have on both the victim of aggression and the perpetrator of aggression. As Veltkamp and Lawson discuss, the two may often times be the same, that is, often the victim of bullying or aggression then becomes a perpetrator. The authors outline a variety of risk factors for both victims and perpetrators that include such variables as the individual, the family, peer groups, community, school, and the potential effects of television and video game playing.

They continue to thoroughly discuss possible interventions that may help both groups of children—victims and perpetrators—and advise that early identification can be a huge benefit when trying to find solutions to victimization. The focus of this section of their chapter is on a wide variety of potential interventions including resiliency concepts, behavior management, parent training, therapy for the children involved, and a well-defined safety plan for the school. Other important topics discussed are legal complexities of victimization issues, what schools can do to help, what parents can do, and a final section on what students can do to help solve the aggression issues that exist in our communities.

In Chap. 10, Drs. Miller and Veltkamp provide a cogent discussion of sexual boundary violations that occur in our school settings—or at least originate there as some of the actual behavior is carried out in a wide variety of locations (trips, homes, back seats of cars, etc.). They recognize that violence in our schools take many forms and that sexual boundary violations is one of many which is traumatic to the young school-aged victims. The purpose of this chapter is to help clarify the spectrum of sex boundary violations, provide a set of triggers for the violations (everything from jokes to inappropriate discussions of personal sex lives with students), discuss profiles of potential victims and perpetrators, review how the victim is exploited, and provide a clear example of boundary exploitation via a legal case study.

Drs. Miller and Veltkamp provide clear policy guidelines for schools in an attempt to help address prevention and intervention strategies. The key once again seems to fall on education, awareness, and a quick response. While a prevention emphasis is stressed, the authors clearly recognize the need to help any student victimized by a sexual boundary violation.

In Chap. 11, Drs. Miller, Holcomb, and Kraus discuss the importance of cliques and cults in the school setting. They outline what constitutes a clique, the value they serve our students (especially our adolescents), the harm they may cause, and how they can lead to bonding with a cult. The latter are typically perceived as much more negative and provide deceptive ways to lure others to them. A well-documented case, with specific aggressive behaviors, is discussed in some detail. The authors outline the case study, provide clear information on what attracts kids to cults, and discuss implications for clinical management.

With respect to the latter, there appear to be three keys: prevention, early detection, and treatment for the victims. With regard to treatment, the authors discuss a variety of potential intervention strategies and focus first on the possible early trauma (neglect, abuse, abandonment) that eventually leads to the attraction to a cult. Another key implication related to treatment is the need and the power of social bonding in our schools (Heatherton & Baumeister, 1991). This need will be met either in a positive way (sports, clubs, extracurricular activities) or via cliques and cults. While the former may be harmless, even sometimes helpful to self-identity, the latter are almost always conduits for further trauma and victimization.

Treatment and Prevention of Violence in the Schools

The next section of this volume focuses on treatment and prevention of violence in our schools. And we start with an exciting and interesting chapter from three practicing school-based educators—a principal, a school psychologist, and a middle school teacher—each highly regarded in the education profession.

Educational administrator Matt Thompson, an elementary principal, outlines for us a variety of strategies that school leaders can use to increase positive relationships (bonding, connectedness), which, in turn, will help ease the need for violent responses to conflict or concerns. His recommendations are as simple as learning the names of each student in the school to a more complicated understanding of school-wide behavior management.

School Psychologist Bobbie Burcham, a psychologist practicing in a high school setting, relates how threat assessments and other effective communication strategies can be used to help prevent violence in the complex world of a high school. Some of her keys seem to revolve around collaborative communication among various staff, prevention when possible, and effective intervention and treatment for students with more intense behavior and emotional needs. The overall need for positive behavior support is thoroughly discussed.

Educator Kathy McLaughlin, a middle school teacher, makes a compelling case that effective teaching is all about relationship building and teaching content effectively—the two seem to go together and allow students to connect or bond to the school. Such bonding seems to reduce the need for violent responses. She describes several strategies for helping kids feel safe in school, protected, and nurtured while at the same time the same strategies are used to enhance learning for all. Teachers and others will find her ideas (as well as those of the other two authors) interesting, effective, and most important—relatively easy to implement.

In Chap. 13, Drs. Yoon and Barton provide a detailed discussion of the various roles of teachers in the prevention of violence and bullying, and they review several school- and classroom-based intervention programs to assist with reducing violence and bullying in the schools. They start with a definition of bullying and then review various characteristics of schools that promote positive student outcomes in terms of academic and social development. The school's climate and core values seem to be critical and how the latter are communicated to all sends a strong message to all concerning whether violence or bullying will be accepted in the school.

The authors further discuss how important the teacher role is as it relates to helping to prevent bullying. Academic success is critical as many aggressive students struggle in school. Managing aggressive behavior falls to the skillful hands of teachers, and they can make a big impact by modeling for all respectful interactions (Elliott, 2001). Other keys seem to be the development of positive, prosocial, nonaggressive environments where caring relationships can flourish, developing a sense of belonging among all students, and making sure that tolerance and respect for individual differences is modeled and taught. The authors conclude with an extensive discussion of several school-wide and classroom-based programs and interventions designed to decrease violence and bullying.

In Chap. 14, Dr. Boxer and his colleagues provide an in-depth and comprehensive discussion of the developmental issues and various concerns related to the primary prevention of aggression and violence in children and adolescents. They recognize and outline the need for a multifaceted approach because of the complexities of the risk factors associated with aggression. And they further discuss how different strategies will be needed for younger children compared to those needed for teens. The authors initially outline three key concerns to be considered in prevention: the multiple risk factors that have been identified with aggression, the form and the function of aggression, and the maintenance of aggression across developmental periods.

The discussion then moves to a deeper understanding of the challenges faced when designing prevention interventions, because of the multiple facets of aggression. Most often a multi-level, multifaceted approach is recommended for programs that address the prevention of aggression. Various forms and functions of aggression are outlined, and the authors present a thorough discussion of a model that is used for predicting aggression in our youth. A major implication for prevention is offered. Prevention practice and developmental research must go together for effective solutions and programs to be further developed.

In Chap. 15, Berger, Rodkin, and Karimpour discuss bullying and victimization from an ecological perspective. They present a multi-level approach to the issues around bullying and victimization, and they recognize a strong need, given the several levels of complexity discussed, for many different levels or types of intervention. Their chapter provides a clear overview and definition of bullying and victimization, and they provide detailed information around several key concepts: prevention and promotion as goals, early adolescence as a key context, a multi-level analysis of bullying issues around the individual, dyad, peer group, and school, and a discussion of intervention guidelines to help reduce bullying in our schools.

These authors discuss prevention in terms of promoting a safe and supportive environment which will assist with the prevention or reduction of aggressive bullying types of behavior. They discuss intervention in terms of multi-level approaches too, and center on the individual victim, the relationship between the victim and the bully, the peer group or classroom level, and the school level. The discussion includes specific implications for each of those four areas, and an outline of specific steps needed to intervene effectively in the reduction of bullying behavior.

In Chap. 16, Psychiatrists Drs. Benedek and Kambam outline and discuss the multifaceted role of the emergency room psychiatrist after a school shooting incident. They provide a case study as an example of all the various needs that are prevalent after such a tragedy occurs, and they use that example as a backdrop to further discuss the importance of the psychiatrist's role. The variety of issues concerning the psychiatrist range from confidentiality concerns to the need to help the media avoid prompting "copy cat" suicides and other aggressive acts.

The authors discuss in some depth other key parts of the role, such as assessment and management of the violent youth who will most likely end up in an emergency room for help and treatment, assisting youth witnesses, helping family members of the perpetrator, working closely with the school system and community members, and as mentioned before, assisting the media with responsible reporting. The authors basically conclude that the psychiatrist's role is not only varied but also critical especially in the aftermath of a violent school tragedy.

In Chap. 17, Dr. Espelage and Dr. Swearer discuss a variety of perspectives on bullying, and the various prevention strategies that appear to be linked to the bullying research. They advocate for a model similar to one used in many schools today—a three-tiered approach to intervention (Positive Behavior Support Model) where interventions are categorized as meeting primary, secondary, or tertiary students' needs based on the extent of need. Primary interventions apply to all students with most (80%) being addressed effectively, secondary apply to at-risk students who need more support (15%), and tertiary apply to high-risk students with intense needs (about 5% of a given school population).

These authors discuss example programs for each type of intervention, and they provide a brief yet cogent review of five different theoretical models or paradigms for explaining behavior and helping us to understand bullying at a deeper level. The paradigms reviewed include social-ecological, social information processing, theory of mind, dominance theory, and attraction theory. The importance of assessment and identifying key influences of bullying was also stressed in this chapter. Those influences centered on the peer groups, family, and school. In addition, key prevention strategies were outlined around teacher training, home–school collaboration, school–community collaboration, and counseling services for a variety of needs. The authors concluded that implementation of effective intervention programs was best achieved with collaboration around the three-tier model.

Several critical management and intervention ideas related to school shootings and high-risk students are explored in Chap. 18 by Dr. Miller, Dr. Weitzel, and clinical psychologist Janet Lane. They present a discussion of "Escape Theory" as a way of understanding what drives a perpetrator to victimize fellow peers (the need to escape perceived painful situations), risk factors related to severe aggression, five case studies of shootings in the United States, the impact of shootings that led to fatalities, diagnostic issues related to students who might be at risk for becoming violent, and several key management and intervention-related issues (U.S. Preventative Services Task Force, 1996; U.S. Department of Education, 2004).

The authors of this chapter provide in-depth discussion of both theoretical issues and practical advice for school administrators and Board of Education. They provide a checklist of behaviors that may help identify potential students who are at risk to commit violent acts, and they outline numerous risk factors found in the school environment that may help identify students in crisis. The case studies, diagnostic issues, and clinical management and school interventions ideas that are outlined lead to a thought-provoking section on recommendations to help reduce violence in our schools. They center on training for school staffs in warning signs, character education, and anger management. And the need to understand identity issues in our students is critical. They also call for more immediate access in the schools to mental health services.

Professors Miller, Kraus, and Veltkamp provide a detailed discussion in Chap. 19 of a study on the impact of character education on violence and bullying in schools. They outline the purpose of the study, explain the methods used, and then thoroughly discuss the results and the many implications for educators and practitioners concerned about school violence. They focused on fourth and fifth graders for intervention with a character education problem behavior prevention program, a summer camp experience, and intervention with parents. Comparison groups were provided, which made the results even more compelling.

These authors focused on three primary results: participants bonded more strongly with teachers than did comparison kids (bonding may reduce violence and bullying), the summer camp experience seemed most potent, and the parent intervention provided more interactions between parents and students. The implications are thoroughly reviewed and include understanding the importance of transitions on youth, and the four domains where most risk factors for violence can be found: the peer group, home, school, and community. A succinct yet thorough chart is provided that outlines the risk factors and protective factors that can be found in each domain. The authors conclude the chapter with a comprehensive series of recommendations for practice for educators and other practitioners concerned about reducing violence in our schools.

In Chap. 20, Drs. Beane, Miller, and Spurling present an in-depth and very comprehensive overview of what an effective Bully Prevention Program needs to look like to be effective in reducing bullying and violence in schools. They use a sample program, the Bully Free Program, as an example to explain and discuss the critical research-based components needed for maximum effectiveness. They provide a clear and comprehensive definition of bullying and explain the various types of bully behavior. Further, they discuss the characteristics of the victimizer and those of the victim, and explain the various consequences that both receive, that is, for being a bully and for being a victim.

In some detail, the authors then explain the essential characteristics and elements of effective Bully Prevention Programs which are research based, and which also include components to respond to current bully behavior (as well as prevention strategies). The reality is that bullying is widespread and observed in all types of school settings. Thus, intervention must focus on both prevention and protective strategies. The Bully Free Program is outlined and the research indicating its effectiveness is reviewed. The keys seem to revolve around awareness, training, systematic intervention, modeling good behavior by adults, and staying focused on the Golden Rule—at all times and communicating it effectively and often to all.

And last but not the least by any means, Drs. Rodney, Srivastava, and Johnson in Chap. 21 provide a comprehensive and thorough discussion of two related studies on the effectiveness of the Family and Community Violence Prevention (FCVP) Program that was designed to address the violence and other risky behaviors experienced by minority students in our communities. They revisit an earlier study and compare it with an expanded later study to review the key findings and critical issues related to this most important topic. They report key findings and results from the first study which were essentially confirmed in the expanded study: participation in the program yielded increased academic performance especially in spelling and math; high math scores tended to indicate less participation in violent and other risky behaviors; more bonding with the school resulted in less violence and risky behaviors; and more exposure to violence led to more violent and risky behaviors by those so exposed (U.S. Department of Education, 2004). A unique finding that demands more explanation and research was that older adolescent girls tended to engage in more violent and risky behavior. In addition, the authors discuss the need for differential curriculum among various minority groups, and the strong protective factor of increased academic performance. One of the strongest risk factors was quite simply the exposure to violent behavior. An in-depth discussion is presented around all of the latter concepts, issues, and concerns.

School Violence and Primary Prevention: The Take Home Message and Lessons Learned

So what have we learned after 20 comprehensive and varied chapters on school violence?

Planning and Prevention for the Healthy School Environment

Numerous high-profile forms of violence in the school setting have led to an atmosphere of fear and apprehension among many students, teachers, administrators, health care professionals, parents, and communities about the safety of their schools. While statistics show that schools, in general, remain safer than their surrounding neighborhoods, every community must take steps to address school violence. In doing so, many questions may arise. Where does a community begin the process of addressing school violence? How can schools prevent or reduce school violence? How can communities plan for handling school violence when it does occur? Should law enforcement include exercises and training as a part of these preparations?

Addressing School Violence

Students, faculty, administrators, health care professionals, parents, and communities can address school violence through three essential steps–planning, practice, and prevention. Prevention refers to taking actions to reduce or prevent school violence from occurring, planning determines what actions to take if school violence does occur, and practice entails rehearsing plans and modifying them when needed.

Prevention Interventions

There are various Web sites and publications available that provide a comprehensive overview of school violence prevention programs and offer various steps communities can take to help prevent violence in their schools. Several organizations encourage communities to establish partnerships between schools and other public agencies. Because school violence remains a community problem, it requires collaboration from all residents, agencies, and businesses. Schools, police, business leaders, and elected officials all must cooperate to address school violence (U.S. Department of Health and Human Services, 2000).

Furthermore, communities are encouraged by several organizations to identify and measure the problem. School officials, working with law enforcement and other community agencies, should collect information that shows the size and scope of violence in their schools. This important step ensures that prevention efforts revolve around the community's specific problems. Communities are encouraged to set goals and measurable objectives. Efforts to encourage school officials to collaborate with parents and students to set and implement goals and objectives for their school violence prevention programs are needed.

Finally, communities are encouraged to identify appropriate research-based programs and strategies. The key to preventing and reducing school violence combines long-term strategies with short-term interventions. Community leaders and school administrators should research and examine various school violence prevention options and select techniques most appropriate for their schools. Such options fall into three broad categories. The first category involves environmental modifications and suggests that police, trained in crime prevention through environmental design, or school security managers, who have attended specialized courses in physical security, audit, or survey each school. These personnel should examine a school's physical environment and recommend modifications to prevent or reduce violence.

The second category includes options for preventing and controlling violence based on school management. For example, this may entail establishing behavior and discipline codes, the use of criminal penalties against selected students, or the placement of problem students into alternative educational institutions.

The final category, education and curriculum-based prevention techniques, could include teaching conflict resolution courses, establishing mentoring programs, developing self-esteem initiatives, or instituting community-oriented policing crime prevention efforts. After reviewing the various options, administrators should work with the entire community to carefully implement the selected prevention measures. Some preventive techniques may require additional resources, outside approval, or long-term planning to prove successful.

In response to the trend in school violence over the last two decades, the World Health Organization (WHO) launched a Global School Health Initiative seeking to mobilize and strengthen health promotion and education activities at the local, national, regional, and global levels. The initiative is designed to improve the health of students, school personnel, families, and other members of the community through schools. The goal of WHO's Global School Health Initiative is to increase the number of schools that can truly be called "Health-Promoting Schools." Although definitions will vary, depending on need and circumstance, a Health-Promoting School can be characterized as a school constantly strengthening its capacity as a healthy setting for living, learning, and working.

The above initiatives represent a good planning start that should help any school, district, and community plan effectively to help reduce the chances of catastrophic school violence. Combined with a well thought out, written, and practiced on a regular basis Emergency Management Plan, as required by many states now, schools will ensure an ongoing process for constantly addressing the complex topic of school violence.

Concluding Comments and Thoughts

Has the new millennium for the twenty-first century witnessed a change in the way we relate to one another? A "culture of hate" has emerged in this new century that is realized in both domestic and foreign realms. The incidence and prevalence of domestic violence, child and adult bullying, school shootings at the middle, high school, and college level, child pornography, and international insurgency in others affairs has yielded a global concern for our innate basic respect for one another. Olweus (2004) has studied this disrespect for one another in several venues and suggests that there are three main features present when bullying occurs: (1) deliberate aggression, (2) an asymmetric power relationship, and (3) the resulting pain, trauma, and debilitating distress in the victim. Olweus (2004) argues that bullying is basically the repeated intimidation of a victim that is intentionally carried out by a more powerful person or group in order to cause physical and/or emotional hurt. Bullying is often a secret activity, and victims are often reluctant to report bullying; therefore, it is difficult to obtain accurate data regarding the incidence of the behavior

(Elliot & Kilpatrick, 1994). However, it is generally agreed that bullying is wide-spread and often underestimated. Beane (1997) suggests that ~3 million bullying incidents per year, or 1,700 per day, are reported in the United States from kinder-garten through 12th-grade students. This means that in every 20 s a child is being harassed, taunted, assaulted, or abused. When Olweus examined more serious cases of bullying, he found that slightly more than 3%, or 18,000 students, were bullied "about once a week" or more frequently, and somewhat less than 2%, or 10,000 students, bullied others at that rate. About 1,000 students were both bully and victim in serious bullying. One of twenty children in Norway was involved in serious bullying (Violence Institute of New Jersey, 2001).

Over the course of time, we have come to realize that outside influences corrupt our inner souls. The question as to why some individuals bully or terrorize have troubled philosophers, behavioral scientists, theologians, legislators, attorneys, and the general public. We want to believe that people are basically good and that inhu-manity to others is the product of a small minority who perpetrate such evil whether in the school setting or in the world community. Zimbardo (2007) revealed for us the reality that those among us who might bully or terrorize are not necessarily sociopaths but ordinary people wherein circumstances turn them into something they might not ordinarily see in themselves. Their victims are dehumanized at one level in the school yard and at another level as in Abu Ghraib and similar settings. Research has revealed this to us through the lessons learned some 35 years ago when Zimbardo and colleagues constructed a mock prison setting only to realize ordinary people began to humiliate, demean, and physically and emotionally abuse their subordinates. Knowing this, what have we been able to accomplish since the original research in providing the guidance toward a more humanitarian world community? What are the dynamics that might explain why we are seeing this frequent inhumanity toward one another? Social psychology suggests that the social stres-sors in our life are linked with escape theory. Escape theory (Baumeister, 1990; Dean & Range, 1996) postulates that peer victimization or bullying is driven by the desire to escape a state of painful self-awareness, characterized by inadequacy, negative affect, and low self-esteem. The emotions associated with this state of self-awareness are focused on the self-perceived failure to achieve acceptance among peers and are often based on rigid self-standards. According to the theory, certain individuals attempt to escape these negative self-perceptions and emotions by narrowing their consciousness to an immediate action, like bullying, which results in irrational cognitions that predominate over normal inhibitions against self-destructive behaviors.

The psychological profile for bullies characterizes people who engage in escape behaviors. According to escape theory, the personality characteristics of bullies which predispose them to episodes of negative self-perceptions affect low self-esteem and high levels of self-awareness. These risk factors set the stage for frequent episodes of acting out against others in the form of bullying accompanied by irrational thoughts, which, in turn, activate the desire to escape. Frequent repetitions of this cycle create high levels of residual negative affect and irrational thinking. Individuals who engage in escape behaviors on a regular basis tend to display more negative affect, irrational thinking, negative self-awareness, unrealistically high self-standards, and low self-esteem. While escape theory does not address how different "escape behaviors" emerge, it does aid in understanding risk factors that that may result in violent behaviors and social stressors. In terms of social trauma, we must examine the influence of how we impact our relationships with others. Whether this is in the home and family, in the work setting, within the social arena, or the world diplomacy stage, social stressors exist and psychology has a critical role to play in providing guidance through research and practice within our global community.

Is there hope for reducing and eliminating school violence? We think so, and we turn to what may at first glance appear to an unlike source for such hope. We return to Zimbardo's The Lucifer Effect (Zimbardo, 2007) as that source for hope. While Zimbardo makes a compelling case for how societal structures and situations (created by men and women) can greatly influence and prompt evil behavior from apparently good people, we can certainly deduce from his work that similar structures are possible to influence and prompt good behavior from good people and even others who may be at risk for engaging in violent, bully types of behavior. And we as educators, mental health experts, health professionals, and simply concerned citizens can work together, collaboratively to build those structures and create those situations so our children and grandchildren will experience far less violence in their future. We are called to do no less, and Zimbardo (2007) summarizes our hope succinctly in this quote from his book:

> And so, the parting message that we might derive from our long journey into the heart of darkness and back again is that heroic acts and the people who engage in them should be celebrated. They form essential links among us; they forge our Human Connection. The evil that persists in our midst must be countered, and eventually overcome, by the greater good in the collective hearts and personal heroic resolve of Everyman and Everywoman. It is not an abstract concept, but, as we are reminded by the Russian poet and former prisoner in Stalin's Gulag Aleksandr Solzhenitsyn: "The line between good and evil is in the center of every human heart (Solzhenitsyn 1973)."

We are called for the sake of our future and our children to be everyday heroes in finding solutions to school violence and bullying. Both will depend on our efforts and willingness to succeed and to be quite simply heroic in the days ahead. There is hope, and the lessons learned in these chapters should provide much guidance and substance to work hard on those structures, initiatives, and interventions needed to be hugely successful.

References

Baumeister, R. F. (1990). Suicide as escape from self. *Psychological Review*, 97, 90–113.

Dean, P. J. & Range, L. M. (1996). The escape theory of suicide and perfectionism in college students. *Death Studies*, 20, 415–424.

Heatherton, T. F. & Baumeister, R. F. (1991). Binge eating as escape from self-awareness. *Psychological Bulletin*, 110, 86–108.

Miller, T. W. (1996). *Theory and Assessment of Stressful Life Events*. Madison, CT: International Universities Press Incorporated.

Beane, A. (1997). The Trauma of Peer Victimization. In T. W. Miller (Ed.), *Children of Trauma*. Madison, CT: International University Press, Inc.

Elliott, D. S. (Ed.) (2001). *Youth Violence: A Report of the Surgeon General*. Atlanta, GA: Office of the Surgeon General.

Olweus, D. (2004). *Bullying at School*. Malden, MA: Blackwell Publishers.

Solzhenitsyn, A. I., (1973). The Gulag Archipelago, 1918–1956. New York: Harper & Row.

U.S. Preventative Services Task Force. (1996). *Guide to Clinical Preventative Services*, 2nd edition. Baltimore, MD: Williams & Wilkins.

U.S. Department of Education. (2004). *2004 Annual Report on School Safety*. Washington, DC: Author.

U.S. Department of Health and Human Services. (2000). *Healthy People 2010*, 2nd edition.

Understanding and Improving Health and Objectives for Improving Health (2 vols.). Washington, DC: U.S. Department of Health and Human Services.

Violence Institute of New Jersey. (2001). *Source Book of Drug and Violence Prevention Programs for Children and Adolescents*.

Zimbardo, P. (2007). *The Lucifer Effect*, p. 488. New York: Random House.

Index

Printed in the United States of America